JBReview

PHARMACY TECHNICIAN EXAM REVIEW GUIDE

Judith L. Neville, CPhT, BA

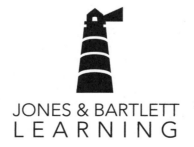

JONES & BARTLETT
LEARNING

World Headquarters
Jones & Bartlett Learning
5 Wall Street
Burlington, MA 01803
978-443-5000
info@jblearning.com
www.jblearning.com

Jones & Bartlett Learning books and products are available through most bookstores and online booksellers. To contact Jones & Bartlett Learning directly, call 800-832-0034, fax 978-443-8000, or visit our website, www.jblearning.com.

Substantial discounts on bulk quantities of Jones & Bartlett Learning publications are available to corporations, professional associations, and other qualified organizations. For details and specific discount information, contact the special sales department at Jones & Bartlett Learning via the above contact information or send an email to specialsales@jblearning.com.

Production Credits
Acquisitions Editor: Katey Birtcher
Editorial Assistant: Teresa Reilly
Associate Production Editor: Jill Morton
Marketing Manager: Grace Richards
Manufacturing and Inventory Control Supervisor: Amy Bacus
Composition: Laserwords Private Limited, Chennai, India
Cover Design: Scott Moden
Rights and Photo Researcher: Sarah Cebulski
Chapter Opener Image: © Evon Lim Seo Ling/ShutterStock, Inc.
Printing and Binding: Courier Companies
Cover Printing: Courier Companies

To order this product, use ISBN: 978-1-4496-4341-6

Library of Congress Cataloging-in-Publication Data
Neville, Judith L.
  Pharmacy technician exam review guide / by Judith L. Neville.
    p. ; cm.
  Includes bibliographical references and index.
  ISBN 978-1-4496-2979-3 — ISBN 1-4496-2979-2
  I. Title.
  [DNLM: 1. Pharmacy—United States—Examination Questions. 2. Certification—United States—Examination Questions. 3. Drug Compounding—United States—Examination Questions. 4. Drug Dosage Calculations—United States—Examination Questions. 5. Pharmacists' Aides—United States. QV 18.2]
    615.1076—dc23
                                                                            2011046409

6048

Printed in the United States of America
16 15 14 13 12   10 9 8 7 6 5 4 3 2 1

In Dedication to Shawn A. Muhr

1984–2011

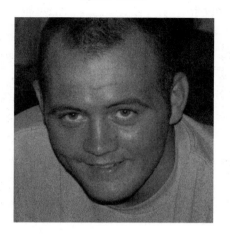

Killed in Action; Afghanistan

So we have the privilege of an education and the freedom to pursue our careers.

Thank you for your service.

Judy

Contents

Chapter 9

Participating in the Administration and Management of Pharmacy 131

Chapter 10

Maintaining Medication Inventory and Repackaging 141

Chapter 11

Hazardous Drugs 153

Chapter 12

Extemporaneous Compounding 161

Chapter 13

Aseptic Technique 169

Chapter 14

Basic Math Review 189

Chapter 15

Measurement Systems and System Conversions 205

Chapter 16

Dosage Calculations 219

Introduction

The goal of this book is to help ease the stress that you might feel in taking the pharmacy technician certification exam. The stress you feel may be associated with the unknown. You may have many unanswered questions: What do I need to know for the exam? Do I know enough from working as a pharmacy technician for 10 years, or do I need to study? How do I sign up to take the exam? How hard is the exam? Why do I need to be certified?

The following chapters will answer these questions and more. I have taught pharmacy technician courses for the past 8 years. I've helped hundreds of students prepare for the national certification exam. Some of these students have never worked as a pharmacy technician. They enroll in a formal training program to prepare for a career and to earn a degree that will help them start a new career as a pharmacy technician.

I have also taught a large number of students who have been pharmacy technicians for more than 20 years. A few of my students own their own pharmacy and work beside their spouse, who is a licensed pharmacist. Some of the students I helped prepare for the exam were taking the exam because they wanted to achieve a personal goal. Many of the students I helped have been mandated by the state to become certified to keep their jobs.

The common thread among all of these students is that they're nervous and they're curious. They're curious about what's on the certification exam. They want to know how to prepare for the exam and what they should study.

THEY'RE NERVOUS, BECAUSE TAKING THIS EXAM IS A DEFINING MOMENT FOR THEM.

"After working as a tech for 10 years, do I know anything?"

"I've been in school for over a year. Have I learned what I need to know?"

"I may lose my job if I can't pass this test!"

"I've been out of school for 15 years! How will I ever be able to study and pass a test!"

The intent of this text is to serve as a guide for the reader on what should be reviewed prior to sitting for the National Pharmacy Technician Certification Exam. This review guide is not for a beginner. Rather, it is designed as a review tool for pharmacy technicians who have been working in the pharmacy field for a number of years and need a review on areas they may be unfamiliar with, and for the pharmacy technician in training who needs a review of coursework prior to taking the exam.

Regardless of whether you have worked as a pharmacy technician for 5 years, 3 months, or are a student in a pharmacy technician training program, there are three areas that pharmacy technicians feel are the most important for them to review and study prior to taking the exam: math, aseptic compounding, and drug classes—brand/generic. For that reason, this textbook will provide a review of all information needed for the certification exam with an emphasis on these common trouble areas.

Abundant practice tests throughout this book and online will help you prepare for the exam. The practice tests are in multiple-choice question format, just like the questions on the certification exam. A detailed answer key is provided with each practice test to help you understand the correct answer choice.

If you are one of those seasoned pharmacy technicians who has been working in the field for a number of years, you have a wealth of practical experience! You're looking for a tool to help you study and to help you review the topics you're a little unsure of. This review book has Task Sheets for each testing topic. The Task Sheet will help you get into that study mode and focus on what you need to know for the exam. Look for helpful tips, study plans, and evaluations on the Task Sheets.

If you are a pharmacy technician in training, you can use this review guide to test your knowledge obtained while in class. Then concentrate on areas that you need to review further.

While this book provides a comprehensive review, an emphasis is placed on the areas of study that technicians desire the most including basic math and pharmacy calculations. To help you study math and pharmacy calculations, this review guide is filled with practice tests. The practice tests are arranged in beginning, intermediate, and advanced levels. Work your way through the test levels to feel comfortable in working pharmacy calculations.

Drug classification is another important area of study. There seems to be an endless number of medications on the market. Each medication has at least two names: brand and generic. Each medication has a certain mode of action and is classified according to that mode of action. You may be very nervous about knowing the medication classes and the brand/generic names of the medications. If you have been working in a retail pharmacy, you might be an expert in generic names of oral medication but will be unfamiliar with IV medications used in the hospital setting. Although a limited number of technicians work with chemotherapy, you are required to know chemotherapy drugs for the exam. This review guide will guide you on which drugs to know for the test, and provide hints on how to memorize drug classifications easily. There are many targeted practice tests to help you check what you've learned. Test-taking tips are included along with tips from certified pharmacy technicians who have successfully taken the exam.

With these tools, content review, and extensive practice tests, you can feel well prepared for the certification exam. Good luck and enjoy this learning process!

About the Author

Judith L. Neville is the program chair for the pharmacy technician department at Vatterott College in Omaha, Nebraska. She also serves as the externship coordinator as well as teaching numerous classes, including aseptic technique, pharmacy practice, medical terminology, pharmacology, and review for the certification exam.

Judy has also taught a number of pharmacy technician certification review classes in southwest Iowa at Iowa Western Community College.

Judy is an expert member of the Institute for the Certification of Pharmacy Technicians (ICPT), assisting with exam-writing for the Exam for the Certification of Pharmacy Technicians (ExCPT).

She is an active member of the Iowa Pharmacy Association (IPA), serving on the Pharmacy Technician Advisory Committee. Judy is a director for the American Association of Pharmacy Technicians (AAPT). She is also an active member of the Nebraska Pharmacy Association (NPA), Pharmacy Technician Educator's Council (PTEC), and American Society of Health-System Pharmacists (ASHP).

She is a certified technician (CPhT) through both certification bodies: ICPT and PTCB.

Along with peer reviews for professional journals and book reviews, Judy has written articles for the *Journal of Pharmacy Technology*. She has authored two college-level pharmacy practice textbooks, *Mosby's Pharmacy Technician Lab Manual* and *Mosby's Pharmacy Management Software for Pharmacy Technicians*.

Reviewers

C. Dorothea Andrews, PharmD, BCPS
Program Director, Pharmacy Technician Training Program
University of Kentucky
Lexington, KY

Sarah Clement, MEd, CPhT
Program Director of Pharmacy Technology
Forsyth Technical Community College
Winston-Salem, NC

Anthony Guerra, PharmD
Chair and Instructor, Pharmacy Technician Program
Des Moines Area Community College
Ankeny, IA

Richard L. Witt
Instructor, Pharmacy Technician Course
Allegany College of Maryland
Cumberland, MD

Why Does Certification Matter?

OBJECTIVES/TOPICS TO COVER:

✓ Describe the differences between certification, registration, and licensure.
✓ List the benefits of pharmacy technician certification.

WHY DOES CERTIFICATION MATTER?

Our country spends more than $177 billion annually on medication errors. Approximately 7000 people lose their lives annually because of prescription errors in the United States.

Studies and statistics show that certified pharmacy technicians are an essential component in reducing medication errors.

1. Certification proves a level of knowledge that the pharmacy technician has obtained.
2. Certification is critical to patient safety. In gaining a standardized level of knowledge, the pharmacy technician will have a broader knowledge base and hence reduce the likelihood of potential medication errors.
3. Certification is a positive step toward demonstrating the professionalism of pharmacy technicians.

On a more personal level, gaining national pharmacy technician certification is a big deal! Certification matters to you, because becoming certified will help you in your employment either to be eligible for a job or to get a promotion.

Certification matters to the employer for a number of reasons.

1. Certification may be required by the State Board of Pharmacy.
2. Certification is thought to be a tool used in selecting more qualified personnel.
3. Employing qualified, competent pharmacy technicians will help ensure medication safety.

Obtaining national certification demonstrates commitment by you, the pharmacy technician. The commitment between you and your employer will increase job satisfaction and will have a positive impact on work-related tasks, thus reducing medication errors.

Every healthcare professional must perform at the highest level of his or her degree. Gaining certification is a giant step toward doing your best in your profession!

A TRUSTED PROFESSION

Pharmacists have been ranked among the most trusted professionals in the country for more than two decades. A 2010 Gallup survey found that most Americans consider pharmacists to have very high honesty and ethical standards. Two other professions came in ahead of pharmacists: nurses and military officers. Grade school teachers and medical doctors came in behind pharmacists. The public sees you, the technician, as an integral part of the pharmacy operations. The trust that the American public has in its pharmacists is conveyed to the entire pharmacy team. It's our professional obligation to achieve our highest standards. Certification helps pharmacy technicians achieve professional goals.

Something to think about: At present, pharmacy technicians perform more than 90% of the daily tasks in pharmacy settings. Yet the education that technicians receive is only about 2% of what a pharmacist receives. Doesn't it make sense to show a baseline level of knowledge for pharmacy technicians through the certification process?

CHASING ZERO

Chasing Zero: Winning the War on Healthcare Harm is a brilliant documentary that explains the intent to teach and guide healthcare professionals to strive for zero medication errors. Actor Dennis Quaid hosts and narrates the documentary.

In 2007, Quaid and his wife's newborn twins were given a massive overdose of the blood thinner heparin. Since the occurrence of this medication error at Cedars-Sinai Medical Center in Los Angles, Quaid has been an advocate for patient safety and has helped educate the public on preventable medication errors. Quaid addressed his support for pharmacy technician certification in a letter to C. K. Mannesse, CEO of the American Society of Health System Pharmacists (ASHP), on December 7, 2009. Quaid wrote, "As pharmacists continue to rely heavily on pharmacy technicians, it is vitally important to ensure that standardized minimum requirements are in place to protect the health and well being of the public."

Take a moment now to link to the documentary at http://www.safetyleaders.org/pages/chasingZeroDocumentary.jsp. Your next 53 minutes of watching this presentation may prove to be the most valuable motivator for you to meet your certification goals.

To link to the Toolbox: http://www.safetyleaders.org/leadersToolbox/home.jsp

WHAT IS THE DIFFERENCE BETWEEN REGISTRATION AND CERTIFICATION?

Certification involves taking an exam to show a level of knowledge. To be certified means that you have passed a test. Registration, on the other hand, is not knowledge based. Registration is signing up with your State Board of Pharmacy. In the same manner that you register for college classes or register your vehicle, most states require pharmacy technicians to be registered. Being registered means that you are on a list of people who are authorized to practice as a pharmacy technician. States have different requirements for registration, or to get on that "list," to practice as a technician. Some states require you to be at least 18 years of age and to have a high school diploma or GED. Some states require a degree in pharmacy technology earned from an accredited college. Whatever the requirements of your state, being registered means that you have met the state's requirements to practice as a technician.

Each State Board of Pharmacy has jurisdiction over the registered pharmacy technician. Since the board has the duty to protect the general public, it is granted the power to undertake disciplinary action against a pharmacy, a pharmacist, or a pharmacy technician in the interest of protecting the public against further harm. The board has the authority to punish the registered individual for committing the wrongful act. Please keep in mind that if a pharmacy technician is *not* legally required to be registered or licensed within the state, the State Board of Pharmacy has no jurisdiction over the individual technician, but does have authority over the pharmacy.

Table 1-1 Pharmacy Regulatory Landscape

Mandatory Certification AZ, LA, TX, WV, WY, ID, IA, MT, NM, OR, UT, WA IL

Recognizes Certification (NH)
  Ratio (AL, ME, NC, CT, KS, MA, MN, NJ, TN, SC)
  Duties (KY, RI)
  1 of multiple options (CA, FL, IN, OH, MD, NV, VA)

Voluntary AK, CO, GA, AR, DE, DC, HI, MI, MS, MO, NE, ND, OK, SD, VT
No Regulation (NY, PA, WI)

Note: MS enacted a certification mandate effective April 2011.
Source: Courtesy of the National Healthcareer Association.

WHAT DOES IT MEAN TO BE LICENSED?

A pharmacist is both registered and licensed. Licensed means that the individual has met educational and testing requirements as well as other state-specific requirements to practice as a pharmacist. For example, a prospective pharmacist generally must earn a PharmD degree to obtain a license.

There are a handful of states that require pharmacy technicians to be licensed. However, the licensing procedures for technicians in these states are virtually the same as registration procedures. Alaska, Arizona, California, Massachusetts, Oregon, Rhode Island, Utah, and Wyoming require a technician to be licensed.

Emily's Law

Most of us have heard about the notable medication error that resulted in the death of a 2-year-old girl named Emily Jerry. Emily was given a parenteral saline solution containing 23% salt when the solution was physician ordered to be 1% salt. The wrong solution was prepared by a pharmacy technician at a Cleveland, Ohio, hospital in 2006. Since the death of his young daughter, Emily Jerry's father has advocated for training and certification for pharmacy technicians. In 2009, Ohio enacted Emily's Law, which requires certification for pharmacy technicians in Ohio. The Ohio Board of Pharmacy recognizes certification through the Institute for the Certification of Pharmacy Technicians (ICPT), the Pharmacy Technician Certification Board (PTCB), or an exam created by the employer that meets the board's requirements and standards.

Government representatives proposed Emily's Act, which called for mandatory pharmacy technician certification not only in Ohio but also in every state. Emily's Act was not enacted into law.

Currently, 13 states require pharmacy technicians to be certified through either PTCB or ICPT. An additional 20 states recognize certification by adjusting pharmacy technician to pharmacist staffing ratios or by allowing additional duties to certified pharmacy technicians. Voluntary certification is mandated in 15 states. As of January 2011, only 3 states did not have regulations regarding the certification of pharmacy technicians. That 48 states now recognize the value of certification for pharmacy technicians is a dramatic increase from 1993 when only 12 states required certification, registration, licensing, or all three for pharm techs (**Table 1-1**).

RESOURCES

1. Mask A, Armstrong R, Hinchcliffe K. NC company invents device to reduce prescription mix-ups. Available at: http://www.wral.com/lifestyles/healthteam/story/8898212/. Accessed February 2011.

2. Jones JM. Nurses Top Honesty and Ethics List for 11th Year. Available at: http://www.gallup.com/poll/145043/Nurses-Top-Honesty-Ethics-List-11-Year.aspx. Accessed February 2011.

3. Sangiacomo M. Ohio governor signs "Emily's Law" forcing standards for pharmacy technicians. Available at: http://blog.cleveland.com/metro/2009/01/emilys_law_enacted_by_gov_stri.html. Accessed January 7, 2009.

4. Emily's Law: Ohio pharmacy technicians and their employers face new state regulations. Jones Day Publication. http://www.jonesday.com/emilys-law-ohio-pharmacy-technicians-and-their-employers-face-new-state-regulations-09-16-2009. Accessed February 2011.

5. Postgraduate Healthcare Education. Prescription errors and their legal consequences: Best practice for prevention. Power-Pak C.E. Available at: http://www.powerpak.com. Accessed February 2011.

6. Institute of Medicine. *To Err Is Human: Building a Safer Heath System*. Kohn LT, Corrigan JM, Donaldson MS, eds. Washington, DC: National Academy Press; 1999:5.

7. National Healthcareer Association: Institute for the Certification of Pharmacy Technicians. Pharmacy Technician Certification (CPhT). Available at: http://www.nhanow.com/pharmacy-technician.aspx. Accessed February 2011.

8. *Chasing Zero: Winning the War on Healthcare Harm* [video]. Silver Spring, MD: Discover Channel/CME; 2010. Available at: http://www.safetyleaders.org/pages/chasingZeroDocumentary.jsp. Accessed February 2011.

TASK SHEET

TOPIC TO REVIEW: REGISTER FOR AN EXAM DATE

Materials

Pharmacy Technician Exam Review Guide

JB Test Prep: Pharmacy Technician Exam Review Guide

To Do List

☐ Study plan in place
☐ Check to see what exam my state recognizes
☐ Register for exam

Prepare

1. Read the section on the certification exam in the review guide.
2. Visit the exam websites: www.ptcb.org and www.icpt.org
3. Contact your state pharmacy board to find out which certification exams are approved in your state: PTCE, ExCPT, or both.
4. Decide which certification exam you will take: PTCE or ExCPT.

Study Plan

No studying at this point, but get a plan in place. How many days a week can you study? How many hours a day? What room of the house is best to study in?

Tips

After you have decided which certification test you will take, register for the exam. Follow the online registration instructions. Pick a testing date that allows you enough study time according to the study plan you have in place.

End of Chapter

Make notes here of questions you have about certification. Find out the answers by rereading the chapter, visiting the testing websites, or calling your state pharmacy board.

All About the Certification Exams

OBJECTIVES/TOPICS TO COVER:

✓ Know the steps to take before registering for the certification exam.
✓ Be familiar with the design of the certification exam.
✓ Evaluate the information to decide which certification exam is best for you.

THE CERTIFICATION EXAMS

Pharmacy technician certification distinguishes you as a professional in your field. The number of certified technicians has grown from a few years ago at an astonishing rate, which shows that the pathway to medication safety is developing.

Two different entities provide a National Certification Exam for pharmacy technicians: (1) the Pharmacy Technician Certification Board (PTCB) administers the Pharmacy Technician Certification Exam (PTCE) and (2) the Institute for the Certification of Pharmacy Technicians (ICPT) administers the Exam for the Certification of Pharmacy Technicians (ExCPT). Before arranging to take the certification exam, it is imperative to check with your State Board of Pharmacy to make sure the state you practice in approves of the PTCE, the ExCPT, or both.

Which Exam Should I Take: PTCE or ExCPT?

The first step is to check with your State Board of Pharmacy to see which exam is approved by your state.

The following states recognize *only* PTCE for certifying pharmacy technicians:

Arizona   Louisiana   Texas   Wyoming

All other states recognize both PTCB and ExCPT for certification of practicing pharmacy technicians.

These listings were current as of November 2010. Pharmacy rules and regulations periodically change. Before registering for your certification exam, please be sure to check with your State Board of Pharmacy for current guidelines on which pharmacy technician certification exam is accepted.

ICPT = ExCPT (the Institute for the Certification of Pharmacy Technicians, which is part of NHA (National Healthcareer Association), administers the Exam for the Certification of Pharmacy Technicians)

PTCB = PTCE (the Pharmacy Technician Certification Board administers the Pharmacy Technician Certification Exam)

Next, look at the similarities and differences in the tests offered by PTCB and ICPT.

How Are the Exams the Same?

Both exams are computer-based. PTCE moved from pencil and paper testing to computer-based testing in 2007. Computer-based testing allowed for quicker test results than the pencil and paper method. It also granted the flexibility to allow more testing days each year.

Computer-based testing means that the test taker will go to a specified site to take the exam on a computer. The exams cannot be taken at home on a personal computer. Test takers travel to a specified location to take the exam. The test taker is monitored by security cameras and by on-site administrators. The testing location is selected when you register for your exam. Again, the exam cannot be taken on a personal computer. You will register for the exam and select the most convenient testing location for you to travel to for the examination.

Both exams are timed. You have two hours to complete the exam.

Both exams have only multiple-choice questions. ExCPT has 110 questions. PTCE has 90 questions: no true/false, no essays, no matching. The exam you take will consist of only multiple-choice questions. While the ExCPT exam has 110 questions, 100 questions are scored or graded, and the other 10 questions are surveyed for possible use on future exams. This holds true for 80 of the 90 questions on the PTCE.

There is a fee for each exam. The fee for ExCPT is $105. PTCE is $129. Registration and payment for the PTCE exam are offered online only. The ExCPT exam registration and payment can be done over the phone or mailed in.

How Is the Exam Scored or Graded?

Both ExCPT and PTCE use a scaled score, which means that the number of questions answered correctly is mathematically converted (scored) and then applied to a pass or fail scale. It's difficult to determine how many questions can be missed to still pass the exam, because not all of the questions have an equal weighting. A question deemed more important in subject matter will have a higher point value than another question.

The passing score on the PTCE is 650. The maximum score is 900, while the lowest score is 300. You will achieve at least a 300 on the PTCE, but it takes a score of 650 or better to pass the exam!

The passing score for the ExCPT is 390, and scores may range from 200 to 500.

When Will I Know If I Passed?

Both PTCE and ExCPT have official pass/fail results available at the exam site as soon as the exam is completed. The pass/fail result will appear on the computer screen and will be printed out for you to have as a record of your results. Certificates and scaled scores will be mailed out within a few weeks of the testing date.

Exam retakes. The ExCPT exam may be taken as many times as necessary to pass. The PTCE may be retaken a maximum of three times. A fee is required for each exam session. PTCB mandates a longer waiting period between retests than ICPT.

Each exam has similar pass rate. As of October 2010, ExCPT had a 72% pass rate. PTCE showed a pass rate of 72% for 2009. (The 2010 pass/fail figures for PTCE were not updated at the time of this printing.)

TESTING GOALS

ICPT and PTCB have similar missions and goals. Among their goals are to enable pharmacy technicians to work more effectively with pharmacists to offer safe and effective patient care and service. A part of their collective vision is to show that certification will recognize pharmacy technicians who are proficient in the knowledge and skills needed to assist pharmacists and to promote high standards of practice for pharmacy technicians.

How Are the Exams Different?

The main difference in the actual exam is the content that the questions focus on. More than half of the ExCPT exam (52%) focuses on the *dispensing process*. The *dispensing process* includes gathering prescription information, preparing and dispensing the prescription, calculations involved in dispensing, business math, aseptic technique, unit dosing, and repackaging. Questions in this category will also cover refill requirements, use of abbreviations, automated dispensing equipment, proper labeling requirements, and proper packaging and storing of medications. The calculation questions in the dispensing process category will involve conversion between units of measure, days supply, and IV drip rates. The business math will focus on markup, pricing, and inventory control. Aseptic technique questions will deal with proper handling of chemotherapy medications, parenteral routes of administration, the use of laminar airflow hoods, and aseptic practices and procedures while compounding.

Although 52% of the ExCPT exam covers the dispensing process, most questions on the PTCB exam fall in the category of *Assisting the Pharmacist in Serving Patients* (66%). Exam questions in this category encompass receiving and processing a medication order, data relating to restricted and investigational drugs, third-party payers, calculations, preparing chemotherapy medications, extemporaneous compounding, storage requirements, record keeping, calibrating equipment, and aseptic technique.

Twenty-five percent of the ExCPT exam is made up of questions that address pharmacy regulations and technician duties. These questions involve labeling of over-the-counter and prescription medications, controlled substance laws and procedures, inventory control, and federal law.

The remaining 23% of the ExCPT exam involves *Drugs and Drug Therapy*. Questions on this topic involve drug classification, brand/generic names, most frequently prescribed drugs, dosage forms, mechanism of action for the drug, and common adverse interactions.

Maintaining Medications and Inventory Control Systems makes up 22% of the content on the PTCB exam. The questions in this category cover home medical equipment (durable medical equipment), stock and inventory, medication disposal, controlled substance and investigation, drug record keeping, repackaging, and quality assurance.

Participating in the Administration and Management of Pharmacy Practice makes up the final 12% of the PTCE. Questions in this category cover HIPAA (Health Insurance Portability and Accountability Act), pharmacy policies and procedures, and compliance regulations.

Table 2-1 summarizes exam categories and content. A detailed listing is outlined in Appendix A.

APPLICATION PROCESS

Just as there are similarities and differences in the exam, there are similarities and differences in applying for the exams. You may choose one exam over the other because of eligibility requirements, application processes, or both. Please read the application process for each exam. Which exam is best for you?

Table 2-1 Exam Content

ExCPT Exam Content	PTCE Exam Content
Dispensing Process 52% of the exam	Assisting the Pharmacist in Serving Patients 66% of the exam
Regulations and Technician Duties 25% of the exam	Maintaining Medication and Inventory Control Systems 22% of the exam
Drugs and Drug Therapy 23% of the exam	Participating in the Administration and Management of Pharmacy Practice 12% of the exam

Am I Eligible to Take the Exam?

To be eligible to take either certification exam, the following criteria may be required:

1. The candidate must be at least 18 years of age.
2. The candidate must have a high school diploma or GED.
3. The candidate must have no felony convictions.
4. The candidate must not have had any license or registration revoked or suspended or any disciplinary actions by a regulatory agency such as a State Health Board or State Board of Pharmacy.

The eligibility requirements for the exams differ somewhat regarding drug-related and felony convictions. If this is an area of concern for you, please read eligibility requirements on the exams' websites. There may be exceptions to the eligibility requirement regarding no felony convictions. Both examination bodies ask that testing candidates write an appeal for consideration if there is a felony conviction on their record. Reading the detailed information on the website will help you make your decision on which exam will work better for you.

> PTCE website: http://www.ptcb.org
>
> ExCPT website: http://www.nhanow.com/pharmacy-technician.aspx

After you determine your eligibility to take the exam, you are ready to apply. The application process is administered a bit differently for each exam.

PTCE Application Process

An online application process is required for the PTCE. Follow the links on the website to apply for the exam. This is a relatively easy process. You will begin by creating an account. It's important for you to use a dependable e-mail address as this is what the PTCB will use to send you the ticket to the test or Authorization to Test (ATT) letter. It's also a good idea to jot down your newly created account password. The password is needed to access account information.

You will need a credit card or an electronic check to pay for the exam at the time of the application.

After the application has been completed and the payment has been received, PTCB will e-mail you, the candidate, an ATT letter. This letter may take a few weeks to arrive, but it's an important document. It will have the instructions on how to schedule your exam and the dates on which you can take your exam. Please respond to your ATT letter right away, because PTCB allows you a limited amount of time to schedule your exam date. Keep your ATT letter in a safe place. This letter is your "ticket" to get into the testing room. You must bring your ATT letter to the testing site on the day of your exam!

Complete your application with the exact name that appears on your government-issued picture ID You will present your government-issued picture ID and your ATT letter at the test site. The names on these two documents must match.

The ATT letter sent to you from PTCB indicates that you are eligible to take the exam. Your next step is to register for your testing date. Please be sure to register for your test date as soon as you receive your ATT letter. PTCB has a 90-day cutoff date from the time you apply for the exam until the time you test.

You may register for your exam date by e-mail or by phone. Your ATT letter will have the e-mail address and phone number to register. You can also find this contact information on the PTCB website. Note that you will be contacting Pearson Vue to schedule your appointment, not PTCB. Pearson Vue is the company that administers the certification exam for PTCB.

ExCPT Application Process

The application process for ExCPT has fewer steps than that of the PTCE. Applicants simply call a toll-free phone number to apply and to schedule a test date. Basic information will be given over the phone when applying for the ExCPT. You will be calling LaserGrade Testing Centers, which is the company that administers the certification exam for ICPT. LaserGrade will help you find the closest and most convenient testing center. Payment for the exam is made at this time by credit card or you may mail in a personal check or money order. One benefit of the ExCPT application process is that candidates can usually take their exam within 24 to 48 hours of registration.

During the application process, alert exam officials to any special needs you may have. Both Pearson Vue and LaserGrade Testing will make special accommodations for candidates who qualify under the American with Disabilities Act.

> Important: Be sure your government-issued picture ID matches the name you gave when registering for your exam.

> Apply for ExCPT: LaserGrade toll-free number 1-800-211-2754
>
> Register for PTCE: PearsonVue toll-free number 1-866-902-0593 or www.pearsonvue.com/ptcb

Can I Change or Cancel My Exam Appointment?

Sometimes candidates get nervous when their test date approaches, and they may decide to move their testing date to a future time. You should make every effort to keep your testing appointment time. However, an emergency may come up that makes it difficult for you to test on the date you selected. Both PTCB and ICPT allow candidates to cancel or to reschedule their exam appointments. Rescheduling must be done at least 24 hours before the testing appointment time to avoid additional fees. If you choose to cancel your appointment, PTCB will allow you to withdraw your application and a full refund will be issued as long as you cancel at least 24 hours before your scheduled appointment time. ICPT will credit your account, and the credit can be used for a future testing date. Detailed rules on rescheduling or canceling your appointment can be found on the exams' websites.

Once you make your appointment, be on time and don't miss your appointment! If you have car trouble or some other problem that prevents you from being on time—go to your appointment late! You will not get a refund if you miss your appointment time. At best, you will arrive late but still be allowed to test and finish on time! No matter what, go to your exam. You may not have enough time to finish the exam, but at least you will have the testing experience and know what to expect the next time you take the exam.

GETTING READY FOR TEST DAY

Make sure you take a computer-based testing tutorial on your home computer before test day. The tutorial shows you how to navigate through the exam, what keyboard keys to use, what the exam screens will look like, how to skip a question, how to go back to a question, how to review your exam questions, and how to use the on-screen calculator. Do this tutorial at home to help relieve anxiety you may have about how computer-based tests work. If you do this tutorial at home, on your testing day all you will have to concentrate on is the actual exam.

> The tutorial for the ExCPT is found at www.psiexams.com
>
> The tutorial for the PTCE is found at www.vue.com/ptcb/

TEST DAY

You have gone through all the steps to determine which test is better for you, determined your eligibility, and applied and registered for your testing date. Now you're ready for the big day!

Studies show that we test better in a familiar surrounding. I recommend that you drive to your testing site before your exam date. Go inside the building, and if you're able to, sit in the room that you'll be testing in. Taking the time for these recommendations will help you gauge the drive time to the testing site. It will help calm your nerves on test day, because you'll be more familiar with where you're going and what your testing environment will be like.

On your actual test day, wear comfortable clothing. You should arrive at your test site at least 20 minutes before your appointment time. Take this time to get your thoughts organized and to use the restroom. Some sites may allow you to begin testing as soon as you arrive so that you may start the test earlier than your appointment time.

When checking in to your testing site, you will be required to show your government-issued picture ID. If you're taking the PTCE, you must also have your ATT letter. Your name on your ATT letter must match your name on your ID. If you're taking the ExCPT, your name on your ID must be the same name given when you registered for your exam over the phone.

You will not be allowed to take any personal belongings into the testing room. I suggest that you go into your testing site empty handed. Depending on the season, you may want to wear a lightweight jacket in case the testing room is chilly. If you have a purse, heavy coat, cell phone, book, or any other personal property, it will have to be stored with the receptionist before going into the testing room.

Do not bring your calculator to the exam! You must use the calculators provided to you by the testing site. On-screen calculators are used, or PTCE offers the option of a handheld calculator. Scratch paper or a dry erase board will also be provided by the testing site. Two suggestions for you or things to watch: If you're issued a dry erase board, make sure your dry erase marker works! Secondly, I suggest you use the on-screen calculator, as the handheld calculators at the testing sites are sometimes unreliable. You will only be given two pieces of scratch paper, which should be sufficient and shouldn't be a problem for you.

You will *not* be able to ask any questions about the exam content. The testing site administrator is there to proctor, or to oversee, the exam, only. The proctor will not be able to answer any questions. Please don't waste any of your testing time trying to ask about or clarify exam content.

Your testing time starts as soon as you walk into the testing room and sit at your computer. There is a tutorial offered before the actual test begins. The tutorial shows you how to navigate through the computer-based testing. You will be able to see an on-screen countdown clock of the remaining time for your exam. I strongly suggest that you do the tutorial at home before your test date. The time you spend on the tutorial may be included in your two-hour time limit. Don't take too long with this tutorial!

Test Taking Tips

- ✓ Set a study schedule to be as prepared as you can be. You'll retain more information if you study in small amounts of time each day rather than "cramming" for the exam the night before. For example, study for 45 minutes and then take a break. Study five times a week for a few weeks before the exam.
- ✓ Take practice tests. Follow-up on missed questions for understanding.
- ✓ Get a study buddy to help you prepare for the exam.
- ✓ Visit the exam site before the day of the test.
- ✓ Don't cram for the exam the night before or the morning of your exam. You're probably not going to learn anything new the morning of the exam. Cramming will only cause you to be more nervous and unsure.
- ✓ Be well rested and alert on test day.
- ✓ Dress comfortably.
- ✓ Read each question carefully. Don't spend too much time on a question. If you're unsure, mark the question to come back to later.
- ✓ If you don't know the answer, eliminate the answers that you know are wrong.
- ✓ Watch the clock and keep track of your time.
- ✓ Never leave a question unanswered.
- ✓ If you are unsure about the correct answer, pick the longer answer choice.
- ✓ Absolutes such as *never*, *always*, and *must* are probably *not* going to be the correct answer.

MORE ABOUT THE EXAM

The exam questions for both PTCE and ExCPT are written by registered pharmacists, certified pharmacy technicians, and pharmacy technician educators. Testing candidates will have a unique test, but each tester will have the same subject matter. The questions encompass knowledge from a variety of work settings. The exam is not specific to one pharmacy setting. Rather, your exam will likely have questions regarding hospital pharmacy, IV compounding, and retail pharmacy. Your exam will most likely have a mix of questions on brand/generic medications, pharmacy calculations, abbreviations, and protocols, for example. You will have to be knowledgeable in all settings to be successful on your exam.

The ExCPT exam is designed for entry-level pharmacy technicians. If you are one of those individuals with many years of practical pharmacy technician experience, the Institute for the Certification of Pharmacy Technicians (ICPT) believes that you deserve to test well! The intent of the ExCPT is *not* to include exam questions to stump the smartest of the smart. The intent *is* to provide a baseline of knowledge for entry-level pharmacy technicians.

Remember, the certification of pharmacy technicians is nationally recognized. What this means is that when you pass the exam, you are then recognized as certified in all states. You don't have to take a new exam if you move to another state. This compares to pharmacists who are mandated to take a state-specific exam for the state that they practice pharmacy in. ICPT and PTCB are recognized in the United States as the authorities in certifying pharmacy technicians.

Some entities may require the certified technician to take an additional test before practicing at that site. For instance, a hospital pharmacy may require the certified technician to take a specific exam on IV Compounding/Aseptic Technique. One of the benefits of the pharmacy technician certification is that it's nationally recognized rather than state specific.

Upon successful completion of the certification exam, you will have the credentialing of CPhT after your name.

STEPS TO BECOMING A CPHT

- ✓ Step 1: Check with your State Board of Pharmacy to determine which exam is approved by your state.
- ✓ Step 2: Look at the similarities and differences in the two exams to determine which certification exam is best for you.
- ✓ Step 3: Make sure you meet the eligibility requirements to take the exam.
- ✓ Step 4: Apply for the exam.
- ✓ Step 5: Choose a testing site and register for a testing date.
- ✓ Step 6: Take the online computer-based testing tutorial at your home computer.
- ✓ Step 7: Prepare for your exam.

CONTACT INFORMATION

Institute for the Certification of Pharmacy Technicians (ICPT)/National Healthcareer Associaion (NHA)
Exam for the Certification of Pharmacy Technicians (ExCPT)
7500 West 160th Street
Stilwell, Kansas 66085
Phone: 800-499-9092
Fax: 913-661-6291
http://www.icpt.org
info@nhanow.com

Pharmacy Technician Certification Board (PTCB)
Pharmacy Technician Certification Exam (PTCE)
2215 Constitution Avenue, NW
Washington, DC 20037-2985
Phone: 800-363-8012
Fax: 202-429-7596
http://www.ptcb.org

Exhibit 2-1 Study Tips from a Certified Tech

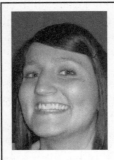

Emma Wickland, CPhT, BS
Story County Hospital
Nevada, Iowa

I said all through high school, "I'll just do it later." Yes, I had a pretty bad case of the studying blues until I was introduced to these techniques in a freshman orientation class.

— Study with a buddy or in a small group! Surrounding yourself with positive thinkers and peers that are dealing with the same obstacles as you will have a good impact on your grades and information retention. I believe the best way to know you understand the material is to be able to explain it to others.
— Note cards work wonders! When studying vocabulary or math conversions, or even studying what certain medications are prescribed for, simply reading through a list won't be enough. I suggest challenging yourself (and friends) to a game of flash cards. It sounds juvenile, but how fast did you learn addition using flash cards?
— An alternative to using note cards is sticky notes. I am partial to sticky notes, mostly because they are so colorful, which makes it more interesting for me.
— Use the teachers and professionals around you to learn all of the real-life knowledge you can. If you don't fully understand something you are reading about, or are interested to learn more, who better to ask for help than the people who deal with those things every day? These healthcare professionals and teachers have been there and done that when it comes to the classes you are taking and intelligence you are after. Not to mention that the 6-plus years of schooling they endured usually means they are passionate about their work and will be more than willing to light that spark in you.

Exhibit 2-2 Study Tips from a Certified Tech

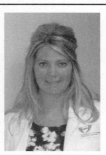

Megan Irlmeier, CPhT, BS-Biology
UNMC Pharmacy Student
Bellevue Medical Center
Bellevue, Nebraska

To prepare for the CPhT exam, I started by looking through the glossary and starring sections that were unfamiliar to me. Since I have worked in the field of pharmacy, I was also able to cross out some sections that I felt I didn't need to study. This allowed me to focus on newer and unfamiliar subjects more than if I were to go through the entire book.

Being unfamiliar with IV preparations and calculations, I started there. It is important to know conversions in this area. Second, if you think about it, the pharmacy field has its own "language." I feel that being knowledgeable about the abbreviations used in pharmacy is a crucial step in understanding many questions. If you don't know what is being asked on the exam because you don't know what an abbreviation stands for, how are you going to be able to answer the question? Along the same lines, knowing the top generics and their brand name is important in being able to answer questions as well.

When taking the certification exam, I felt it was beneficial to go through the introduction, because I had not taken a computer-based exam before. This portion of the test was not timed, and the program showed me how to use the calculator, how to flag questions to go back to, and how to see if there were any unanswered questions. I was also able to calm my nerves a bit during the tutorial. On that note, knowing how to flag questions is useful when you are unable to figure out a question. Since the exam was timed, I found it best to answer the questions I knew and save the harder questions for the end by flagging them. This allows you to manage your time for the questions that may require more time. Before submitting the exam, make sure all the questions have been answered. Last, but not least, if you are someone that gets anxious when others are "waiting to see" how you do on the exam, don't tell anyone you are taking it. Surprise them after the exam when you find out you have passed, because you will!

RESOURCES

1. Institute for the Certification of Pharmacy Technicians. *ExCPT Candidate's Guide: Exam for the Certification of Pharmacy Technicians*. Available at: register.nhanow.com/pics/.../ExCPT%20 Candidate%20Handbook.pdf. Accessed February 2011.
2. National Healthcareer Association: Institute for the Certification of Pharmacy Technicians. Pharmacy Technician Certification (CPhT). Available at: http://www.nhanow.com/pharmacy-technician.aspx. Accessed February 2011.
3. Pharmacy Technician Certification Board Website. http://www.ptcb.org. Accessed February 2011.

TASK SHEET

TOPIC TO REVIEW: PROCESSING PRESCRIPTION ORDERS

Materials

Pharmacy Technician Exam Review Guide

JB Test Prep: Pharmacy Technician Exam Review Guide

Prepare

1. Read the section on processing orders.
2. Take practice test at the end of the chapter.

To Do List

☐ Get a study buddy
☐ Read chapter
☐ Complete test
☐ Review missed questions

Study Plan

Make your own study plan for this chapter. Write down pages you will read and the practice test you'll take by the end of the week.

1. Read pages_____ on _____(date).
2. Take end of chapter practice test on_____(date).

Tips

Get a study buddy! If math is your weakness but your coworker's or classmate's strong point, team up with them to help you prepare for your exam. If you are most familiar with retail pharmacy procedures, for instance, team up with a pharm tech who is accustomed to IV pharmacy. Becoming study buddies will help you learn from each other's strong points. Your IV study buddy will help you learn commonly prescribed parenteral medications, while you, the retail expert, will share your expertise in insurance billing.

End of Chapter

List what you need to review.

Processing Prescription Orders

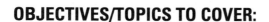

OBJECTIVES/TOPICS TO COVER:

- ✓ Formulate the correct procedures in processing prescription orders.
- ✓ Recognize patient profile data.
- ✓ Know how to assist with medication therapy management.
- ✓ Understand the proper use of pharmacy automation.

PROCESSING PRESCRIPTION ORDERS

Prescriptions may be presented to the pharmacy by fax, telephone, mail, electronic prescribing via computer, or in person. The procedure for processing prescriptions or medication orders differs from setting to setting. Mail-order pharmacy prescription processing will differ from home infusion pharmacy. Nuclear pharmacy prescription processing will differ from compounding pharmacies. Processing a prescription in the acute care or hospital setting is different from accepting and processing a prescription in the retail or ambulatory pharmacy.

An ambulatory pharmacy is a pharmacy that the patient can walk into or ambulate (ambulate means to walk) into to have a prescription filled. Another name for ambulatory pharmacy is retail pharmacy, or outpatient pharmacy.

An acute care pharmacy may also be called an inpatient pharmacy or hospital pharmacy. These terms may all be used interchangeably.

Ambulatory Pharmacy

Step 1: Receive the Prescription

The first step in processing the retail/ambulatory prescription is to receive the prescription. A paper prescription is called a hard copy. You will get a hard copy from the customer dropping off the prescription or from a fax sent from the physician's office. The physician's office may also call in a new prescription to the pharmacy. When the prescription is phoned in, the pharmacy technician will write down the patient's name, medication name, and all other directions as relayed by the physician's office. This prescription information written down by the pharmacy technician will now become the hard copy. It's very important for the technician to write legibly. Repeating the prescription directions back to the physician's office will help ensure accuracy. Although there is no federal law governing phoned-in prescriptions, some states will not allow pharmacy technicians to accept phoned-in *new* prescriptions.

The retail pharmacy may also receive an e-prescription (electronic). The e-prescription will be received on the pharmacy computer directly from the physician's data entry device. The e-prescription may be printed off or retained in the electronic format.

Step 2: Check the Prescription for Completeness

The following information must appear on the prescription according to federal pharmacy law (see **Figure 3-1**). State pharmacy laws may vary on prescription requirements. The certification exam will test you on requirements per federal law.

- **a.** Patient's full name
- **b.** Date written
- **c.** Name of medication
- **d.** Strength, dose, and dosage form
- **e.** Administration route
- **f.** Signa
- **g.** Quantity to dispense
- **h.** Refill information
- **i.** Prescriber's signature
- **j.** Prescriber's name

Schedule II prescriptions have additional information requirements:

- **a.** Prescriber's Drug Enforcement Agency (DEA) number
- **b.** Prescriber's address
- **c.** Patient's address

Signa is short for signatura, not to be confused with signature. Signa means directions for dispensing and for patient use. Signatura may also be abbreviated as S or as Sig.

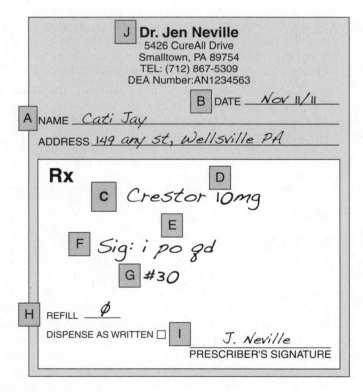

Figure 3-1 Prescription

At the time of prescription drop-off, the technician will be able to ask the patient questions to gather needed information for the patient profile.

- ✓ Patient's date of birth (DOB)
- ✓ Patient's full name if not written on prescription
- ✓ Patient's gender: Do not assume the patient's gender by name, alone. Many names are unisex.
- ✓ Any known drug allergies
- ✓ Whether the patient is taking any other medications: prescribed medications, over the counter (OTC), herbals, and vitamins
- ✓ Source of payment

Step 3: Interpret the Prescription and Check to Be Sure the Prescription Is Accurate

Read the prescription in its entirety. Does the drug ordered make sense for the patient's medical condition? Is the dosing schedule indicative of the prescribed medication? Does the strength coincide with the patient's age? Is the length of therapy and quantity to dispense sensible? Take this time to confirm the following:

- ✓ The prescription is authentic—check for possible forgery.
- ✓ Does the pharmacy have this medication in stock?

We must be 100% certain when interpreting and transcribing prescriptions. If you're unsure of what the prescription says, ask another technician to help you interpret it. It's important to *not* give your opinion of what the prescription says. Giving your opinion may sway the other technician to see the order as you do, rather than taking a fresh look. Any questionable prescriptions should be brought to the attention of your pharmacist. Your questions may be a result of misinterpreting the prescriber's handwriting or misreading an abbreviation.

Step 4: Enter Data

This step allows new prescription information to be entered into the computer. Data entry is critical to get reimbursement from the insurance company. Patient information, insurance information, and prescription information must all be entered correctly.

Some pharmacies will have the pharmacist enter new prescriptions as a safeguard to check for allergies, drug–drug interactions, and other alerts specific to the newly prescribed medication. Many pharmacies allow technicians to enter new prescriptions. Pharmacy computer software will present a series of warning dialogue boxes to alert the pharmacist of potential risks associated with the new medication. When entering new prescriptions, carefully read each warning and let your pharmacist know of any potential problems associated with the prescribed medication.

Dispense as Written (DAW)

The prescriber may indicate dispense as written (DAW) on the prescription. DAW means that the medication the pharmacy dispenses to the patient must be the exact medication that is written on the script (see **Table 3-1**). No generic substitution or otherwise pharmaceutical equivalents may be dispensed. Prescription pads may have a DAW signature line or a check box for the prescriber to specify DAW to the pharmacy.

Third-party payers have guidelines on how medication claims are paid. DAW codes help payers determine whether the medication is eligible for full reimbursement or whether the patient will be responsible for partial payment.

DAW codes are universal for all pharmacies and payers. Although you will not need to memorize the codes, and you will probably not be tested on which code means what, it's good to know that DAW codes exist and that the reason for the codes is to ensure proper reimbursement.

Most prescriptions processed will be entered as DAW Code 0. This means that the prescriber will allow the generic equivalent to be dispensed. DAW Code 0 is probably the default code preset in the pharmacy's software program, as this is the most common DAW code used in data entry.

Table 3-1 Dispense as Written (DAW) Codes

DAW Code 0	No DAW indicated
DAW Code 1	DAW: Prescriber states that brand name drug is medically necessary
DAW Code 2	Patient requests brand name
DAW Code 3	Pharmacist selects brand name
DAW Code 4	Generic equivalent is not stocked in the pharmacy
DAW Code 5	Pharmacy uses this brand as generic but realizes it will be reimbursed at the generic rate
DAW Code 6	Override
DAW Code 7	Brand drug is mandated by law
DAW Code 8	Generic not available from manufacturer

DAW Code 1 is used when the prescriber indicates DAW on the prescription—no substitution allowed.

Days Supply

Days supply must be calculated and entered in the computer for each prescription. Days supply is a very important figure, as this is how third parties will reimburse the pharmacy. If the wrong days supply is calculated and entered in the system, the pharmacy will not receive the correct amount of reimbursement from the insurance company (third-party payer).

To calculate days supply:

Total Quantity Dispensed ÷ Total Quantity Taken per Day

Example: The patient is to have 30 tablets and takes 1 tablet per day.

$$30 \div 1 = 30 \quad \text{The days supply is 30.}$$

Example: The prescription is for 60 tablets to be dispensed. The patient takes 4 tablets per day.

$$60 \div 4 = 15 \quad \text{The days supply is 15.}$$

Step 5: Adjudication

Adjudication is the online process in which a claim is sent to the insurance company and the insurance company accepts the claim for payment. The label for the medication is generated and automatically printed.

In the event that a claim is rejected by the insurance company, the technician will work to resolve any rejected claims. After the medication label is printed, the technician will perform an important check by matching the label against the hard copy prescription. A check is performed to make sure the right medication, the right dose, the correct patient, and other directions have been accurately transcribed and entered into the computer. Patient directions on the label should be in a clear, simple, and to-the-point sentence. Terms used on the label should be commonly known to the patient. Do not use unfamiliar words, abbreviations, or other medical lingo.

Label

Federal pharmacy law requires the following information to be on the prescription product label (see **Figure 3-2**):

    a. Pharmacy name, address, and telephone number
    b. Patient name

    c. Prescriber's name
    d. Medication name
    e. Strength of medication
    f. Directions for use in easy-to-understand terms
    g. Quantity dispensed
    h. Date the prescription was filled or refilled
    i. Prescription number
    j. Any cautionary statements
    k. The initials or name of the dispensing pharmacist

Step 6: Select Medication for Dispensing

The importance of this step is to be sure the correct medication is pulled from the shelf for dispensing. Stock bottles are similar in appearance. Sound-alike and look-alike names also contribute to dispensing errors. The best way to make sure the correct medication is selected for dispensing is to compare the National Drug Code (NDC) number on the stock bottle selected with the NDC number on the computer-generated label. The numbers must match to ensure correct dispensing.

Technicians may work in a pharmacy that uses handheld scanners. The technician will scan the barcode or NDC number on the computer-generated label and then scan the selected stock bottle. The handheld scanner will alarm if the NDC numbers do not match, therefore signifying the wrong drug has been selected for dispensing.

Step 7: Count/Measure Medication for Dispensing

The quantity to be dispensed is printed on the computer-generated medication label. Count or measure the correct quantity, and then initial the label next to the quantity. Initialing serves two purposes: (1) it serves as a second check for the technician to make sure the correct amount was dispensed; and (2) it allows the pharmacist to see which technician counted or measured the medication.

Mark an X on the stock bottle to indicate it has been opened. This simple step helps with inventory control.

This is another good checkpoint to ensure the correct medication is being dispensed. Before dispensing the medication, check to make sure the stock bottle NDC number matches the NDC number on the computer-generated label (see **Figure 3-3**).

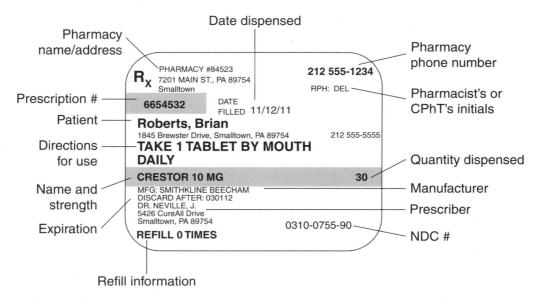

Figure 3-2 Rx Label

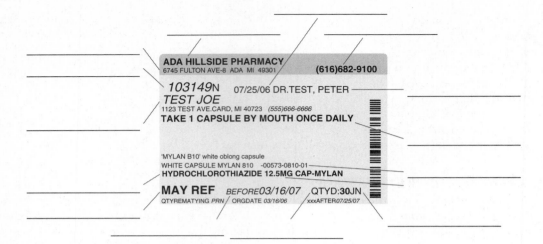

ADA HILLSIDE PHARMACY
6745 FULTON AVE-8 ADA MI 49301   **(616)682-9100**

*103149*N   07/25/06 DR.TEST, PETER
TEST JOE
1123 TEST AVE.CARD, MI 40723 *(555)666-6666*
TAKE 1 CAPSULE BY MOUTH ONCE DAILY

'MYLAN B10' white oblong capsule
WHITE CAPSULE MYLAN 810 -00573-0810-01
HYDROCHLOROTHIAZIDE 12.5MG CAP-MYLAN

MAY REF *BEFORE03/16/07* QTYD:**30**JN
QTYREMATYING *PRN* ORGDATE *03/16/06* xxxAFTER07/25/07

Figure 3-3 Vial Label for Practice

Medication vials must have safety (childproof) lids unless a customer-documented request for easy-open lids is on file at the pharmacy. There are exceptions to the safety lid law which are outlined in the child resistant packaging federal pharmacy law.

Step 8: Affix the Label to the Vial or Container

Take care to apply the vial label straight and neat. You may apply clear adhesive tape over the label. Clear tape will protect the paper label from spills. It's important for the label to remain on the bottle so that the patient has the dosing instructions and so the name of the patient is identified. Clear adhesive tape will also deter label tampering.

Medication Containers

An ambulatory pharmacy will dispense medications in a variety of containers. It's best to apply the label directly to the actual container that holds the medicine. For example, an inhaler may be dispensed to the customer in the manufacturer's box. Apply the label directly to the inhaler, rather than to the box. The patient may throw the box away, leaving the inhaler unidentified and leaving the patient with no administration instructions.

- ✓ Vial: amber in color to block out direct light for better storage
- ✓ Oval: also referred to as ointment jar used to dispense semisolids such as creams and ointments
- ✓ Bottle: used to dispense liquid solutions
- ✓ Tube: used to dispense semi-solids
- ✓ Manufacturer's pre-packaged containers: for inhalers, eye/ear drops, and aerosols

Auxiliary and Warning Labels

Apply auxiliary and warning labels to the vial or container. Auxiliary labels give additional instructions to the patient. Warning labels call out specific warnings to patients. Please don't confuse *auxiliary*, which means supplemental or additional, with *axillary*, which is the medical term for armpit (see **Figure 3-4**).

A section of the computer-generated label is applied to the back side of the hard-copy prescription. The label applied to the back side of the hard copy serves as a lasting record of the prescription number, dispensed medication, patient instructions, and quantity dispensed.

> Prescription number is also known as Serial number

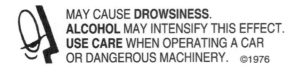

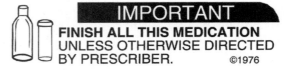

Figure 3-4 Auxiliary and Warning Labels

Source: © Pharmex/Precision Dynamics Corporation. Pharmex Original Copyrighted Warning Labels were copied/printed with authorization by Precision Dynamics Corporation.

Step 9: Place Items for Pharmacist Check

The prescription order must be checked before it leaves the pharmacy. To check the medication, the pharmacist will need to see the original hard-copy prescription, the stock bottle, and the computer-generated label.

Tech Check Tech

A small group of states, including California, Minnesota, Iowa, and Texas, have sanctioned a tech check tech practice. While most states authorize tech check tech programs only in hospital and clinical pharmacy, the checking process in retail pharmacy could also include a step of tech check tech.

Tech check tech practices allow one technician to make the final check of another technician's work. The technicians who take part in the tech check tech program have to go through specialized training. Tech check tech programs help free up the pharmacists' time to do more counseling and patient-centered medication therapy management (MTM).

Step 10: Provide the Patient with HIPAA Information and Teaching Sheets

First-time customers to the pharmacy will need a copy of HIPAA, or Health Insurance Portability and Accountability Act, regulations and will need to sign off that they have received a copy of the regulations.

It's especially important for patients getting a new medication to receive a teaching sheet. The teaching sheet gives information on their new medication, such as why they are taking the medication, side effects, whether the medication should be taken on an empty stomach or with food, and when their physician should be contacted because of an adverse reaction. The teaching sheets work hand in hand with counseling the patient will receive from the pharmacist.

Some medications need to be dispensed with a package insert (PI). Federal law mandates hormones, including oral contraceptives, to be dispensed with the patient package insert (PPI) provided by the manufacturer. Other medications with dangerous side effects, such as Accutane, may also be dispensed with a PPI. The PPI is a leaflet that details information on the medication. Indication for use, serious adverse reactions, side effects, and precautions are among the detailed in the PPI.

Step 11: Complete Transaction: Pharmacist Provides Counseling

Complete the transaction by checking the patient out at the point of sale (POS) or cash register. It's not uncommon for the patient who is receiving a routine refill to want to speak with the pharmacist. Make sure to ask all patients if they have any questions about their medication. If they do have a question, direct them to the pharmacist for counseling.

It must be the pharmacist, not the technician, who offers counseling to all patients receiving a new medication. Counseling should also be offered to patients who have a dosage change or a change in administration instructions. Patient counseling provided by the pharmacist is an important step in preventing medication errors. During consultation, the pharmacist will talk with the patient about how to take the medicine, when to take the medicine, and why the medicine was prescribed. Consultation is a checkpoint in making sure the correct medication is going to the correct patient.

A pharmacy technician must never provide consultation to the patient[1]. Counseling is the sole responsibility of the pharmacist. A distinguishing factor between the pharmacy technician and the pharmacist is that only the pharmacist may provide patient counseling. The technician works with the drug product, such as counting, while the pharmacist is the expert on drug knowledge, such as side effects.

The patient has a right to refuse counseling offered by the pharmacist. Patients may be pressed for time or a caregiver may pick up the medication rather than the patient. Suggest that the patient phone the pharmacy when the time is more convenient for them to receive counseling.

Step 12: File Hard Copy and Return to Stock (RTS)

The steps in dispensing a retail prescription continue after the patient has left the pharmacy with the medication. The final step is a sort of cleanup step in which the hard copy is filed and the stock bottle is returned to stock. Prescription hard copies are filed by prescription number. The prescription number was assigned to the hard copy after adjudication.

Returning stock bottles back to the shelf is also known as return to stock (RTS). Filing the hard copy and putting the stock bottles back on the shelf are two final checkpoints completed as time allows. Most often the pharmacy procedure is to file the hard copies at the end of the day. RTS is done when prescription processing time allows.

Acute Care Pharmacy

Step 1: Receive the Medication Order

A prescription is referred to as a medication order in the acute care pharmacy setting. Acute care, or hospital, pharmacies may receive a paper order by fax, by pneumatic tube, or by a runner. A runner is a hospital employee who acts as a type of mail carrier, or messenger, delivering materials and supplies to different departments in the hospital. The runner picks up the order from the nurses' station and delivers the order to the pharmacy.

Pneumatic tubes are used to "tube" orders to the pharmacy from different departments in the hospital. Pneumatic tubes used in the hospital are similar to the pneumatic tubes used in drive-through banking.

A nurse or physician may call in an emergency, or STAT, order to the pharmacy. An order that is called in is called a verbal order. Although the order is called in, it will be followed up with a paper medication order.

Many hospital pharmacies are paperless. This means the pharmacy will receive all medication orders electronically via computer.

Step 2: Check for Completeness

Medication orders should include the following information. A medication order is depicted in **Figure 3-5**:

    a. Patient name
    b. Patient's medical record number
    c. Patient's date of birth (DOB)
    d. Patient's height and weight
    e. Location of patient/room number
    f. Known allergies
    g. Diagnosis
    h. Gender
    i. Physician's name
    j. Date and time order written

---

[1] Pharmacy technicians working on a military base may have authority to provide certain aspects of patient counseling. Air Force pharmacy technicians are called apprentices. Army pharmacy technicians are called specialists.

    k. Authorizing signature (physician or nurse)

    l. Medications ordered to include:

       ◦ Medication name, strength, dosage form, dosing schedule, route of administration, administration instructions

Step 3: Prioritize Orders (Triage)

Once the order is received in the pharmacy, it's triaged. Triage is categorizing orders to determine which ones need to be acted on first and which orders are less urgent and can be filled later.

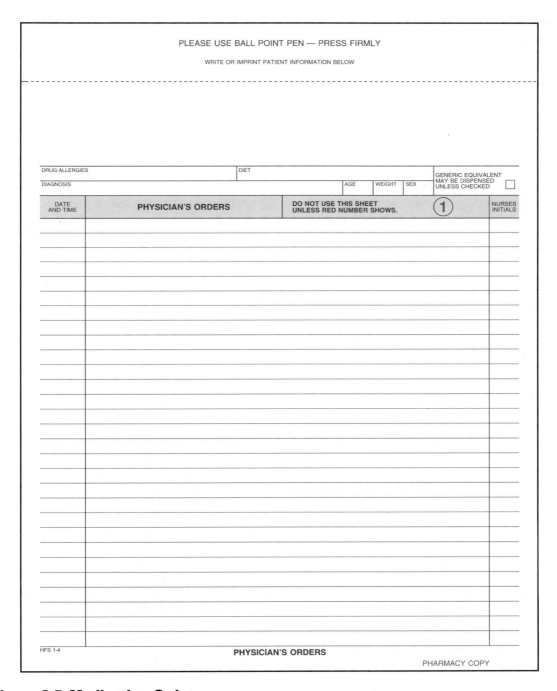

Figure 3-5 Medication Order

Prioritizing orders is an important step in hospital pharmacy. For instance, a patient may need a medication prior to surgery. If the patient doesn't receive the medication on time, the surgery team could be left waiting, causing a backup in the surgery schedule for the day.

Many patient conditions exist where time is paramount in filling the medication order. A STAT order must be delivered to the patient care unit within 15 minutes. ASAP orders and NOW orders will also come into the hospital pharmacy. ASAP and NOW orders should be processed with more urgency than a routine order. When working with STAT, ASAP, and NOW orders, it's important to be quick and, equally important, to be accurate! Some institutions may require STAT orders to be hand-delivered.

Step 4: Enter Data

After receiving the medication order and triaging it, the order is entered into the computer. In most hospital pharmacies, the pharmacist enters the orders. Many considerations are made when inputting medication orders in the hospital setting. Pharmacists will monitor lab values, potential drug–drug interactions, dosing regimens, and other patient data related to medication therapy.

If the hospital pharmacy procedures allow the pharmacy technician to enter data, then a pharmacist will verify the data entry.

Step 5: Dispense

Many hospital pharmacies have some type of automated dispensing machines or robotics in place. Patient data is entered in the computer, and the robot is then queued to dispense the medication order. Even with robots, manual order filling will still be needed in the hospital.

Pharmacy technicians fill medication orders according to computer-generated labels. Labels in the hospital setting look different from prescription labels applied to vials in the retail pharmacy setting. Hospital labels are smaller and more concise. The hospital label has a barcode that the pharm tech scans to match the barcode on the medication. Barcoding technology helps ensure the correct medication is pulled from the shelf.

Medications are unit dosed in the hospital setting. Unit dose means that the medications are individually packaged rather than shelved in stock bottles (**Figure 3-6**). Unit dose packaging is labeled with the drug name and strength, the expiration date and lot number, and a barcode. Unit dose is crucial in the hospital setting as this allows the medication to be identifiable until the tablet reaches the patient's mouth. Because the unit dose medication is individually packaged, it can be

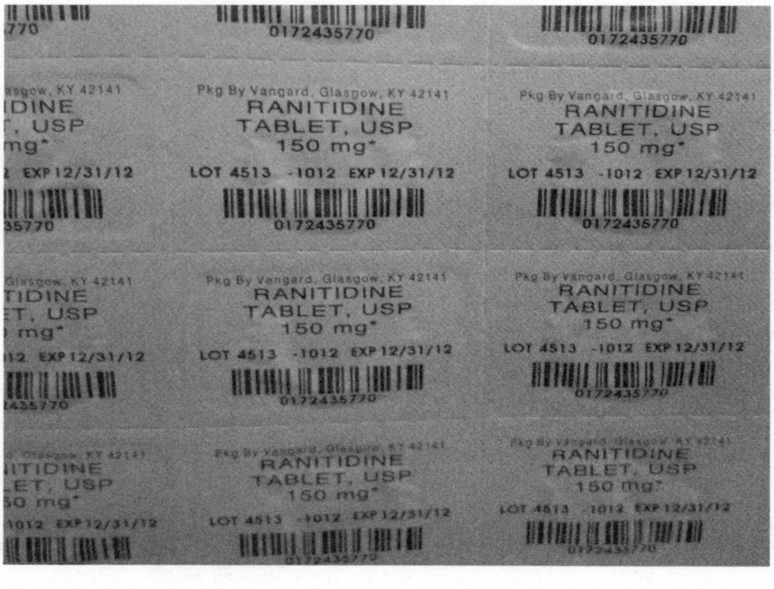

Figure 3-6 Unit Dose Medication

returned to stock if there is an order change, thus saving money for the patient, the hospital, and the insurance carrier.

Routine medication orders are filled for a 24-hour time period in hospital pharmacy. Dosages can change, medications can be added or discontinued, and patients may be discharged to go home. Filling medication carts or patient drawers in a 24-hour cycle is an efficient workflow pattern.

IV compounding is also completed at this dispensing step. The technician uses a compounding sheet as a guide in preparing the IV medication order. The compounding sheet is derived from the physician's order. The final IV product is labeled and placed for pharmacists' check.

Step 6: Place for Pharmacist Check

All medication orders must be checked before leaving the pharmacy. A handful of states use the tech check tech system for inpatient/hospital pharmacy. Otherwise, a pharmacist must perform the final check on medication orders before leaving the pharmacy. STAT orders, IV, medications dispensed from the robotics—all medications need a final verification check before leaving the pharmacy.

Step 7: Deliver to Patient Care Unit

Medications will be hand-delivered or can be "tubed" to the patient care area. Delivering medications by pneumatic tube systems is convenient, but some medications cannot be tubed. Do not use the pneumatic tube for these situations:

- ✓ Product exceeds tube size so that product can't be secured or padded
- ✓ Items are too heavy
- ✓ "Do not shake" medications
- ✓ Hazardous medications such as chemotherapy and radiopharmaceuticals
- ✓ Glass bottles
- ✓ CII's
- ✓ Expensive medications
- ✓ Explosive or flammable items

PATIENT PROFILE

Both acute care and ambulatory pharmacies maintain a database of patient information. When a patient is new to the facility, information will be obtained to create a profile. The technician will assist the pharmacist in asking the patient questions to help complete the profile. Patient contact is more frequent in the ambulatory setting, which helps in keeping the profile up to date. Much of the patient profile information needed in the acute care pharmacy can be obtained from the patient chart. Nursing will gather the patient's weight; admissions will have demographic information. It is the technician's responsibility to keep the profile updated at each recurrent patient visit.

The benefit of having an accurate and up-to-date patient profile is to better serve the patient. The pharmacist can check for drug–drug interactions and possible medication duplication. The pharmacist will be able to see a broader picture of possible reasons for noncompliance. The patient profile is a building block to medication therapy management (MTM).

The patient profile contains the following information:

- ✓ Patient name
- ✓ Demographic information
- ✓ Medical record number
- ✓ Date of birth (DOB), height, weight, diagnosis
- ✓ Lab/test results (also blood pressure [BP], blood glucose)
- ✓ Allergies
- ✓ Primary physician
- ✓ Medications and regimen (including over the counter [OTC])
- ✓ Date of hospital admission

   ✓ Insurance information
   ✓ History of adverse reactions
   ✓ Interactions
   ✓ Special considerations for patient (easy-open lids, hard of hearing)

ASSISTING WITH MEDICATION THERAPY MANAGEMENT

The passage of Medicare Modernization Act of 2003 mandated medication therapy management (MTM). The government created MTM in an effort to reduce healthcare costs associated with medications. The intent of MTM is that pharmacists review patients' medication history to check for inconsistencies. Patients who have a greater need for MTM are those who use multiple meds, have multiple diseases, or have excessive medication costs.

Medication compliance, or making sure patients are taking their medication as instructed, is one goal of MTM. Making sure prescribed medications are used correctly, discontinuing duplicate drugs, or changing a patient from a brand medication to the generic not only will control costs but also will serve the patient in better therapy outcomes. An accurate and up-to-date patient profile helps the pharmacist to manage the patient's medication regimen. Patients should have an annual comprehensive medication review by a pharmacist. This patient-centered meeting might be an in-person meeting, a telephone call, or web camera exchange.

The pharmacy technician assists the pharmacist in medication therapy management by collecting and recording patient data. Data are obtained from patients and healthcare providers. A wider range of patient profile information is desired for MTM. The more information gathered, the more effective the pharmacist can be with MTM. Demographic, medical, administrative, lifestyle, and economic information are gathered for MTM (see **Figure 3-7**).

Besides gathering patient profile information, another important part of MTM for the technician is assisting the pharmacist in patient care activities. Blood pressure monitoring, immunizations, and flu shots are three areas of patient care activities. Some states certify pharmacists to administer immunizations and flu shots. One way the pharmacy technician will assist the pharmacist in administering immunizations or flu shots is by registering the patient and by helping the patient to complete required paperwork.

The pharmacy technician may perform administrative duties to collect reimbursement from insurance carriers and from patients for MTM services. Insurance claims require special coding called current procedural terminology (CPT). The exact CPT codes must be entered correctly on the insurance claim form in order for the company to process the claim. Once the claim is processed, the pharmacy will be paid for MTM services. A pharmacy technician with knowledge in CPT codes and with training in insurance claim processing is an asset to the pharmacy team.

What Is Nonadherence?

The term *nonadherence* refers to a patient who does not take his or her medication as prescribed. Examples of medication nonadherence, or noncompliance, are taking less than the prescribed dose, taking someone else's medicine, not filling the prescription, or stopping the medication before the supply runs out (antibiotics).

Poor adherence, or nonadherence, may be detrimental to the patient's health. Pharmacy technicians can play a role in improving adherence by making sure the patient receives counseling from the pharmacist.

PHARMACY AUTOMATION

Pharmacy automation is designed to reduce medication error and to increase productivity. Automation can be found in all pharmacy settings.

   ✓ Automated prescription dispensing systems
   ✓ Automated point of care dispensing machines

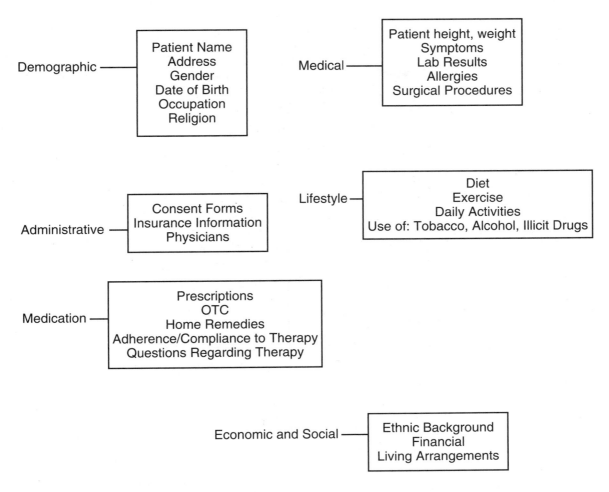

Figure 3-7 MTM Information Gathered

- ✓ Barcoding
- ✓ Automated cart fill machines
- ✓ Robots to deliver products

An automated machine may also be called a robot. An automated machine, or robot, stores medications. It will then dispense the medicine when a computer prompts it to. It's the pharmacy technician's responsibility to maintain the inventory in the machines/robots and to help maintain the machines.

Pharmacy automation will not take away the pharmacy technician's role in the pharmacy. Rather, automation will shift the work pattern to provide time for other pharmacy duties. While automation is a hefty initial investment, the increased productivity and reduction in errors will dramatically outweigh the costs. The U.S. Food and Drug Administration (FDA) estimates barcode technology alone will save $93 billion over the next 20 years.

Automated Prescription Dispensing System

Automated prescription dispensing systems count out tablets, put the tablets in a vial, put the lid on the vial, and apply the label to the vial (see **Figure 3-8**)!

Automated Point of Care Dispensing Machine

The point of care automated machines are located in specialized departments throughout the hospital. These automated dispensing devices (ADD) will be stocked with the medication needs of that specific

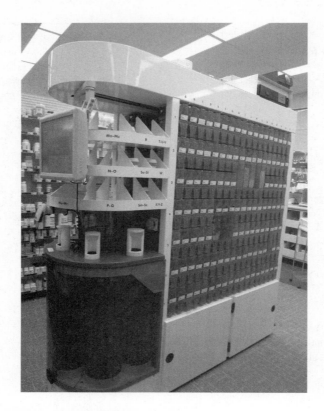

Figure 3-8 Parata Robotic Dispensing System

department. The ADD in the cardiac unit will be stocked with cardiac-specific medications; the ADD in the emergency department (ED) will be stocked with the medications most needed for that department. The benefit of automated point of care dispensing machines is that they allow medications to be stored and dispensed near the point of care. The machines keep inventory reports and track health-care personnel who remove medication from the cabinet (see **Figures 3-9**, **3-10**, and **3-11**).

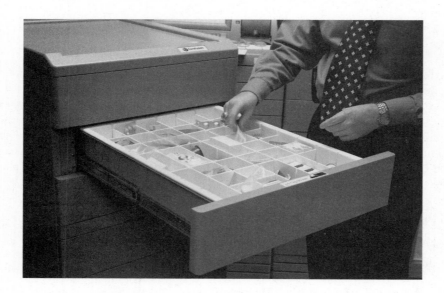

Figure 3-9 The Pyxis MedStation™ system is an automated dispensing cabinet supporting the decentralized medication management process by providing an added safety precaution for high risk medications of diversion

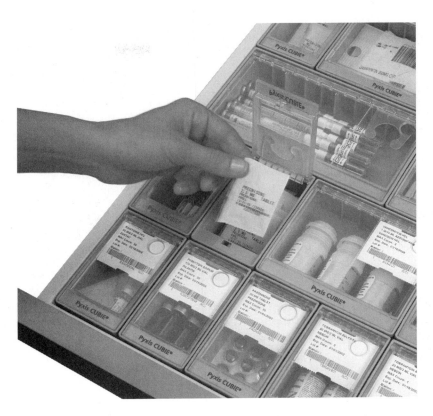

Figure 3-10 The Cubie® Replenishment system helps address medication management challenges by focusing on the security of the process of filling, delivering and removing medications at the Pyxis MedStation™ system or the Pyxis SpecialtyStation™ system

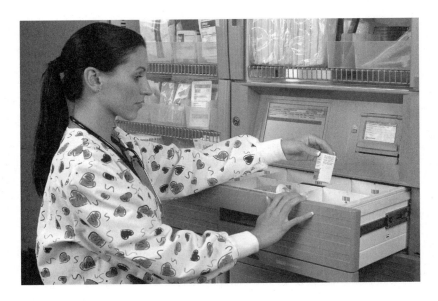

Figure 3-11 An automated system that tracks both medications and supplies, the Pyxis SpecialtyStation™ system helps ensure products are always available and charges are accounted for while helping to increase pharmacy and nursing efficiencies and time spent on patient care

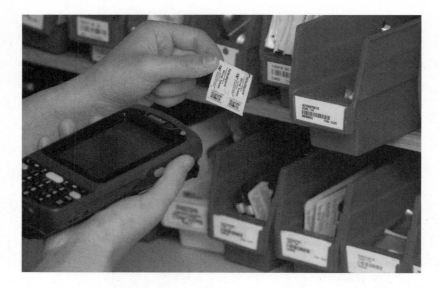

Figure 3-12 The Pyxis PARx® system effeciently and accurately automates the procedure by utilizing barcode-scanning technology to track medication handling, review, and delivery from the pharmacy to the Pyxis MedStation™ system

Barcoding

In an effort to reduce medication errors, the FDA issued a ruling that requires certain prescription packaging to have a National Drug Code (NDC) barcode. The NDC contains the medication name and dose. The lot number and expiration date may also be presented on the packaging, but these are less important pieces of information when dealing with medication errors.

A handheld, wireless scanner is used for barcoding technology. The pharmacy technician can verify that the correct medication is being pulled from the shelf by scanning the barcode on the packaging. Barcoding technology alerts the tech if the wrong drug has been pulled. Some hospitals take barcoding technology a step further in that the nursing team will also scan the medication's barcode before administering the medication to the patient. First, the patient's identification bracelet is scanned, and then the barcode on the unit dose packaging is scanned. Barcoding technology alerts the nurse if the wrong drug has been chosen (see **Figure 3-12**).

This is your checklist to make sure you understand what you need to know for the certification exam. Review chapter content if there is a topic you're uncertain of.
I know:

√	...the information needed to make up a complete prescription (ambulatory and acute care)
	...systems for checking prescriptions
	...how to correctly calculate days supply
	...the steps to follow to ensure correct medication distribution
	...labeling requirements
	...why auxiliary labels are used
	...DAW codes
	...my work as a pharmacy technician must be checked by a pharmacist unless my practice site makes use of a "tech check tech" program.
	...only a pharmacist may council the patient

	...information needed for a patient profile
	...the pharmacy technician's role in MTM
	...the use of automated dispensing devices

RESOURCES

1. Appropriate Utilization of Dispense as Written (DAW) Codes. Available at: http://www.medicaid. state.al.us/documents/program-RX/DAW_Codes_2-26-09.pdf. Accessed February 2011.
2. US Department of Health and Human Services. US Food and Drug Administration. http://www. fda.gov. Accessed January 2011.
3. Peak A. Delivering medications via pneumatic tube systems. *Hosp Pharm*. 2003;38(3):287–290.
4. The United States Pharmacopeial Convention 2011. *Pharm Forum*. 2011;37(1).
5. Reiss BS, Hall GD. *Guide to Federal Pharmacy Law*. 4th ed. Delmar, NY: Apothecary Press; 2004.
6. Williams, H. Federal Requirements for Pharmacy Technicians working on a Military Base. Available at: http://www.ehow.com/list_7510155_federal-technicians-working-military-base.html. Accessed January 2011.

CHAPTER 3

MULTIPLE CHOICE

Identify the choice that best completes the statement or answers the question.

_____ **1.** The next step after receiving a prescription in an ambulatory pharmacy is to

a. calculate the days supply for the prescription

b. check the prescription for completeness

c. enter the prescription information into the database

d. select the medication needed to fulfill the prescription

_____ **2.** According to federal pharmacy law, what information must appear on an ambulatory prescription?

a. patient's full name, name of medication, pharmacy name

b. patient's full name, name of medication, date dispensed

c. patient's full name, name of medication, date written

d. patient's full name, name of medication, manufacturer name

_____ **3.** The patient's profile will include

a. DOB, drug allergies, gender

b. patient's full name, drug allergies, marital status

c. patient's gender, drug allergies, place of employment

d. prescribed medications, OTC medications, level of education

_____ **4.** When interpreting the prescription, check

a. if the prescribed medication is on the patient's insurance plan

b. the prescription for possible forgery by phoning the prescriber

c. with the pharmacist to be sure required information is included

d. that the dosing schedule is customary for the prescribed medication

_____ **5.** The purpose of a DAW code is to

a. ensure proper third-party reimbursement

b. direct the technician on which medication to dispense

c. alert the prescriber to potential interactions

d. allow the pharmacist to dispense an alternative medication

_____ **6.** The patient is to have a quantity of 60 tablets and is to take 2 tablets a day. What is the days supply?

a. 2

b. 60

c. 30

d. 15

_____ **7.** The ambulatory prescription label must contain

a. pharmacy name, patient name, prescription number

b. prescription number, quantity dispensed, manufacturer

c. manufacturer, prescriber's name, medication name

d. medication name, directions for use, generic and brand name of medication

_____ **8.** The hard copy is the

a. label for the vial

b. electronic prescription saved to the computer hard drive

c. paper copy of the prescription

d. copy of the original prescription returned to the patient for record keeping

_____ **9.** A PPI (patient package insert)

a. provides instructions to the patient

b. lists additional drug information to the patient

c. lists emergency contact information to the patient

d. provides billing information for the patient

_____ **10.** Patient counseling

a. may be provided by the technician for OTC products

b. is the sole responsibility of the pharmacist

c. may be provided by the technician if the pharmacist is not available

d. may be provided by the insurance carrier

ANSWER SECTION

1. B

The first step is to receive the prescription. The second step is to check the prescription for completeness. The third step is to interpret the prescription.

2. C

Information that must appear on the prescription:

    Patient's full name

    Date written

    Name of medication

    Strength, dose, dosage form

    Administration route

    Signa

    Quantity to dispense

    Refill information

Prescriber's signature

Prescriber's name

3. A

The patient profile will include:

DOB

Full name

Gender

Drug allergies

Medications the patient is taking: prescribed medications, OTC medications, herbals, vitamins
Source of payment

4. D

Things to check for during interpretation:

Does the drug make sense for the patient's condition?

Is the dosing schedule indicative of the prescribed medicine?

Does the strength make sense for the patient's age?

Is the length of therapy sensible?

Is the quantity to dispense sensible?

5. A

6. C

Total Quantity Dispensed ÷ Total Quantity Taken per Day 60 ÷ 2 = 30

7. A

Label must include:

Pharmacy name and address

Patient name

Prescriber's name

Medication name

Strength of medication

Directions for use

Quantity dispensed

Date filled

Prescription number

Caution statements

8. C

Hard copy is the original paper copy of the prescription order; it can be faxed, computer generated, or handwritten.

9. B

The patient package insert is mandated for some medications. It gives detailed information about the drug.

10. B

The technician may never counsel. This is the sole job of the pharmacist.

TASK SHEET

TOPIC TO REVIEW: ASSISTING THE PHARMACIST WITH SERVICE PATIENTS

Materials

Pharmacy Technician Exam Review Guide

JB Test Prep: Pharmacy Technician Exam Review Guide

Prepare

1. Read the section on assisting the pharmacist with serving patients.
2. Take practice test at the end of the chapter.

Study Plan

1. Read pages_____ on _____(date).
2. Take end of chapter practice test on_____(date).

Tips

1. Learn more about Medicare by visiting the website http://www.medicare.gov.
2. Look at your own third-party insurance information. What medications are on your formulary? Are there payment tiers? What is your deductible for prescription medications?

End of Chapter

List what you need to review.

Assisting the Pharmacist in Serving Patients

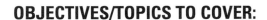

OBJECTIVES/TOPICS TO COVER:

✓ Identify investigational drug data procedures.
✓ Know third-party payers and review claim processing.

INVESTIGATIONAL DRUG DATA

Investigational, or experimental, drugs, in most cases, have not yet been approved for market by the U.S. Food and Drug Administration (FDA). These drugs are listed as Investigational New Drugs (IND) by the FDA. The exception to the rule is that sometimes a drug can be on the market but listed as IND because it is being tested for a different disease condition than originally approved.

IND status is a step in getting the drug to market. After the FDA has approved IND status, the drug is tested on humans for safety and effectiveness. This is where the pharmacy technician's responsibilities come into play.

The pharmacy technician can assist the pharmacist with:

✓ Preparation of drug
✓ Special record keeping
✓ Special procedures
✓ Protocols

There are two reasons someone would take an experimental or investigational drug. First, a physician may request IND for a patient with a serious disease or condition for which approved drugs aren't working. The physician may feel the patient could benefit from the investigational drug because of promising early study results. Compassionate use is an expanded access program the FDA offers to allow seriously ill patients the use of investigational drugs.

The second reason is that an individual desires to participate in a clinical trial. In a clinical trial, the participant is enrolled in a controlled study that involves a blind study or a double-blind study. A placebo, or "sugar" pill, containing no active medication, is given to a group of participants, while the actual IND is given to another group of participants. In a blind study, participants have no idea whether they are getting the actual medication or the placebo. They're "blind" to what they're receiving. Researchers document observations and outcomes. The difference in a double-blind study is that neither the participant *nor* the researcher knows which group of participants is receiving the placebo or the actual medication. Double-blind studies are thought to be more accurate, as there are no predispositions or expectations from the researcher that may interfere with observations and data outcome.

Preparation of Drug

The pharmacy technician will often assist the pharmacist in compounding and preparing the IND as well as the placebo to be administered to the study participants. Don't mix up the two! Your pharmacy will have protocols in place to ensure proper dispensing.

Special Record Keeping

Investigational drugs may pose unknown risks to patients. Therefore, special record-keeping procedures are required. Similar to record keeping for controlled drugs, investigational drugs require strict inventory control and accountability. The technician will assist the pharmacist in keeping dispensing records, documenting adverse events, and recording unintended side effects.

Special Procedures and Protocol

Protocol means to follow a set of rules and a procedure. IND protocol must be closely followed to ensure accuracy. Careful preparation of the drug and meticulous record keeping are imperative steps in order for the drug to reach the market. After clinical trials are satisfactorily completed, the drug company will file with the FDA for a New Drug Application (NDA). IND is an exciting area for the pharmacy technician to assist the pharmacist. What a rewarding feeling to know that you've been a part of bringing a new drug to the market!

> IND Protocol: Borrowing or lending investigational drugs is prohibited.

> Something to Think About: On average, pharmaceutical companies spend $802 million to get an IND to market.

THIRD-PARTY PAYERS

Direct payment is when patients pay the pharmacy 100% of their bill from their own funds or bank account. Patients may make *direct payment*, also known as out-of-pocket expense, if they don't have insurance or if their insurance doesn't cover the medication or service.

Third-party payer refers to the entity that makes full or partial payment to the pharmacy for medication and services. The patient is the first party, the pharmacy is the second party, and the third party is a nondirect payer, most often the insurance company. The pharmacy technician is expected to assist the pharmacist in processing third-party payer claims.

Government Payment

Third-party payers are categorized as either government payment or nongovernmental payment. Government payment originates from:

- ✓ Medicare
- ✓ Medicaid
- ✓ Workers' Compensation
- ✓ Military Health Plans

Medicare and Medicaid were established in 1965 through the Social Security Administration. In 2001, Centers for Medicare and Medicaid Services took over management of the two government-run programs.

Medicare

Medicare is an insurance program run by the federal government. Individuals eligible for Medicare benefits are:

- ✓ Age 65 years and older
- ✓ Individuals younger than 65 years with certain disabilities
- ✓ Patients of any age with end-stage renal disease

Medicare insurance coverage is broken down into four different parts:

- ✓ Part A: Insurance coverage for inpatient hospital stays, skilled nursing facilities (SNF), home health care, and hospice. Think of Medicare Part A as that part of the patient's Medicare insurance that helps to pay for hospital stays and other levels of care. Most patients don't have to pay a monthly fee, or *premium*, for Medicare Part A.
- ✓ Part B: Insurance coverage for certain injectable drugs; physician fees; outpatient hospital care; home medical equipment (HME), also known as durable medical equipment, prosthetics, orthotics, and supplies (DMEPOS); physical therapy (PT); and occupational therapy (OT). The best way to think of Medicare Part B is medical insurance for office visits. Patients will be responsible for a monthly premium for Medicare Part B coverage.
- ✓ Part C: Also known as Medicare Advantage. The individual must be enrolled in Medicare Parts A and B to be eligible for Part C. Medicare Advantage, or Part C, is insurance coverage offered by private companies. The patient may choose to enroll in Medicare Advantage because there is extra insurance coverage available. A Medicare Advantage plan provides all of Part A (hospital insurance) and Part B (medical insurance) plus extra coverage such as vision, hearing, and dental. Most Medicare Advantage plans will also include Medicare prescription drug coverage (Part D). Part C was formerly known as Medicare Choice. Think of Medicare Part C this way: Patients who choose to enroll in and pay for this coverage will have the advantage of extra insurance coverage, or Medicare Advantage.
- ✓ Part D: Insurance coverage for prescription drugs. Part D was added to Medicare coverage after the passage of the Medicare Modernization Act (MMA) of 2003. Effective in 2006, this voluntary program allows patients to purchase drug coverage through a private insurance policy. The patient's monthly premium will vary depending on which prescription drug plan (PDP) they enroll in. Pharmacy technicians working in a retail setting will assist the pharmacist in helping Medicare beneficiaries find a Part D prescription drug coverage plan that fits their needs. Open enrollment for coordination of Part D benefits runs October 15 – December 7. Think of Medicare Part D as prescription drug coverage.

Medicare Part D

As a pharmacy technician, you will deal most often with Part D coverage. For the sake of preparing for your certification exam, this review guide will focus on Medicare Part D.

The Affordable Care Act was passed in 2010. It includes legislation to help make prescription drugs more affordable for people using Medicare insurance. You may hear the phrase "close the Medicare Part D prescription drug coverage gap." What this means is that there is a gap, or an area, at which Medicare participants lack prescription drug coverage. If the Medicare participants are in the gap, or area of no coverage, they must pay 100% of their medication costs until they have reached the next tier, or fee schedule, in their insurance coverage. During this gap, some Medicare participants may go without medication, because they don't have the income to pay the full cost of prescribed drugs. In 2010, in recognition of this hardship, the government mailed a $250 rebate check to most people who reached their coverage gap.

People who are in the Medicare Part D coverage gap may also be eligible to receive a 50% discount on certain applicable drugs. In addition to the 50% discount, in 2001, the federal government gradually began to subsidize, or to discount, all other drugs covered under the Part D plan beginning with a 7% subsidy. This 7% government subsidy is planned to climb to a 75% subsidy by 2020.

To simplify and summarize this information:

✓ The coverage gap, most commonly known as the donut hole, is when the Medicare Part D prescription drug plan reaches its limit in covering the cost of prescription medication and the insured is responsible for paying 100% of drug costs. The coverage gap for 2011 is $2840–$4550.

Table 4-1 summarizes true out of pocket (TrOOP) expenses for a Medicare beneficiary. A Medicare beneficiary is an individual who receives benefits or insurance coverage through Medicare.

The beneficiary's yearly deductible, copayments, and coverage gap costs all count as out-of-pocket spending to help get out of the coverage gap. There are drug plans available that offer some coverage during the gap.

We can offer suggestions at a pharmacy level to help patients lower their drug costs while they are in the coverage gap. Patients may be able to switch to a generic medication or change to a lower-cost medication with the same therapeutic outcome. The pharmacy technician can assist the pharmacist by helping patients search for patient assistance programs and state programs that may help to lower their drug costs.

> Explanation of Benefits (EOB): Medicare beneficiaries receive this notice each month to show the amount of prescription drug costs funded by the manufacturer, the government, and/or out-of-pocket expenses.

✓ Affordable Care Act allows for financial assistance for those patients who have reached their Medicare Part D coverage gap or donut hole.

Table 4-1 TrOOP Expenses for Medicare Beneficiary

Annual Patient Spending for Medication Prescription Drug Coverage Plan with a deductible of $250:	% Patient Pays	Total Patient Pays	TrOOP
If the patient spends between **$0–$250** per year on prescription medications . . .	. . . the patient is responsible for **100%** of the costs. . . .	. . . so the patient's total costs are **100% of up to $250**. . . .	. . . the patient's true out of pocket expenses are up to **$250**.
If the patient spends between **$250.01–$2840** a year on prescription medications. . .	. . . and the prescription drug coverage plan has a **25%** copay. . .	. . . the patient pays **25%** of each dollar over **$250** plus the deductible of $250 . . .	. . . the patient's true out of pocket expense for spending **$2840** a year is **$897.50**
If the patient spends more than **$2840** and less than **$4550**,	Coverage Gap begins. Patient is responsible for 100% of prescription medication drug costs between **$2840** and **$4550**.		For **$4550** in spending: $4550 −$2840 _____ $1710 plus $897.50 from deductible and copay **$2607.50**
Above **$4550**	Catastrophic Coverage Begins		

Note: TrOOP, true out of pocket.

The following is a list of steps outlined in the Affordable Care Act to provide financial assistance for most Medicare Part D participants who have reached their plan limitations in prescription drug coverage. These steps will only apply when the beneficiary has reached the coverage gap, or donut hole:

1. $250 onetime rebate check mailed to Medicare Plan D beneficiaries in 2010
2. 50% discount on certain applicable drugs
3. 7% increase in coverage for all other covered Part D drugs

✓ Applicable drugs are generic and/or brand-name drugs and vaccines covered by Medicare Part D prescription drug coverage plans. The Centers for Medicare and Medicaid Services has a published listing of drug manufacturers that have agreed to coverage gap discounts. This listing of applicable drugs *is not* needed for your certification exam, but some of you currently working in the field as a pharmacy technician may find the listing helpful (http://www.cms.gov/prescriptiondrugcovgenin).

Example of coverage for an applicable drug. Mr. Tony Johnson reaches his coverage gap. He goes to his local pharmacy to fill a prescription for an applicable drug. The price of the medication is $80. He will receive a 50% discount off the drug cost. He will pay $40 plus a small dispensing fee. Even though Mr. Johnson paid $40 plus a dispensing fee, he will be able to count the full medication cost ($80 plus dispensing fee) toward his out-of-pocket spending, which will help him get out of his coverage gap faster.

Example of coverage for other covered drugs. Mr. Tony Johnson reaches his coverage gap. He goes to his local pharmacy to fill a prescription for a medication that is covered by Medicare Part D but is not part of the 50% discount program (applicable drug). The price for Mr. Johnson's covered medication is $35 plus a small dispensing fee of $2. Mr. Johnson's bill of $37 will be discounted by 7%. He will pay $34.41, and only the $34.41 will count toward his out-of-pocket spending to help him get out of his coverage gap.

Sometimes patients may have insurance coverage through Medicare and another private insurance company. In most cases, Medicare is the primary payer. When billing for prescription medication, supplies, and services, bill Medicare first. The other private insurance company is billed if Medicare doesn't pay on or cover the service. The other private insurance company is called the *secondary payer*.

Medicaid

Although Medicare is run by the federal government, Medicaid is a state-run program *overseen* by the federal government. Medicaid policies may vary from state to state, but mostly, Medicaid has similar guidelines in every state. Medicaid is health insurance that helps many people who can't afford medical care pay for some or all of their medical bills. If eligibility requirements are met, Medicaid is available to:

✓ Low-income adults and their families
✓ Immigrant children
✓ Pregnant women
✓ Children and teenagers
✓ Individuals who are aged, blind, and/or have certain disabilities

The patient may pay a small part of the medication cost (copayment) at the time the prescription is picked up from the pharmacy. After the insurance claim is submitted, the state reimburses the pharmacy for prescription medications at a maximum allowable cost (MAC), which is based on the usual and customary (U&C) price for the medication. The state conducts a periodic survey with drug manufacturers to determine the U&C product prices.

Some individuals are eligible for both Medicare and Medicaid (dual eligible). These people pay no premium or deductible but will have a $1–$3 copay. The copay is waived for nursing home patients.

Workers' Compensation

Workers' compensation involves compensation for employees who are accidentally injured on the job. An injured worker will have no copay for prescription medications. The pharmacy will work with the injured worker's employer to send claims in for full reimbursement.

Military Health Plans

TRICARE is the health insurance plan that serves uniformed service members, retirees, and their families worldwide. It's a managed care program with network providers. Patients may have copays.

Civilian Health and Medical Program of the Veterans Administration, commonly referred to as CHAMPVA, is health insurance for family members of totally and permanently disabled veterans. CHAMPVA is also available to eligible beneficiaries younger than age 65 years.

Nongovernmental Payment

Private health insurance and patient assistance programs are two examples of nongovernmental payers. Patient assistance programs are offered by drug manufacturers to help patients afford medication. An example of this is the drug manufacturer AstraZeneca, which has a prescription drug discount program called RxAssist to help reduce medication costs for patients.

Private health insurance is most often a managed care program categorized as

✓ Health maintenance organizations (HMO)
✓ Preferred provider organizations (PPO)
✓ Point of service (POS)

Managed care programs grew out of the need to control healthcare costs in the late 1970s and early 1980s. Health maintenance organization (HMO) is the most common type of private health insurance. HMO insurance plans offer comprehensive healthcare by network providers. A *network provider* is an entity such as a physician or hospital that has signed an agreement with the insurance company to provide healthcare services at a specified rate of reimbursement. HMO plans are usually less expensive for the patient, but the downside is that there may be a limited number of physicians and/or medical services available. If the patient goes out of network, the service may not be covered at all by insurance. A well-known HMO is Blue Cross and Blue Shield.

Preferred provider organizations (PPO) offer specialized healthcare in and out of network. A PPO has many of the same aspects as a HMO. Just like an HMO, agreements are made between the PPO and the providers for a specified amount of reimbursement for services. Unlike the HMO, if the patient decides to go out of network a PPO plan will help pay costs. The PPO patient may likely pay a little higher premium than an HMO plan but will be able to see his or her physician of choice. An HMO requires that a patient see an in-network primary care physician of their choice who will then refer the patient to a specialist. A PPO allows a patient to see a specialist without a referral. A well-known PPO is Humana.

Point of service (POS) plans mix HMO and PPO characteristics. An in-network primary physician is assigned to or chosen by the patient. The primary care physician, referred to as the patient's point of service, can make referrals to specialists who are outside to the network. This allows more freedom of choice than an HMO plan. Another benefit of a POS plan is lower copays. A well-known POS provider is CIGNA.

CAPITATION FEE

Some third-party payers reimburse the pharmacy in the form of a monthly fee called a capitation fee. The capitation fee is a flat fee set by the third-party payer and is paid to the pharmacy each month whether or not patients covered under that insurance plan receive prescriptions during that month. The pharmacy in return must dispense prescriptions for the patients covered under that insurance plan, even if the prescription costs rise above the set capitation fee.

ONLINE ADJUDICATION

Accurate and complete data entry is critical to getting reimbursement from the third-party payer. Patient information, insurance information, and prescription information must be entered in the pharmacy computer with attention to detail.

Assisting the pharmacist with denied or rejected claims is a much-appreciated task for the pharmacy technician. Rejected claims can most often be resolved by phoning the insurance help desk. When a claim is rejected, an error code and an explanation appears on the computer screen. The error codes are universal codes: "prescriber not covered" is error code 71. You may be familiar with error codes if you've been working in retail pharmacy. When preparing for the certification exam, you won't need to know the actual error code, but you should be familiar with common reasons for rejected claims.

- ✓ *Invalid patient date of birth (DOB), gender, or person code.* Each covered patient is assigned a person code by the insurance company. The policyholder or cardholder is person code 00, for instance. The patient's DOB, gender, or person code may have been keyed in wrong or the patient may have given the wrong information. In most cases, this is an easy fix by simply correcting the information on the patient profile and resubmitting the claim.
- ✓ *Expired coverage.* The patient no longer has valid coverage with this insurance plan. Ask the patient whether he or she has a new, updated insurance card. The claim can be resubmitted after updating the insurance plan information. If there is no new insurance coverage, a claim cannot be submitted, and the patient will have to pay full price for the medication out of pocket.
- ✓ *Prescribed quantity exceeds limits of insurance plan.* Much of the time insurance companies will pay for a one-month supply of medication. This is a cost management technique based on the premise that the prescriber may alter dosages, strengths, or medications. There won't be as much waste with a prescription change of a one-month supply versus a three-month supply. The claim can be resubmitted by either reducing the quantity to fill or by explaining the patient's need for a greater supply.
- ✓ *Refill too early.* On average, insurance will pay to refill a prescription five to seven days before the medication runs out. The refill point varies, depending on the supply the patient is receiving. A greater supply warrants an earlier refill date. The pharmacy technician should alert the pharmacist for patient counseling if a "refill too early" rejection appears. The patient may be taking the medication incorrectly and may need guidance on how to take the medication. However, there may be a plausible reason for an early refill: a change in dosage or supply is needed early because of vacation plans. In that case, the pharmacy technician will be issued and override code by the insurance company. The override code will authorize adjudication of the claim. *Adjudication* is when the third-party payers reimburse the pharmacy for the cost of the drug plus a dispensing fee.
- ✓ *Prescriber not covered.* The prescriber is not in the insurance company's network, so insurance will not pay on the claim. The patient will have to pay out of pocket for this prescription.
- ✓ *NDC not covered.* The National Drug Code (NDC) number signifies the medication name, manufacturer, and packaging. "NDC not covered" means the insurance company will not reimburse for the medication selected to fill the prescription. The pharmacist will choose an alternate generic or may need to call the prescriber for a therapeutic equivalent that's covered under the patient's insurance formulary. Sometimes a prior authorization (PA) is needed on certain medications and pharmacy services. A *prior authorization* is a procedure originating with a request from the prescriber, ending with the insurance company granting or authorizing a nonformulary medication to be dispensed to the patient. The pharmacy technician frequently assists the pharmacists in preparing PA paperwork.

Effective May 2007, the Health Insurance Portability and Accountability Act (HIPAA) requires all pharmacies to have a National Provider Identifier (NPI) number for all electronic transactions. The NPI number is a unique 10-digit identification number used in administration and financial transactions. The pharmacy must include the NPI number when billing for medications and related services.

PAPER CLAIMS

Some pharmacy supplies, services, and medications may require paper claims rather than online adjudication. Two paper claim forms that are used by all third-party payers are the Universal Claim Form (UCF) and the CMS-1500. The CMS-1500 is the standard claim form used to bill Medicare and Medicaid. Items that may need a UCF are walkers and other durable medical equipment (DME) and clinical services. Codes are used on paper claim forms to clarify the service that seeks reimbursement. For instance, the code used for face-to-face medication therapy management (MTM) is CPT code 99605. HCPCS (pronounced hicpics) are commonly used for billing DME.

- ✓ Common Procedural Terminology (CPT) codes
- ✓ International Classification of Diseases, 9th edition (ICD-9) codes
- ✓ Healthcare Common Procedure Coding System (HCPCS) codes

PBM COMPANIES

Pharmacy benefits management (PBM) companies handle reimbursement and drug utilization review (DUR) for numerous insurance companies. Although the main purpose for a PBM company is to process and pay on prescription drug claims, the PBM company is also valuable to negotiate discounts with drug manufacturers. The negotiated discounts are passed on to the patients by referencing the medications in the insurance provider's formulary. A *formulary* is a preferred list of drugs that the patient may use to treat the disease. Express Scripts is a well-known PBM company.

INSURANCE FRAUD

Insurance fraud involves billing for services that were not provided. An example of this would be billing the insurance company for medication therapy management (MTM) when the service was not provided. Perhaps the patient missed the MTM appointment, but services were inadvertently billed. Even though it was unintentional, it is still fraud.

Other examples of possible insurance fraud would be billing the patient's insurance company for a full 30-day supply of medication when only a partial-fill of 20 tablets was dispensed to the patient. Again, this could have been an unintentional error, but possible fraudulent activities take place when the patient forgets to pick up the remaining 10 tablets that have already been billed to the insurance company.

Billing the insurance company for a brand medication when the prescription was filled with a generic is yet another example of insurance fraud.

The pharmacy technician must use best practices and procedures to reduce improper claim adjudication. Suspected misconduct should be reported to the pharmacy manager.

340B PROGRAM

The 340B Program was first established by federal law in 1992 to reduce the cost of drugs for covered entities through discounts from drug manufacturers. The savings for the covered entity (hospital) is then passed along to patients.

The Affordable Care Act increases patient access to discounted drugs by allowing more entities to be eligible to enroll in the 340B program. The Affordable Care Act allows 340B eligibility for freestanding cancer centers, critical access hospitals, sole community hospitals, and rural referral centers.

This is your checklist to make sure you understand what you need to know for the certification exam. Review chapter content if there is a topic you're uncertain of.
I know:

√	...the regulations to follow when working with investigational drugs.
	...the procedure to process third party claims.
	...the importance of accurate data entry when processing claims for adjudication.
	...reasons for rejected claims.
	...the use of a NPI number.

RESOURCES

1. US Department of Health and Human Services. US Food and Drug Administration Website. http://www.fda.gov. Accessed January 2011.
2. Medicare.gov. The Official US Government Site for Medicare. Available at: http://www.medicare.gov. Accessed February 2011.
3. US Department of Health and Human Services. Centers for Medicare and Medicaid Services Website. http://www.cms.gov. Accessed February 2011.

CHAPTER 4

MULTIPLE CHOICE

Identify the choice that best completes the statement or answers the question.

____ **1.** Medications that are used by some patients but have not yet been approved for market by the FDA are:

a. investigational new drugs (IND)   c. priority medications (PM)

b. test drugs (TD)   d. illegal drug applications

____ **2.** A tablet containing no active medication is termed a

a. blind tablet   c. placebo

b. double-blind   d. study tablet

____ **3.** The pharmacy technician will assist in Compassionate Use Programs by

a. compounding and prescribing the IND   c. providing one-on-one healthcare to the patient

b. using special record keeping procedures   d. counseling the patient on special procedures

____ **4.** The pharmacy's set of rules and procedures is termed

a. pharmacy state law   c. protocol

b. pharmacy federal law   d. handbook

_____ **5.** Out-of-pocket expense is also termed

a. direct payment

b. third-party payment

c. manufacturer payment

d. government payment

_____ **6.** The third-party payer may be

a. the patient

b. the pharmacy

c. the patient's insurance carrier

d. the patient's guardian

_____ **7.** Medicare beneficiaries are

a. patients 65 years and younger

b. individuals younger than 65 years with no disabilities

c. patients 65 years and older

d. individuals younger than 65 years who are free of renal disease

_____ **8.** What Medicare part provides prescription drug coverage?

a. Part A

b. Part B

c. Part C

d. Part D

_____ **9.** The donut hole is

a. a period of time when Medicare prescription drug coverage reaches a limit

b. also termed communication gap

c. a time frame when Medicare pays 100% of prescription drug expenses

d. a period of time when Medicaid prescription drug coverage reaches a limit

_____ **10.** The third-party payer that is billed first is termed

a. secondary payer

b. primary payer

c. first in line

d. out of pocket

ANSWER SECTION

1. A
2. C
3. B
4. C
5. A
6. C
7. C
8. D
9. A
10. B

TASK SHEET

TOPIC TO REVIEW: PHARMACOLOGY FOR PHARMACY TECHNICIANS

Materials

Pharmacy Technician Exam Review Guide

JB Test Prep: Pharmacy Technician Exam Review Guide

Prepare

1. Read the section pharmacology.
2. Take practice test at the end of the chapter.

Study Plan

1. Read pages_____ on _____(date).
2. Make flash cards using http://quizlet.com.
3. Take end-of-chapter practice test on_____(date).
4. Ask a coworker to help you review brand/generic.

Tips

1. Study only the drugs you're not familiar with. Start by learning the top 10 drugs and move on to learn more after you have memorized the top 10.
2. Look at the endings of the generic drug names to help you remember what drug class they belong to.
3. Memorable icons may help you recall drug side effects such as those used in the chapter. Make up your own images for drug classes, side effects, or top-selling drugs.

End of Chapter

List what you need to review.

Pharmacology for Pharmacy Technicians

OBJECTIVES/TOPICS TO COVER:

- ✓ Identify the general principles of pharmacology.
- ✓ Explain basic drug classification.
- ✓ Identify common IV drugs.
- ✓ Identify common chemotherapy drugs.
- ✓ Recall top prescribed drugs.
- ✓ Recognize radiopharmaceuticals.
- ✓ Recognize and understand procedures when working with restricted drugs (RD).

PRINCIPLES OF PHARMACOLOGY

Pharmacokinetics is the movement of the drug through the body. It is what the BODY does to the drug. The four steps of pharmacokinetics are

- Absorption
- Distribution
- Metabolism
- Elimination

Absorption

First, the drug is administered or absorbed into the bloodstream. Absorption can happen through intravenous (IV) injection when the drug is absorbed directly into the bloodstream. Absorption can happen orally in which the drug is administered in the mouth and then passes through the esophagus and into the stomach. Some other routes of absorption are

- ✓ Topically: through the skin
- ✓ Sublingual (SL): under the tongue
- ✓ Buccal: between the cheek and gum
- ✓ Enteral: into the intestine
- ✓ Ophthalmic: into the eye
- ✓ Otic: into the ear
- ✓ Rectal
- ✓ Vaginal

- ✓ Intramuscular (IM)
- ✓ Intrathecal (IT): into the fluid surrounding the spinal cord
- ✓ Intra-articular: into the joint
- ✓ Subcutaneous (SQ): under the skin into the subcutaneous tissue
- ✓ Intradermal (ID): under the skin into the dermis layer
- ✓ Transdermal: over the skin such as a patch
- ✓ Implant
- ✓ Inhalation: either through the nose or inhaled through the mouth

Each route has specific purposes, advantages, and disadvantages.

Distribution

After the drug is absorbed into the bloodstream, distribution takes place wherein the drug travels to the intended site of action. The drug uses the bloodstream as a vehicle to get to where it needs to be. The drug leaves the bloodstream when it reaches the tissue that has an affinity (or attraction) for the drug. Once the drug is at the intended site of action, the drug leaves the bloodstream and moves into the body tissue. Some drugs leave the bloodstream very slowly, because they bind tightly to proteins circulating in the blood. Others leave the bloodstream quickly and enter tissue, because they are less tightly bound to blood proteins.

Some drugs act locally, which means the drug is absorbed and stays at the site of the absorption. An example of a local-acting medication is a topical cream applied to a minor burn to relieve pain.

Some drugs are systemic, which means the drug will affect the whole body system rather than have just a local effect on a certain area of the body. Drugs go through the distribution process whether the drug is local acting or systemic.

Metabolism

Metabolism is where the magic takes place. This is the pharmacokinetic process in which the active ingredient in the drug changes into the chemical form (*metabolite*) that binds with the body to do what it is intended to do. After the process of metabolism changes the drug into a metabolite, the metabolite then goes to work to produce the desired effect on the body. Most of the drug metabolism takes place in the liver.

You should be familiar with the *first pass effect*. This is the process in which the liver metabolizes oral medications. The medication reaches the liver for absorption and metabolism "first." Some drug routes, such as IV administration and suppositories, bypass the liver and the first pass effect, thus leaving a higher concentration of active drug for circulation.

A *prodrug* is administered in an inactive form and when metabolized changes into an active form. Prodrugs are designed to reach their intended site of action with more precision. Many chemotherapy drugs are prodrugs.

Elimination

Elimination is when drugs leave the body. The kidneys eliminate most drugs in urine. Other means of elimination are through defecation, perspiration, breast milk, and exhalation.

Pharmacokinetics of a drug depends on patient-related factors as well as on the drug's chemical properties. Some patient-related factors are age, weight, and gender. For example, metabolism is markedly slower in elderly patients, which results in slower elimination of the drug.

PHARMACODYNAMICS

Pharmacodynamics is what the drug does to the body. Reducing cholesterol and pain relief are examples of drugs' therapeutic effects or pharmacodynamics. Nausea and diarrhea are examples of drug side effects. Patient-related factors affect both pharmacokinetics and pharmacodynamics.

Pharmacology Terms

Here are some terms and definitions you should be familiar with for your certification exam:

Half-Life (T ½): Length of time for drug levels in the blood to decrease by one half. Half-life is important to determine the amount of active drug in the body to help maintain therapeutic drug levels.

Therapeutic Index (TI): Ratio of effective dose to the lethal dose. A drug with a narrow therapeutic index such as Digoxin with a 2:3 TI is not as safe as a drug with a wider therapeutic index range such as 2:10. Medications with a narrow therapeutic index require patient monitoring and careful dosing.

Bioavailability: The amount of drug available at the site of action. An oral medication will lose some of the active drug when it goes through the first pass effect in the liver. The greater the bioavailability, the more the active drug is available to do what it's intended to do. A high bioavailability is desirable.

Synergistic Effect: When two or more drugs are administered at the same time and produce effects that are greater than the effect that would have occurred if the drugs were administered alone.

Onset of Action: The time it takes for a drug to reach the concentration necessary to produce the therapeutic effect.

Therapeutic Substitution

When a pharmacists needs to substitute a medication or suggest a substitution to the prescriber, the drug's active ingredient and therapeutic outcome of the drug therapy is considered. A medication may be referred to as a bioequivalent, a pharmaceutical alternative, a pharmaceutical equivalent, a therapeutic duplication, a therapeutic alternative, or a therapeutic equivalent. You should be familiar with the differences in these terms.

Bioequivalence: Generic drug manufacturers must run studies to prove their generic medication releases the same amounts of the active drug into the bloodstream at the same speed as the original drug. A bioequivalent drug has the same chemical equivalent of drug concentration in the blood as the original brand-name drug. Not all generic drugs are bioequivalent to the original brand-name drug. Also, generic drugs will have the same active ingredient as the original drug but may have different inactive ingredients. The different inactive ingredients may cause possible adverse reactions for a patient who has been switched from brand to generic.

Pharmaceutical Alternative: The medication has the same active ingredient as another drug, but the strength and dosage forms may be different.

Pharmaceutical Equivalent: The medication has the identical amount of active ingredient (strength and concentration) as another drug. It has the same dosage form but may have different inactive ingredients.

Therapeutic Alternative: This medication contains different active ingredient than another drug but produces the same therapeutic outcome.

Therapeutic Duplication: Two different medications have similar therapeutic effects and may belong to the same therapeutic class.

Therapeutic Equivalent: Medication that is a pharmaceutical equivalent and bioequivalent to another drug and can be expected to have the same outcomes as another drug when administered to patients under the conditions specified in the labeling.

Therapeutic equivalence codes or ratings are used to evaluate whether one medication is equivalent to another medication. Therapeutic codes/ratings are assigned by the U.S. Food and Drug Administration. You can find the codes/ratings listed in *Orange Book*, a pharmacy reference book.

"A" Codes: Medications are bioequivalent. Substitution is permitted between medications with an AA rating and an AB rating.

"B" Codes: The FDA considers medications not to be therapeutically equivalent to other pharmaceutically equivalent products. Substitution is not permitted between medications with B ratings, such as BC rating and BN rating.

Side Effects

With all types of medications, the patient must weigh the benefits of taking the medication against the possible risks and side effects. *Side effects* are undesired effects of the medication and may vary from one person to another. Some may assume that common side effects occur more than half of the time. The truth is that common side effects occur in only 1% to 10% of patients.

Almost any drug can cause an *adverse reaction*. An adverse reaction can be a mild side effect, such as an upset stomach, or it can be a very serious reaction that causes the patient harm.

Sometimes a medication has an unexpected side effect, or an *idiosyncratic reaction*. An idiosyncratic reaction is an unusual and unpredicted adverse reaction to the medication.

Pharmacogenomics is a new twenty-first-century term that means genetic information from the patient is used to identify his or her response to medication therapy. Hopes are that an increased use of genetic testing and *biomarkers* (drugs given to a patient as a means to examine organ function or other aspects of health) may improve safety and efficacy and reduce side effects.

DRUG INTERACTIONS

There are two types of drug interactions:

✓ Drug–Drug Interactions
✓ Drug–Food Interactions

Patients who take more than one drug at a time may be at risk of a *drug–drug interaction* (see **Table 5-1**). Taking multiple drugs, whether the drugs are over the counter (OTC), herbals, or prescription, could affect the distribution of the drug and either increase or decrease the therapeutic effects of one or more of the medications. A well-known drug–drug interaction is taking an OTC antihistamine while taking a prescription sedative. The OTC antihistamine (used for a runny nose) can interact with the therapeutic effect of the prescription sedative and increase the level of drowsiness. Sometimes combination drugs may be prescribed to *mitigate* the severity of a side effect. For instance, an antiemetic may be prescribed for a patient receiving chemotherapy drugs.

Drug–food interactions are not uncommon. There are hundreds of food and drinks such as chocolate, beverages containing caffeine, and grapefruit that have the potential to interact with certain medications. Consequences of a drug–food interaction may be a delayed onset or an enhanced absorption of the drug

DRUG CLASSIFICATION

Drugs are grouped, or "classed," together when the drugs have similar activities or when the drugs are used for the same type of disorder. Medications in the same class have the same mechanism of action, the same intended response, and generally the same side effects. The therapeutic classification of a medication may depend on how the medication affects the nervous system and then, in turn, how the nervous system responds to the drug.

A medication may be listed in different therapeutic classifications, depending on the reference book; there is no one official or standard classification system used in pharmacy. To make classifications a bit more challenging, classification schemes have grown significantly as different types of receptors have been discovered. *Receptors* are parts of the blood (protein) that the drug chemical attaches to. When simplified the receptor is sometimes referred to as the lock and the drug is the key.

Table 5-1 Common Drug–Drug Interactions

OTC NSAIDs such as: aspirin, ibuprofen, naproxen OTC analgesics such as: acetaminophen	Rx Anticoagulants such as: warfarin	Increases blood-thinning effect of anticoagulants
aspirin	insulin	Increases the blood sugar–lowering effects of insulin
aspirin	Rx antiseizure medications such as: phenytoin, valproic acid	Leads to increased antiseizure drug levels in blood
OTC antihistamines such as: diphenhydramine chlorpheniramine brompheniramine	Rx sedatives, muscle relaxers, antianxiety such as: alprazolam, temazepam, lorazepam, diazepam	Increases depressant effects such as sleepiness
Decongestant: pseudoephedrine	Stimulants	May increase side effects
	High blood pressure meds	Reduces effects
	Monoamine oxidase inhibitors (MAOIs)	May cause dangerous increases in blood pressure
Cough medicines such as: dextromethorphan	MAOIs	May cause *Serotonin Syndrome*, which is a potentially life-threatening condition caused by an excess of drug in the body
	Sedatives	Increases sedative effects
Herbal: St. John's Wort	MAOIs and SSRIs	Increases effects
	lanoxin, lovastatin, sildenofil	Reduces effects
Antacids	Many	Decreases effects
Antibiotics	Birth control pills	May make birth control less effective

Common Drug–Food Interactions

Grapefruit	Certain blood pressure lowering medications buspirone	Increases drug levels in blood, which may contribute to increased chance of side effects
Chocolate	MAOIs	Raises blood pressure
Licorice	Digoxin HCTZ spironolactone	May reduce effects
Alcohol	Many medications	May either increase or decrease the effects of the medication

Note: NSAIDs, nonsteroidal anti-inflammatory drugs.
This table is not all inclusive. Patients should always consult with the pharmacist if they have questions about interactions.

Unfortunately, there is no clear-cut method to categorizing drugs. Drugs have different uses and may "float" between therapeutic classes. Beta blockers are a class of drugs that are used primarily in the cardiovascular system to treat high blood pressure. However, beta blockers may also be used as an antianxiety drug for someone with stage-fright symptoms. The beta blocker will work to help decrease heart palpitations.

Origin of Drugs

Drugs come from three different sources. Drugs derived from a plant or animal are of a *natural* origin. Drugs can be a man-made copy of a naturally occurring drug. Man-made drugs prepared in a laboratory are called *synthetic* drugs. Drugs can also be a combination of natural and synthetic, termed *semisynthetic* drugs.

Generations of Medications

As research evolves, new drugs are discovered and new drug generations are determined. Each new generation of medicine will have some type of benefit or different nuance from the generation before it. For instance, the second generation of antihistamines has less drowsiness side effects than the first generation. The second and third generations of antidepressants have fewer side effects than the first generation. The second-generation cephalosporin antibiotics kill more bacteria than the first generation.

Cardiovascular Drugs

Cardiovascular drugs affect the heart. This is the most widely prescribed class of medications. Because these drugs are frequently prescribed, odds are your certification exam will have a question or questions pertaining to this class. The cardiovascular drug class has many subclasses such as beta blockers, calcium channel blockers (CCB), vasodilators, antihypertensives, and angiotensin converting enzymes (ACE) inhibitors. Study the generic name endings to help you remember medications in each class (see **Tables 5-2** to **5-6**).

> Beta Blockers commonly end in –olol. Example: aten*olol* or metopr*olol*
>
> Calcium Channel Blockers commonly end in –tiazem. Example: dil*tiazem*

Anti-infectives

Most germs fall into two broad categories: bacteria or virus. An anti-infective medication will interfere with cell replication to stop the infection. Some antibiotics are effective only against limited types of bacteria. Others, known as *broad-spectrum* antibiotics, are effective against a wide range of bacteria.

Gastrointestinal Agents

The gastrointestinal (GI) system is commonly called the digestive system. Organs and accessory organs in the GI system are those that aid in eating and digesting food, such as the stomach, large intestine, small intestine, liver, gall bladder, and esophagus or throat.

Antidiarrheals, a GI agent subclass, work to stop diarrhea. The prefix "anti-" means *against*. There are two main types of antidiarrheal medications. One acts as an adsorbent, while the other works to slow down the contractions of the bowel muscles so that the fecal matter is expelled more slowly.

Another GI agent subclass is laxatives. There are different types of laxatives: stimulant, bulk forming, and stool softeners. Stimulant laxatives work by stimulating the bowel wall to contract and push the fecal matter out. Bulk-forming laxatives work by increasing the bulk or size of the feces to help promote a bowel movement. Stool softeners act by adding more liquid to the fecal matter, which lubricates the feces and helps with evacuation.

Laxatives may be taken by mouth or may be administered directly into the rectum as suppositories or enemas. Laxatives should not be taken on a regular basis. Using laxatives too often may cause a *rebound effect*, which is when the symptoms being treated return in a more severe manner after the medicine is stopped.

Nervous System

The two branches of our nervous system are the autonomic nervous system (ANS) and the central nervous system (CNS). There are many drug subclasses in the central nervous system.

Table 5-2 Drugs

	Drug Class	Example of Medication in the Drug Class	How the Drug Works	Side Effects	Common Ending
Cardiovascular Drugs	**Antiarrhythmics** Subclasses may include Beta Blockers and Calcium Channel Blockers (CCB)	amiodarone sotalol (Betapace)	Controls irregularities of heartbeat	Dizziness Nausea Photosensitivity	Beta Blockers: -alol, -olol
	Glycosides	digoxin (Lanoxin)	Treatment of congestive heart failure and irregular heart beat	Abdominal pain Confusion Depression Dizziness Headache Nausea	
	Vasodilators	isosorbide nitroglycerin verapamil	Relaxes the blood vessels or dilates the vessels to allow blood to flow through easier	Anxiety Dizziness Headache Hypotension (low blood pressure)	-dil -pamil
	Antihypertensives Subclasses include diuretics (commonly called water pills), Beta Blockers, Calcium Channel Blockers (CCB), angiotensin-converting enzyme (ACE) inhibitors	ACE: enalapril ACE: captopril Beta Blocker: atenolol Beta Blocker: metoprolol CCB: amlodipine CCB: diltiazem CCB: nifedipine Diuretic: furosemide Diuretic: hydrochlorothiazide (HCTZ) doxazosyn (Cardura)	Lowers blood pressure	Diarrhea Dizziness Fatigue Flushing Headache Insomnia Lightheadedness Bradycardia (slow heart beat) Diuretic: dehydration	ACE: -pril Beta Blocker: -alol and -olol CCB: -ipine -tiazem Diuretics: -thiazide ACE: -sartan -azosin
Respiratory System Drugs	**Antihistamines**	chlorpheniramine diphenhydramine cetirizine (Zyrtec) fexofenadine	Used primarily to counteract the effects of histamine, one of the chemicals involved in allergic reactions	Blurred vision Confusion Drowsiness	
	Bronchodilators	salmeterol (Serevent) clenbuterol (Spiropent) pirbuterol (Maxair)	Opens up or dilates the bronchial tubes within the lungs Bronchodilators ease breathing in diseases such as asthma	Nervousness Restlessness Bad taste in mouth Coughing Dizziness Drowsiness	-terol

(continues)

Table 5-2 (Continued)

	Drug Class	Example of Medication in the Drug Class	How the Drug Works	Side Effects	Common Ending
Respiratory System Drugs	**Cough suppressants** Also called antitussives	codeine dextromethorphan	Suppress coughing reflex	Dizziness Drowsiness Stomach upset	
	Decongestants	pseudoephedrine phenylephrine	Helps to relieve nasal stuffiness	Restlessness Anxiety Nervousness Weakness	
	Expectorants subclass of mucolytic	guaifenesin	Promotes coughing to eliminate phlegm from the respiratory tract	Nausea Diarrhea Drowsiness	
Central Nervous System (CNS) Drugs	**Anticonvulsants** Subclass: hydantoin	clonazepam valproic acid topiramate (Topamax) phenotoin	Prevent epileptic seizures	Abdominal pain Blurred vision Anorexia Fatigue Headache	-toin
	Antidepressants Subclasses include selective serotonin reuptake inhibitors (SSRIs), tricyclic, monoamine oxidase inhibitors (MAOIs), serotonin noradrenaline reuptake inhibitors (SNRI), noradrenaline dopamine reuptake inhibitors (NA/DRI)	SSRI: citalopram (Celexa) SSRI: escitalopram (Lexapro) Tricyclic-amitriptyline Tricyclic-imipramine Tricyclic-nortriptyline MAOI-phenelzine (Nardil)	Mood lifting	Anorexia Anxiety Constipation/diarrhea Dizziness Dry mouth Insomnia Blurred vision Confusion	-pramine -oxetine -azepam
	Antianxiety (also called anxiolytic) Subclasses include benzodiazepines, azapirones May also be referred to as sedatives	alprazolam diazepam lorazepam clonazepam Azapirone: buspirone (BuSpar) only drug in this class	Calms nervousness, relaxes muscles	Change in appetite Blurred vision Drowsiness Memory impairment	-azepam
	Antipsychotics May be listed as typical and atypical Sometimes called tranquilizers or neuroleptics Subclasses include thienobenzodiazepines, phenothiazines	haloperidol chlorpromazine (Thorazine) aripiprazole (Abilify) clozapine risperidone olanzapine (Zyprexa)	Used to treat symptoms of severe psychiatric disorders such as schizophrenia and bipolar disorder	Blurred vision Confusion Dizziness Drowsiness Agitation Anxiety Constipation	-peridol -azine

Table 5-2 (Continued)

	Drug Class	Example of Medication in the Drug Class	How the Drug Works	Side Effects	Common Ending
Central Nervous System (CNS) Drugs	**Cholinesterase Inhibitors**	donepezil (Aricept) galantamine (Reminyl) rivastigmine (Exelon)	Alzheimer's disease agents that prevent the breakdown of acetylcholine, a chemical that is important for memory, thinking, and reasoning	Abdominal pain Anorexia Diarrhea Dizziness Headache Nausea and vomiting	
	Anti-Parkinson agents	amantadine carbidopa levodopa robinirole (Requip)	Relieves muscle stiffness, tremors, weakness	Abnormal/ excessive dreaming Anorexia Confusion Constipation/ diarrhea	
	Tranquilizes/ hypnotics Sometimes called sleepers	clorazepate flurazepam (Dalmane) phentobarbital triazolam zolpidem (Ambien)	Calming or sedative effect Lower dose is sedative and higher dose is sleeper	Abnormal dreams Confusion Drowsiness Hangover effect Headache	
	Amphetamine stimulants Nonstimulant	Stimulants: amphetamine salts (Adderall) methylphenidate (Ritalin, Concerta) Nonstimulant: atomoxetine (Stratterra)	Treatment of attention deficit hyperactivity disorder (ADHD)	Increased blood pressure Insomnia Irritability Weight loss	
	Analgesics can be narcotic or nonnarcotic including the subclass of triptans	acetaminophen (APAP) Important to know (you will likely see on the exam): APAP maximum dose is 4,000 mg within a 24-hour period hydrocodone morphine meperidine Triptans: sumatriptan (Imitrex), rizatriptan (Maxalt), naratriptan (Amerge), zolmitriptan (Zomig)	Narcotic: Severe pain relief Nonnarcotic: mild pain relief Triptans used for migraine headache relief	Constipation Dizziness Drowsiness Confusion Dry mouth	-adol -triptan

(continues)

Table 5-2 (Continued)

	Drug Class	Example of Medication in the Drug Class	How the Drug Works	Side Effects	Common Ending
Central Nervous System (CNS) Drugs	**Antipyretics**	acetaminophen (APAP) ibuprofen (IBU) aspirin (ASA)	Drugs that reduce fever	Drowsiness Nausea Itching	
	Anesthetics can be categorized as local or general	Local: bupivacaine (Marcaine) benozocaine procaine General: propofol (Diprivan) desflurane: inhalation	Local anesthetics may be used as topical pain relievers by blocking nerve impulses, used as a nerve block for epidurals. General anesthetics bring a loss of consciousness for surgery.	Numbness Tingly feeling Nerve damage	-caine
	Anti-inflammatory Subclasses include NSAIDs, Cox-II inhibitors, salicylates	aspirin (ASA) ibuprofen (IBU) indomethacin diclofenac	Reduces inflammation	Abdominal pain Constipation/ diarrhea Dizziness Edema (fluid retention)	-profen -nidap
Anti-Infectives	**Antibacterials** Belongs to a larger class called antibiotics	levofloxacin cefdinir azithromycin valaciclovir penicillin	Fights bacterial infection	Allergic reactions Photosensitivity Dizziness Headache	-sulfa -kacin -mycin -cillin -cycline -oxacin
	Antifungals	clotrimazole	Treats fungal infections	Dermatologic reactions Itching	-conazole
	Immuno-suppressives	cyclosporine (Neoral or Sandimmune) azathioprine (Imuran) prednisolone	Prevents or reduces the body's normal reaction to invasion by disease or by foreign tissues. Used to treat autoimmune diseases where the body's defenses work abnormally and attack its own tissues. Helps to prevent rejection of organ transplants, HIV.	Hypertension Hyperglycemia Body is more vulnerable to infections.	
	Antivirals	amantadine (Symmetrel) oseltamivir (Tamiflu)	Used to treat viral infections or to provide temporary protection against infections such as influenza	Nervousness Anxiety Agitation Difficulty sleeping	-mantadine

Table 5-2 (Continued)

	Drug Class	Example of Medication in the Drug Class	How the Drug Works	Side Effects	Common Ending
Gastrointestinal (GI) Agents	**Antacids**	calcium carbonate aluminum hydroxide magnesium hydroxide	Relieve indigestion and heartburn by neutralizing stomach acid	Abdominal cramps Constipation/ diarrhea	
	Antidiarrheals	bismuth subsalicylate diphenoxylate and atropine (Lomotil/ Lonox) lopermide	Relief of diarrhea	Abdominal distention Anxiety Constipation Drowsiness Dry mouth	
	Antiemetics	ondansetron (Zofran) meclizine prochlorperazine	Treat nausea and vomiting	Blurred vision Constipation/ diarrhea Dizziness Drowsiness	
	Proton Pump Inhibitors (PPIs) Histamine Receptor (H2) Blockers	omeprazole famotidine cimetidine esomeprazole	Helps relieve gastroesophageal reflux disease (GERD), peptic ulcers by reducing stomach acid	Constipation Headache Nausea Discoloration of tongue	-tidine -prazole
	Laxatives	bisacodyl cascara sagrada docusate sodium magnesium citrate	Increase the frequency and ease of bowel movements	Abdominal cramping Bloating Diarrhea Flatulence	
Endocrine System/Hormones	**Female Hormones:** estrogens and progesterone **Male Hormones:** testosterone	conjugated estrogens (Premarin) estradiol progesterone anabolic steroids	Treat menstrual and menopausal disorders. Hormone replacement therapy (HRT). Used as oral contraceptives. Estrogens may be used to treat cancer of the breast or prostate. Testosterone given to men for disorders of the testes and may be used to treat breast cancer. Anabolic steroids used for body building.	Abdominal pain Back pain Breast pain Depression Flu-like symptoms Headache Nausea Vaginal bleeding	

(continues)

Table 5-2 (Continued)

	Drug Class	Example of Medication in the Drug Class	How the Drug Works	Side Effects	Common Ending
Endocrine System/Hormones	**Contraceptives**	Many combinations of estrogen and progestin available: Yaz, Alesse, Nordette	Prevent pregnancy. Treat symptoms of premenstrual syndrome (PMS).	Weight gain Acne Breakthrough bleeding Depression	
	Antihyperlipidemic Also called statin drugs or cholesterol lowering drugs	atorvastatin gemfibrozil (Lopid) lovastatin simvastatin ezetimibe (Zetia)	Lowers the fat level in the blood	Abdominal pain Constipation/ diarrhea Indigestion Flatulence Muscle cramps	-statin -fibrate
	Diabetic Agents	Many types of insulin Oral medications: glyburide, glipizide, metformin	Helps control blood sugar levels	Edema Hypoglycemia (low blood sugar)	
	Corticosteroids	cortisone dexamethasone (Decadron) prednisolone	Hormonal preparations that are used primarily for inflammation in arthritis or asthma	Appetite change Edema Headache Insomnia	
Cytotoxic Musculo/Skeletol Agents	**Biophosphonates**	alendronate (Fosamox) risedronate (Actonel)	Helps with osteoporosis	Abdominal pain constipation	
	Muscle Relaxants	baclofen carisoprodol (Soma) cyclobenzaprine	Relieves muscle spasm. Antianxiety drugs also have a muscle-relaxant action.	Blurred vision Confusion Dizziness Drowsiness Dry mouth	
	Antineoplastics	fluorouracil-5-FU or f5U (Adrucil, Carac, Efudex, Fluoroplex) estramustine (Emcyt, Estracit) nelarabine prednimustine	Drugs that kill or damage cells. Drugs used to treat cancer. May also be used as immunosuppressives.	Diarrhea Nausea and vomiting Loss of appetite	-rubicin -mustine -arabine
Hemotologic Agents	**Anticoagulants and Thrombolytics**	heparin enoxaparin (Lovenox) clopidogrel (Plavix) warfarin	Anticoagulants prevent blood from clotting. Thrombolytics help dissolve and disperse blood clots.	Abdominal pain Constipation Dizziness Bleeding Headache	

Benzodiazepines are the principal class of medications used to treat anxiety, panic attacks, and insomnia. Benzodiazepines, sometimes called benzos, are used more widely than barbiturates because they are safer and the side effects are less noticeable. Even though benzodiazepines are listed as a Class IV scheduled drug, there is less risk of eventual physical dependence than barbiturates.

Benzodiazepines commonly end in –epam or –olam. Example: clonaz*epam*

Example: alpraz*olam*

Antidepressants are a large class of drugs acting on the central nervous system. Antidepressants have many subclasses with the tricyclic antidepressants (TCAs) being the oldest class. Other subclasses are selective serotonin reuptake inhibitors (SSRI) and monoamine oxidase inhibitors (MAOI). Serotonin noradrenaline reuptake inhibitors (SNRI) and noradrenaline dopamine reuptake inhibitors (NA/DRI) are second- and third-generation antidepressants with fewer side effects. Examples of second- and third-generation antidepressants are buproprion (Wellbutrin), mirtazapine (Remeron), and venlafaxine (Effexor). All antidepressant classes have the same therapeutic outcome but are prescribed for tolerance of side effects.

The information on Table 5-2 is not comprehensive. It is intended to highlight side effects, drug classification and uses, and drug names.

Table 5-3 Commonly Prescribed IV Medications

Generic Name	Pronunciation	Trade Name	Indications
heparin	he-pə-rən		Anticoagulant
enoxoparin	ee nox AP a rin	Lovenox	Anticoagulant
hydrocortisone	hye dro KORT i zone	Solu-Cortef	Steroid
dexamethasone	dex a METH a sone	Decadron	Steroid
methylprednisolone	METH il pred NIS oh lone	Solu-Medrol	Steroid
adenosine	ah-den′o-sēn	Adenocard	Acute cardiovascular
dobutamine	doe BUE ta meen	Dobutrex	Cardiovascular
dopamine	DOE-pa-meen	Intropin	Cardiovascular
nitroglycerin	NYE troe GLIS er in	Tridil	Cardiovascular
lidocaine	LYE doe kane	Xylocaine	Cardiovascular or anesthetic
atropine	AT roe peen	AtroPen	Emergency: cardiovascular
nitroprusside	nye troe PRUS ide	Nipride, Nitorpress	Cardiovascular
norepinephrine	nor ep i NEF rin	Levophed	Cardiovascular
filgrastime	fil gra′ stim	Neupogen	Colony stimulating: Used in conjunction with chemotherapy to stimulate white blood cell production
azathioprine	ay za THYE oh preen	Imuran	Immunosuppressive
cyclosporine	SYE kloe SPOR een	Sandimmune	Immunosuppressive
tobramycin	toe bra MY sin	Nebcin	Anti-infective
doxycycline	DOX i SYE kleen	Vibramycin	Anti-infective: Tetracycline class

(continues)

Table 5-3 (Continued)

Generic Name	Pronunciation	Trade Name	Indications
minocycline	mye no SYE kleen	Minocin	Anti-infective: Tetracycline class
cefotaxime	SEF oh TAX eem	Claforan	Anti-infective: Cephalosporin class
cefazolin	sef A zoe lin	Ancef, Kefzol	Anti-infective: Cephalosporin class
ceftriaxone	SEF trye AX one	Rocephin	Anti-infective: Cephalosporin class
ciprofloxacin	SIP roe FLOX a sin	Cipro	Anti-infective: Quinolone class
ampicillin/ sulbactam	am pi SIL in and sul BAK tam	Unasyn	Anti-infective: Penicillin class
piperacillin/ tazobactam	pi PER a sil in and tay zoe BAK tam	Zosyn	Anti-infective: Penicillin Class
gentamicin	JEN-tuh-MY-sin	Geramycin	Anti-infective
imipenem/cilastatin	IM i PEN em and SYE la STAT in	Primaxin	Anti-infective
levofloxacin	leev oh FLOX a sin	Levaquin	Anti-infective
metronidozole	me troe NI da zole	Flagyl	Anti-infective
vancomycin	VAN koe MYE sin	Vancocin	Anti-infective
clindamycin	klin da MYE sin	Cleocin	Anti-infective
foscarnet	fos KAR net	Foscavir	Antiviral
ganciclovir	gan SYE kloe veer	Cytovene	Antiviral
acyclovir	a SYE klo veer	Zovirax	Antiviral
fluconazole	floo KOE na zole	Diflucan	Antifungal
fentanyl	FEN ta nil	Sublimaze	Analgesic
ondansetron	on DAN se tron	Zofran	Antinausea
epinephrine	EP i NEF rin	Adrenalin	Emergency: Allergic reactions
midazolam	mid-AY-zoe-lam	Versed	Sedative
propofol	PROE-poe-fol	Diprivan	Sedative
famotidine	fam OH ti deen	Pepcid	Histamine (H2) antagonist
ranitidine	ra NI ti deen	Zantac	Histamine (H2) antagonist
cimetidine	sye ME ti deen	Tagamet	Histamine (H2) antagonist
fosphenytoin	fos FEN i toyn	Cerebyx	Anticonvulsant
phenytoin	FEN i toyn	Dilantin	Anticonvulsant
vecuronium	VEK ue ROE nee um	Nocuron	Muscle relaxer: Administered before general anesthesia to prepare for surgery
calcium gluconate magnesium sulfate potassium: chloride/phosphate/ acetate sodium: bicarbonate/ chloride/acetate			Electrolytes

Table 5-4 Commonly Prescribed Chemotherapy Medications

Brand Name	Generic Name
Blenoxane	bleomycin
Cerubidine	daunorubicin
Xeloda	capecitabine
Platinol	cisplatin
VePesid	etoposide
Mustargen	meclorethamine
Purinethol	mercaptopurinem
Leukeran	chlorambucil
Cytoxan	cyclophosphamide
Adriamycin	doxorubicin
5-FU, Efudex	fluorouracil
Alkeran	melphalan
Trexall	methotrexate
Eloxatin	oxaliplatin

Table 5-5 Common Medications Used in the Hospital

Brand Name	Generic Name	Medical Use
Lovenox	enoxoparin	Anticoagulant
Aranesp	darbepoetin alfa	Treats anemia
Procrit	epoetin alfa	Treats anemia
Revlimid	lenalidomide	Treats anemia, multiple myeloma
Neulasta	pegfilgrastim	Promotes growth of white blood cells (WBC) to fight against infection Used in conjunction with chemotherapy
Remicade	infliximab	Rheumatoid arthritis, psoriatic arthritis, ulcerative colitis, Crohn's disease
Rituxan	rituximab	Cancer treatment
Levaquin	levofloxacin	Antibiotic
Avastin	bevacizumab	Cancer treatment
Zosyn	piperacillin and tazobactam	Antibiotic
Neupogen	filgrastim	Promotes growth of white blood cells (WBC) to fight against infection
Eloxatin	oxaliplatin	Chemotherapy
Diprivan	propofol	Sedative

(continues)

Table 5-5 (Continued)

Brand Name	Generic Name	Medical Use
Omnipaque	iohexol	Radiopharmaceutical Diagnostic contrast medium
Integrilin	eptifibatide	Anticoagulant
Advair Diskus	fluticasone and salmeterol	Treatment of asthma, chronic obstructive pulmonary disorder (COPD)
Sodium chloride	sodium chloride	Used as diluent for IV medications
Zyvox	linezolid	Antibiotic
Herceptin	trastuzumab	Cancer treatment
Protonix oral Protonix IV	pantoprazole	Proton pump inhibitor (PPI) decreases stomach acid production
Taxotere	docetaxel	Cancer treatment
Angiomax	bivalirudin	Anticoagulant
Thrombin-JMI	thrombin	Helps to control bleeding
Cancidas	caspofungin	Antifungal for internal organs
Ultane	sevoflurane	General anesthetic
Seroquel	quetiapine	Antipsychotic
Carimune NF Nanofiltered	human immune globulin g	Treatment of hepatitis A virus
Gemzar	gemcitabine	Cancer treatment
Erbitux	cetuximab	Cancer treatment
Visipaque	iodixanol	Radiopharmaceutical Contrast medium
Primaxin	imipenem and cilastatin	Antibiotic
Simvastatin	simvastatin	Reduces bad cholesterol
Gammagard S/D Gamunex	immune globulin	Treatment of immune deficiency disorders
morphine sulfate	morphine sulfate	Narcotic analgesic
vancomycin HCl	vancomycin HCl	Antibiotic
Nexium	esomeprazole	Proton pump inhibitor (PPI) decreases stomach acid production
Plavix	clopidogrel	Anticoagulant
Zometa	zoledronic acid	Biophosphonate to treat bone cancer
Camptosar	irinotecan	Cancer treatment
Risperdal	risperidone	Antipsychotic
Zyprexa	olanzapine	Antipsychotic
Lupron Depot	leuprolide	Prostate cancer treatment

Table 5-5 (Continued)

Brand Name	Generic Name	Medical Use
Prevacid	lansoprazole	Proton pump inhibitor (PPI) decreases stomach acid production
Azithromycin	azithromycin	Antibiotic
Lipitor	atorvastatin	Reduces levels of bad cholesterol
Cubicin	daptomycin	Antibiotic
Suprane	desflurane	General anesthetic
Normal Saline Flush	sodium chloride	IV administration to keep IV line from becoming blocked and to "flush" IV medication through the line

Table 5-6 Drug Acronyms

Suffix Acronym	Meaning	Example
DS	Double strength	Bactrim DS
CC	Coat core (an external coating and an internal core)	Adalat CC
HFA	Hydroflouroalkane	Advair HFA
PM	Nighttime	Tylenol PM
ES	Extra strength	Vicodin ES
XR or XL	Extended release	Augmentin XR
AR	Acid reducer	Axid AR
SR	Sustained release	Wellbutrin SR
CD	Controlled delivery	Cardizem CD
ER	Extended release	Depakote ER
TTS	Transdermal therapeutic system	Catapress TTS
CR	Controlled release	Oxycontin CR
D	Decongestant	Clarinex D
EC	Enteric coated	EC-Naprosyn
LA	Long acting	Detrol LA
DM	dextromethorphan	Robitussin DM
PF	Preservative free	HypoTears PF

Study suggestion: Study the ending of the generic names to help you remember which drug class they're in or the medical purpose of the medication.

RADIOPHARMACEUTICALS

Nuclear pharmacies are specialized pharmacies that dispense radiopharmaceuticals. Radiopharmaceuticals are medications used for diagnostic purposes or to treat certain diseases (see **Table 5-7**).

When radiopharmaceuticals are used to help diagnose medical problems, only small amounts are administered to the patient. The radiopharmaceutical then passes through, or is taken up by,

Table 5-7 Examples of Radiopharmaceuticals

Drug Name	Use
Iodine-131	1. Diagnosis 2. Treatment of cancer (CA)
Technetium	Diagnosis
Cobalt-60	Radiation therapy for cancer (CA)

an organ of the body (which organ depends on which radiopharmaceutical is used and how it has been given). Then the radioactivity is detected and pictures are produced by special imaging equipment. These pictures allow the nuclear medicine doctor to study how the organ is working and to detect cancer or tumors that may be present in the organ. The contrast medium used for a computerized tomography (CT) scan, for instance, is a radiopharmaceutical. Radiopharmaceuticals may be given to the patient orally or by injection.

Some radiopharmaceuticals are used in larger amounts to treat certain kinds of cancer and other diseases. In those cases, the radioactive agent is taken up in the cancerous area and destroys the affected tissue.

Handle radiopharmaceuticals with care. The rule when working with radiopharmaceuticals is distance and speed. The technician should perform compounding steps as quickly as possible. The less time spent working with the product, the less chance of exposure. The technician may also use tongs or forceps to handle the radiopharmaceutical vials. Long-handled forceps help to create a greater distance between the product and the technician's body.

Many special procedures at nuclear pharmacies are unique and are not found at other types of pharmacy setting. From processing and delivering orders to storing and disposing of medication, the nuclear pharmacy technician requires specialized training. An agency called the Nuclear Regulatory Commission (NRC) inspects nuclear pharmacies for quality control of radiopharmaceuticals.

The amount of radioactivity of a radiopharmaceutical is expressed in units called becquerels or curies. Generally, the radiopharmaceuticals administered to patients have short half-lives to minimize the radiation dose and the risk of prolonged exposure. In most cases, radiopharmaceuticals decay to stable elements within minutes, hours, or days, allowing patients to be released from the hospital in a relatively short time.

RESTRICTED DRUGS (RD)

Restricted drugs (RD) are rarely used medications that have limited therapeutic outcomes. The use of restricted drugs requires postmarketing restrictions, because of their severe side effects (see **Table 5-8**). Accutane (isotretinoin) is a medication indicated for treating severe acne. Because Accutane (isotretinoin) has been known to cause severe birth defects and spontaneous abortion, it is listed as a restricted drug.

Prior to 2005, SMART, a risk management program, was used as a *System to Manage Accutane Related Teratogenicity*. The SMART program, administered by Roche the manufacturer of Accutane, mandated yellow *Accutane Qualification* stickers. A yellow sticker on the hard copy prescription signified to the pharmacist that the patient had received a pregnancy test, was not pregnant, and was therefore eligible to take Accutane.

The SMART program has since been replaced by the iPLEDGE program. The patient, the physician, and the pharmacy must all adhere to special guidelines for using and dispensing a restricted drug in the iPLEDGE program as well as other restricted drug programs, such as the *Clozapine Prescription Access System* (CPAS) and the *System for Thalidomide Education and Prescribing Safety* (S.T.E.P.S.).

Table 5-8 Restricted Drugs

Drug Name	Indications	Side Effects	Distribution Guidelines
Generic: isotretinoin EYE-soe-TRET-i-noin Brand: Accutane, Amnesteem, Claravis, Sotret	1. Acute acne	1. Adverse effects on fetal development (Teratogenicity) 2. Spontaneous abortion 3. Suicidal thoughts or behavior	1. Prescribers must be registered with iPLEDGE program 2. iPLEDGE program enrollment for both male and female patients 3. Pregnancy testing; two negative results before therapy begins and monthly testing thereafter 4. Electronic system to track pregnancy testing and registered users 5. Patient agreement 6. Patient must pick up prescription within 7 days after office visit/ prescription written
Generic: thalidomide Brand: Thalomid	1. Acute erythema nodosum leprosum (ENL)	1. Teratogenicity	1. Pharmacy, prescriber, and patient must be registered with S.T.E.P.S. program 2. Patient consent 3. Pregnancy testing 4. Patient counseling: brochure and video on side effects 5. Limited quantity dispensed 6. No phoned-in prescriptions
Generic: clozapine Brand: Clozaril	1. Severe Schizophrenia	1. Seizures 2. Myocarditis 3. Severe reduction in white blood cells (WBC) (Agranulocytosis)	1. Patient registered with CPAS™ or other restricted drug program offered by the drug manufacturer 2. Requires lab test prior to dispensing; Acceptable WBC and absolute neutrophil count (ANC) (routinely monitored) 3. Limited quantity dispensed
Generic: alosetron Brand: Lotronex	1. Female severe-chronic irritable bowel syndrome (IBS)	1. Reduced blood flow to the intestines (ischemic colitis) 2. Severe constipation	1. Written Rx, only; no telephone, faxed, or electronic prescriptions 2. Yellow prescribing program sticker 3. Medication guide given with every fill 4. Patient agreement

Study Tip: Use memorable icons to help remember common side effects for drugs. See **Table 5-9**.

THE DO'S AND DON'TS OF DISPENSING

Tablet Splitting

Pharmacy technicians commonly split tablets to reduce patient costs and to provide the correct dose. For example, a 50-mg tablet may be split or broken in half to provide the prescribed 25-mg dose.

Table 5-9 Common Drug Side Effects

Mediation Use/Class	Common Side Effects
High Blood Pressure Medications: **Beta Blockers** **Calcium Channel Blockers (CCB)** **Angiotension Converting Enzyme (ACE) inhibitors** **Vasodilators**	Headache Feeling tired Dizziness Upset stomach
Diuretics commonly called 'water pills'	Dizziness Headache Upset Stomach Frequent urination
High cholesterol medications: **Statins** **Fibrates** **Sequestrants**	Headache Upset stomach Gas Dizziness Diarrhea Constipation
Analgesics commonly called pain killers	Constipation Dizziness Headache Feeling tired Upset stomach Nausea/vomiting Dry mouth
Antibiotic	Diarrhea Nausea/vomiting Dizziness Headache Upset stomach Constipation Gas
PPI	Constipation Diarrhea Nausea/vomiting Headache
Antipsychotics	Feeling tired Dizziness Constipation Dry mouth Weight gain
Antidepressants	Constipation Dizziness Feeling tired Diarrhea Dry mouth Headache Decreased sexual desire

Splitting tablets saves money, because the 50-mg tablet may cost the same as the lower-strength tablet; thus, the customer gets two tablets for the price of one. In some cases, the pharmacy may not stock the lower dose of medication, so a higher-strength tablet is split to get the correct dose.

Tablet splitting can lead to medication errors. Even when a tablet is scored and split well, there can still be crumbling and uneven pieces. Rather than expecting the patient to split their own tablets, it's advised to have pharmacy personnel split the tablet. A patient can become easily confused about the split tablets and how they should be taken! Follow through with telling the patient that the tablets have been split and why the pharmacy split them rather than giving a full tablet. Pharmacy technicians working in a hospital pharmacy should split the tablets for nursing to administer to the patient.

1. Make sure the tablet is suitable to be split. Most extended release (ER) or sustained release (SR) tablets cannot be split. Splitting a time-released tablet may interfere with the diffusion properties of the medication.
2. Small tablets or tablets that break into tiny pieces should not be split. The dosing will be inaccurate.
3. Most enteric-coated tablets should not be split. The coating benefits are destroyed when the tablet is split.

Confusing Names

The Institute for Safe Medication Practices (ISMP) publishes a list on sound-alike/look-alike drug names. An example of sound-alike medications are Taxol and Paxil. A serious medication error would occur if Taxol, a cancer medication, were dispensed in place of Paxil, an antidepressant. To work toward eliminating medication-dispensing errors, scanning the National Drug Code (NDC) number of the medication is a necessary step. Another step to help reduce medication errors in sound-alike/look-alike drug names is for the manufacturer to make the labeling easier to read. Look-alike drug names are distinguished from one another by the use of tall man lettering. Tall man lettering is uppercase letters mixed with lowercase letters to call attention to the difference in the drug names; buPROPion is confused with busPIRone.

Not only do medication names look alike but packaging looks alike too. Stock bottles lining the pharmacy shelves have the same appearance. The technician might easily grab the wrong bottle from the shelf. Adding color to the white stock bottles or to the labels may help in distinguishing medications. Keep in mind, though, a colorblind person must take extra steps to ensure proper dispensing.

Crushing Tablets

There are times when a patient may not be able to swallow an oral tablet. Crushing the tablet and then sprinkling it on food is an option for administration. Not all oral medication is suitable for crushing. A time-released medication's chemical properties may be destroyed if the tablet is crushed. Avoid crushing time-release tablets and enteric-coated tablets. Prepare for your certification exam by memorizing the brand and generic names of top selling prescription drugs (**Table 5-10** and **Table 5-11**).

Table 5-10 Top-Selling Prescription Drugs

Drug Class	Brand Name	Generic Name Pronunciation	Medical Use	Dosage
1. Antihyperlipidemic	Lipitor	atorvastatin (a TOR va sta tin)	Cholesterol lowering	Oral tablets, once a day
2. Proton Pump Inhibitor (PPI)	Nexium	esomeprazole (ee so MEP ra zol)	Decrease acid production in stomach	Oral capsules taken at least one hour before a meal
3. Anticoagulant	Plavix	clopidogrel (kloe PID oh grel)	Keeps blood from clotting	Oral tablet
4. Respiratory Steroid	Advair	fluticasone and salmeterol (floo TIK a sone, sal ME te rol)	Asthma, COPD	Diskus

(continues)

Table 5-10 (Continued)

Drug Class	Brand Name	Generic Name Pronunciation	Medical Use	Dosage
5. Antipsychotic	Seroquel	quetiapine (kwe TYE a peen)	Schizophrenia	Oral tablets, XR
6. Antipsychotic	Abilify	aripiprazole (AR i PIP ra zole)	Schizophrenia, bipolar, treats irritability and mood swings	Oral tab
7. Respiratory agent	Singulair	montelukast (mon te LOO kast)	Asthma, allergy symptoms	Oral tab, chewable tab
8. Narcotic Analgesic	OxyContin	oxycodone (ox i KOE done)	Moderate to severe pain reliever	Oral tab
9. Diabetic	Actos	pioglitazone (PYE o GLIT a zone)	Helps control blood sugar	Oral tab
10. Proton Pump Inhibitor (PPI)	Prevacid	lansoprazole (lan SOE pra zol)	Decrease acid production in stomach	Oral tab
11. Antidepressant: Selective Serotonin and Norepinephrine Reuptake Inhibitors (SSNRIs)	Cymbalta	duloxetine (du LOX e teen)	Treats major depressive disorder and general anxiety disorder	Oral capsule Delayed release
12. Antidepressant: Serotonin-Norepinephrine Reuptake Inhibitor (SNRI)	Effexor XR	venlafaxine (VEN-la-FAX-een)	Depression, panic disorder, anxiety disorder	Oral tab
13. Antidepressant: Selective Serotonin Reuptake Inhibitors (SSRIs)	Lexapro	escitalopram (EE si TAL o pram)	Anxiety, major depressive disorder	Oral tab
14. Antihyperlipidemic	Crestor	rosuvastatin (roe SOO va sta tin)	Reduces levels of bad cholesterol	Oral tab Film coated
15. Antipsychotic	Zyprexa	olanzapine (oh LANZ a peen)	Schizophrenia, bipolar	Oral tab
16. Antiviral	Valtrex	valacyclovir (val a SYE kloe veer)	Slows the growth or spread of herpes virus	Oral tab Film coated
17. Alpha-adrenergic blockers	Flomax	tamsulosin (tam soo LOE sin)	Improves urination in men with enlarged prostate	Oral capsule

Table 5-10 (Continued)

Drug Class	Brand Name	Generic Name Pronunciation	Medical Use	Dosage
18. Endocrine System/ Hormone/Diabetic	Lantus	insulin glargine (IN soo lin GLAR jeen)	Long-acting insulin that lowers levels of sugar in blood	Injection
19. Anticonvulsant	Lyrica	pregabalin (pre GAB a lin)	Controls seizures	Oral capsule, solution
20. Nonsteroidal Anti-inflammatory Drugs (NSAID)	Celebrex	celecoxib (oral) (SEL e KOX ib)	Reduces inflammation and pain	Oral capsule
21. Antibiotic Fluoroquinolones (flor-o-KWIN-o-lones).	Levaquin	levofloxacin (leev oh FLOX a sin)	Treats bacterial infections	Oral tab, solution Injection
22. Central Nervous System Agent	Aricept	donepezil (doe NEP e zil)	Treats mild to moderate dementia caused by Alzheimer's disease	Oral tab Film coated Oral disintegrating tab
23. Respiratory Agent: Bronchodilator	Spiriva	tiotropium inhalation (tye oh TROE pee um)	Enlarges airway to allow for easier breathing	Comes as a capsule containing dry powder, which is inhaled through the mouth using an inhaler
24. Cardiovascular Agent angiotensin II receptor antagonist	Diovan	valsartan (val SAR tan)	High blood pressure Heart failure	Oral tab Film coated
25. Cardiovascular Agent Combination Drug: angiotensin II receptor blocker and diuretic	Diovan HCT	valsartan/ hydrochlorothiazide (val-SAR-tan/HYE-droe-KLOR-oh-THYE-a-zide)	High blood pressure	Oral tab Film coated
26. Antihyperlipidemic "Fibrate" Class	Tricor	fenofibrate (FEN oh FYE brate)	Helps reduce cholesterol in the blood	Oral tab
27. Central Nervous System Agent: Stimulant	Concerta	methylphenidate (METH il FEN i date)	Used to treat attention deficit disorder (ADD) and attention deficit hyperactivity disorder (ADHD)	Oral tab Extended release
28. Endocrine/Diabetic	Januvia	sitagliptin (SI ta glip tin)	Helps control blood sugar levels in blood	Oral tab Film coated

(continues)

Table 5-10 (Continued)

Drug Class	Brand Name	Generic Name Pronunciation	Medical Use	Dosage
29. **Antihyperlipidemic**	Vytorin	ezetimibe and simvastatin (ez ET i mibe and SIM va stat in)	Reduces levels of bad cholesterol while increasing levels of good cholesterol in the blood	Oral tab
30. **Central Nervous System Agent Stimulant**	Adderall XR	amphetamine/ dextroamphetamine am-FET-a-meen/ DEX-troe-am-FET-a-meen	Treating attention deficit hyperactivity disorder (ADHD)	Oral capsule
31. **Anticoagulant**	Lovenox	enoxaparin (ee nox AP a rin)	Prevents formation of blood clots	Injection
32. **Antiviral**	Atripla	efavirenz, emtricitabine, and tenofovir (ef AV ir enz, em trye SYE ta been, and ten OF oh vir)	Prevents human immunodeficiency virus (HIV) from reproducing	Oral tab Film coated
33. **Antihyperlipidemic**	Zetia	ezetimibe (ez ET i mibe)	Treats high cholesterol	Oral tab
34. **Proton Pump Inhibitor (PPI)**	Aciphex	rabeprazole (ra BEP ra zole)	Decrease acid production in stomach	Oral delayed release tab
35. **Sedative Hypnotic**	Ambien CR	zolpidem (zole-PI-dem)	Insomnia	Oral extended release tab
36. **Phosphodiesterase (PDE) Inhibitors**	Viagra	sildenafil (oral) (sil DEN uh fil)	Erectile dysfunction	Oral tab
37. **Anticonvulsant**	Topamax	topiramate (toe PYRE a mate)	Treat seizures	Oral tab Coated Oral capsule Coated pellets
38. **Local Anesthetic**	Lidoderm	lidocaine topical (LYE doe kane TOP i kal)	Used to relieve postshingles pain used to reduce pain or discomfort caused by skin irritations such as sunburn, insect bites	Patch
39. **Respiratory System Bronchodilator**	ProAir HFA	albuteral (al-BUE-ter-ol)	Asthma	Metered aerosol
40. **Endocrine System/ Hormone Diabetes**	NovoLog	insulin aspart (IN su lin AS part)	Fast-acting insulin to lower sugar levels in blood	Injection

Table 5-10 (Continued)

Drug Class	Brand Name	Generic Name Pronunciation	Medical Use	Dosage
41. Central Nervous System Agent	Suboxone	buprenorphine and naloxone (byoo PREH nor feen and NAH lox own)	Treatment of opiod addiction	Sublingual (SL) Injection
42. Respiratory System Agent	Nasonex	mometasone (moe MET a sone)	Treat and prevent nasal congestion, runny nose, allergy symptoms	Nasal inhalation
43. Central Nervous System Agent	Provigil	modafinil (moe DAF i nil)	Treats excessive sleepiness	Oral tab
44. Antipsychotic	Geodon	ziprasidone (zi PRAY si done)	Schizophrenia Bipolar	Oral capsules Injection
45. Antiviral	Truvada	emtricitabine and tenofovir (em trye SYE ta been and ten OF oh vir)	Prevents human immunodeficiency virus (HIV) from reproducing	Oral tab Film coated
46. Sedative hypnotic	Lunesta	eszopiclone (es ZOE PIK lone)	Insomnia	Oral tab Coated
47. Endocrine System Agent/Hormone Diabetes	Humalog	insulin lispro (IN soo lin LISS pro)	Lowers levels of sugar in the blood. Fast-acting insulin usually given together with another long-acting insulin.	Injection
48. Antihyperlipidemic	Niaspan	niacin (nicotinic acid) (NYE a sin (NIK oh TIN ik AS id))	Helps to reduce bad cholesterol (LDL) and to increase good cholesterol (HDL)	Oral tab Film coated Extended release
49. Urinary System Agent cholinergic receptor blocker	Detrol LA	tolterodine (tol-TER-oh-deen)	Treats overactive bladder	Oral extended release capsule
50. Hormone Contraceptive	Yaz	drospirenone and ethinyl estradiol (dro SPY re nown, ETH in il, ESS tra dy ol)	Contraceptive to prevent pregnancy	Oral tab

Note: Remember to make dosage adjustments for patient age or health.

Drug classes are a bit like family trees with new generations and offspring. The following charts diagram broad drug classes branching into their more specific subclasses (see **Figures 5-1** to **5-5**).

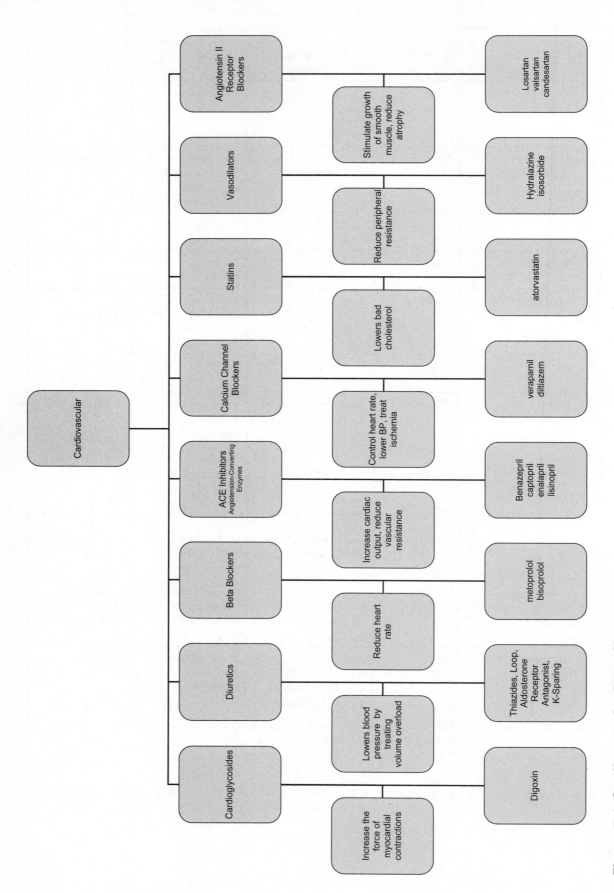

Figure 5-1 Cardiovascular Drug Classes

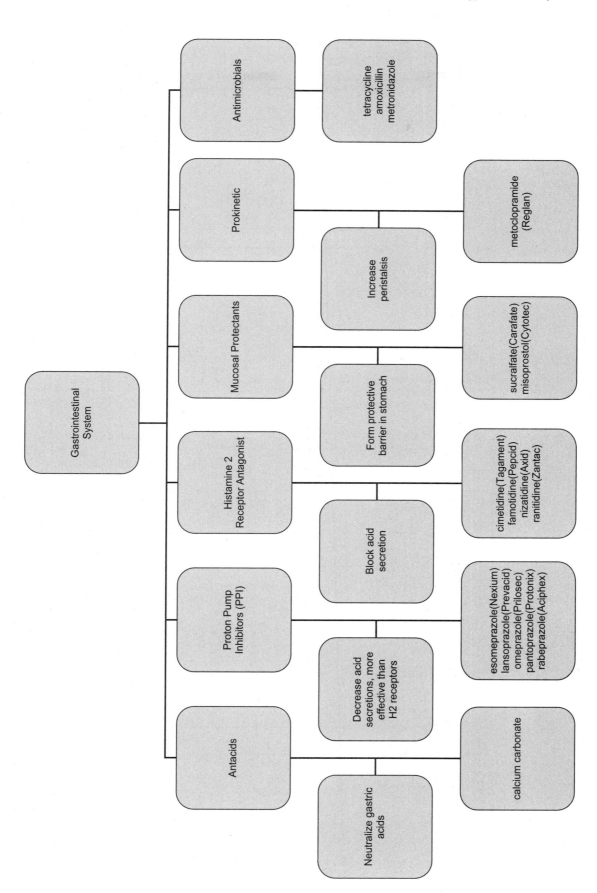

Figure 5-2 Gastrointestinal System Drug Classes

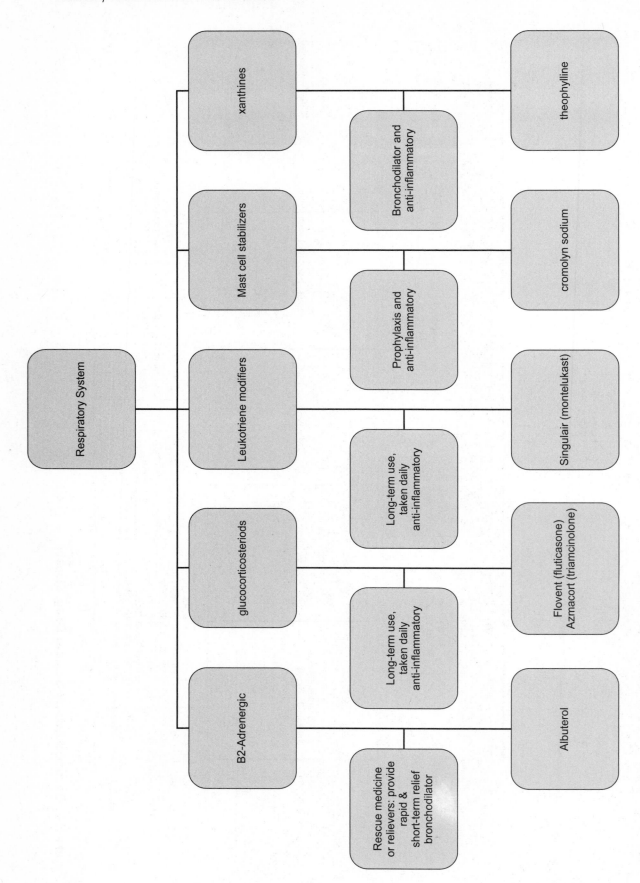

Figure 5-3 Respiratory System Drug Class

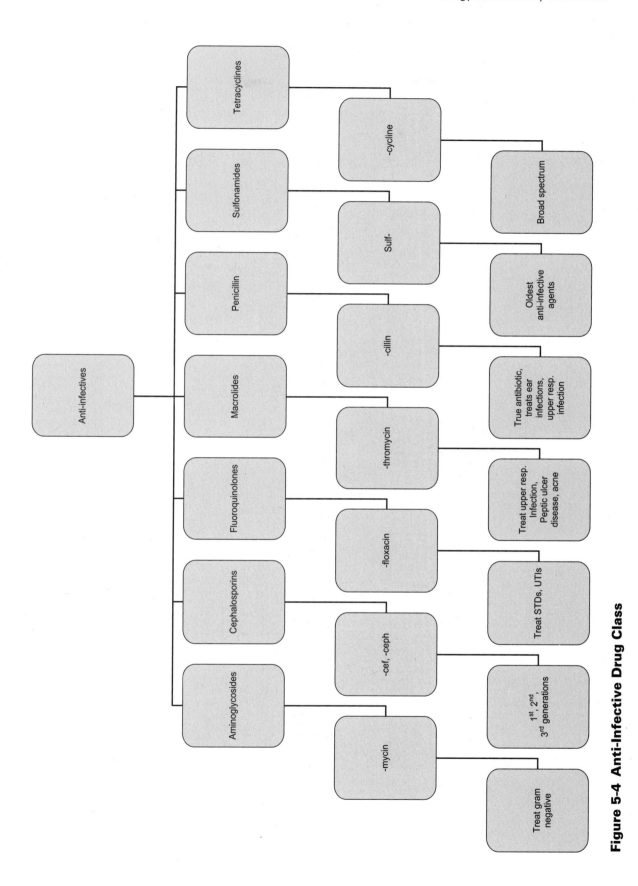

Figure 5-4 Anti-Infective Drug Class

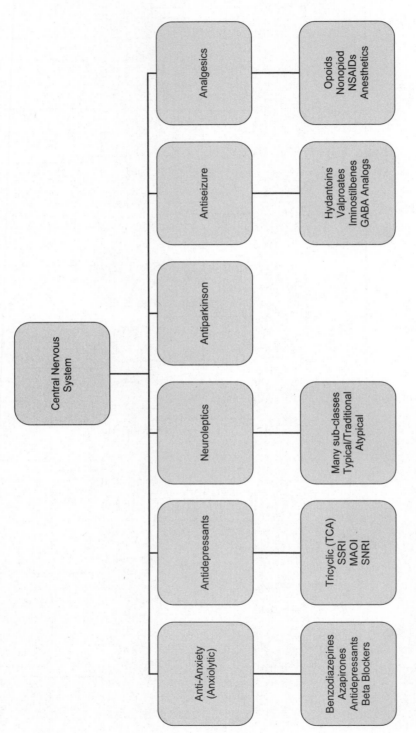

Figure 5-5 Central Nervous System Drug Class

Table 5-11 Top-Selling Over-the-Counter Drugs

Private label oral analgesic tablets	Aleve—Tylenol—Bayer—Tylenol PM
Private label oral cold/allergy/sinus tablets	Claritin—Benadryl—Claritin D—Mucinex—Airborne
Private label mineral supplements	Osteo Bi Flex
Oral antacid tablets	Prilosec OTC
NSAID oral tablets	Advil
Private label first aid topical ointments/antiseptics	Neosporin Plus
Antismoking gum	Nicorette
Private label multivitamins	Centrum Silver
Private label laxative oral tablets	Metamucil
Private label antacid oral tablets	Zantac—Tums EX
Private label one and two letter oral vitamins	Vitamin C

This is your checklist to make sure you understand what you need to know for the certification exam. Review chapter content if there is a topic of which you're uncertain. I know:

√	
	…the differences in the therapeutic drug classes.
	…the most common OTC drugs.
	…indications for the most common Rx and OTC drugs.
	…brand and generic names of the most common drugs.
	…the common side effects of the most common drugs.
	…basic drug–drug interactions and drug–food interactions.
	…how to avoid mix-ups in sound-alike, look-alike drugs.
	…procedures to follow to avoid medication errors.
	…the routes of administration and absorption.
	…rules regarding drug substitutions.

RESOURCES

1. Drug Information Online [information for chart taken from website]. Available at: www.drugs.com. Accessed February 13, 2011.
2. Porter RS, eds. *The Merck Manual of Medical Information* [home edition]. Whitehouse Station, NJ: Merck Sharp & Dohme Corp.; 2004–2010. Available at: http://www.MerckManuals.com/home. Accessed February 13, 2011.
3. Wolters Kluwer Health. Top 200 Drugs Used in Hospitals in 2007. Available at: http://drugtopics.modernmedicine.com/drugtopics/data/articlestandard//drugtopics/262008/526563/article.pdf. Accessed February 18, 2011.
4. Martin B. Health literacy: strategies to improve communication. *Pharm Today*. November 2010:38.
5. US Nuclear Regulatory Commission Website. Radiopharmaceutical. Available at: http://www.nrc.gov/reading-rm/basic-ref/glossary/radiopharmaceutical.html. Accessed February 14, 2011.
6. Thomson Healthcare Inc. Radiopharmaceutical [oral route]. Available at: http://www.mayoclinic.com/health/drug-information/DR602307. Accessed February 14, 2011.

7. Posey LM. Pharmacy's top 10 news stories of 2010. Available at: http://www.pharmacist.com/AM/Template.cfm?Section=Pharmacy_News&template=/CM/ContentDisplay.cfm&ContentID=24973. Accessed February 2011.

CHAPTER 5

MULTIPLE CHOICE

Identify the choice that best completes the statement or answers the question.

_____ **1.** The steps of pharmacokinetics are

a. taking, absorbing, eliminating

b. absorbing, movement, metabolize, synthesize

c. absorb, distribute, metabolize, eliminate

d. intake, absorb, metabolize, excrete

_____ **2.** Routes of absorption include

a. IV, IM, SL

b. tablet, lozenge, capsule

c. BID, QD, TID

d. CR, XL, SR

_____ **3.** Sublingual (SL) means the medication is

a. inhaled

b. placed under the tongue

c. placed between the cheek and gum

d. injected under the skin

_____ **4.** A medication that may affect the whole body rather than staying at the site of action is

a. nondistributed

b. local

c. systemic

d. prodrug

_____ **5.** Most of the drug metabolism takes place

a. in the mouth

b. in the liver

c. while the patient is sleeping

d. before meals

_____ **6.** The first pass effect involves what body organ?

a. liver

b. mouth

c. stomach

d. spleen

_____ **7.** Most drugs are eliminated by what body organ?

a. liver

b. kidneys

c. stomach

d. spleen

_____ **8.** What the drug does to the body is termed

a. pharmacokinetics

b. pharmacodynamics

c. pharmacology

d. pharmacogenomics

____ **9.** Bioavailability is

a. the available amount of therapy time

c. the amount of drug available at the site of action

b. new life made available through medication therapy

d. the available dosage forms

___ **10.** The same chemical equivalent of active ingredient is released into the bloodstream as the comparable drug:

a. therapeutic alternative

c. bioavailability

b. therapeutic duplication

d. bioequivalent

___ **11.** Medication that contains a different active ingredient than another drug, but produces the same therapeutic outcome:

a. therapeutic equivalent

c. pharmaceutical equivalent

b. therapeutic alternative

d. pharmaceutical alternative

___ **12.** Megan had an unusual and unpredicted reaction to her new medication. She experienced a(n)

a. idiosyncratic reaction

c. adverse reaction

b. side effect

d. therapeutic outcome

___ **13.** Types of drug interactions involve

a. drug–drug/drug–food

c. drug–food/drug–dosage

b. drug–drug/drug–activity

d. drug–dosage/drug–drink

___ **14.** Patients who take more than one drug at a time may be at risk of a_____ interaction.

a. drug–activity

c. drug–drug

b. drug–food

d. drug–dosage

___ **15.** A delayed onset or an enhanced absorption of the drug may be consequences of a _____ interaction.

a. drug–food

c. drug–activity

b. drug–dosage

d. drug–drink

___ **16.** NSAIDs should not be taken with which other prescription?

a. sedatives

c. antibiotics

b. anticoagulants

d. antidepressants

___ **17.** Which drug class has potential for drug–drug interactions with a wide range of medications?

a. antitussives

c. antacids

b. NSAIDs

d. CCB

___ **18.** To ensure protection, a patient using birth control pills should use another method of birth control while taking

a. sedatives

c. antihistamines

b. antidepressants

d. antibiotics

___ **19.** Alcohol interacts with many medications by

a. producing a sedative effect

b. producing a stimulant effect

c. increasing or decreasing the effects of the medication

d. increasing the blood concentration

___ **20.** Man-made drugs prepared in a laboratory are

a. natural

b. biologics

c. synthetic

d. seminatural

___ **21.** The most widely prescribed class of medications:

a. cardiovascular

b. antibiotics

c. antidepressants

d. PPIs

___ **22.** Antibiotics that are effective against a wide range of bacteria:

a. broad spectrum

b. wide spectrum

c. broad range

d. wide range

___ **23.** The prefix "anti-" means

a. before

b. after

c. against

d. normal

___ **24.** The symptoms that Jennifer was being treated for returned in a more severe form after discontinuing the medication. She may have experienced

a. reuptake

b. a drug–drug interaction

c. a plateau

d. a rebound affect

___ **25.** The oldest class or generation of antidepressants:

a. MAOI

b. SSRI

c. benzos

d. tricyclic

___ **26.** ACE inhibitors commonly end in

a. "olol"

b. "pril"

c. "ipine"

d. "mycin"

___ **27.** Guaifenesin promotes coughing. It is an

a. expectorant

b. antitussive

c. antihistamine

d. acute bronchodilator

___ **28.** Antianxiety medications may also be referred to as

a. antipsychotics

b. stimulants

c. anxiolytics

d. antidepressants

___ **29.** What is the generic of Aricept?

a. rivastigmine

b. galantamine

c. donepezil

d. olanzapine

___ **30.** Acetaminophen:

a. ASA

c. NSAID

b. APAP

d. ACE

___ **31.** The maximum dose of acetaminophen within a 24-hour period is

a. 4000 g

c. 4 mg

b. 4000 mg

d. 400 g

___ **32.** Cati was prescribed methylphenidate. What might her diagnosis be?

a. CHF

c. diarrhea

b. ADHD

d. rheumatoid arthritis

___ **33.** IBU is an antipyretic; helping to

a. relieve constipation

c. reduce fever

b. fight bacteria

d. relieve heartburn

___ **34.** NSAIDs help

a. eliminate headaches

c. cure irregular heart beat

b. sleeplessness

d. reduce inflammation

___ **35.** What drug class treats nausea and vomiting?

a. PPIs

c. laxatives

b. antiemetics

d. corticosteriods

___ **36.** Which medication was Emma prescribed to help with her stiff neck?

a. cyclobenzaprine

c. meclizine

b. metformin

d. warfarin

___ **37.** Which IV medication helps with nausea?

a. Zantac (ranitidine)

c. Zofran (ondansetron)

b. Zovirax (acyclovir)

d. Zosyn (piperacillin/tazobactam)

___ **38.** Radiopharmaceuticals are medications

a. used to diagnose

c. that are high in demand and short in supply

b. that have not yet been FDA approved

d. used to treat alopecia

___ **39.** Enrollment in distribution programs and special guidelines must be followed to dispense

a. radiopharmaceuticals

c. reproductive therapy drugs

b. restricted drugs

d. hazardous drugs

___ **40.** These tablets should not be split:

a. scored tablets

c. large tablets

b. time release tablets

d. expensive tablets

ANSWER SECTION

1. C

2. A

3. B

4. C

5. B

6. A

7. B

8. B

9. C

10. D

11. B

12. A

13. A

14. C

15. A

16. B

17. C

18. D

19. C

20. C

21. A

22. A

23. C

24. D

25. D

26. B

27. A

28. C

29. C

30. B

31. B

32. B

33. C

34. D

35. B

36. A

37. C

38. A

39. B

40. B

TASK SHEET

TOPIC TO REVIEW: ABBREVIATIONS

Materials

Pharmacy Technician Exam Review Guide

JB Test Prep: Pharmacy Technician Exam Review Guide

Prepare

1. Read about abbreviations.
2. Take practice test at the end of the chapter.

Study Plan

1. Read pages_____ on _____(date).
2. Make flash cards using quizlet.com.
3. Take end of chapter practice test on_____(date).
4. Ask a coworker to help you review abbreviations.

Tips

1. Study only the abbreviations you're not familiar with.
2. Ask coworkers or classmates how they remember an abbreviation. Hearing their way of remembering may help you.

End of Chapter

List what you need to review.

Abbreviations

OBJECTIVES/TOPICS TO COVER:

- ✓ Know common abbreviations used in pharmacy practice.
- ✓ Recognize error prone abbreviations.

WHERE DO PHARMACY ABBREVIATIONS ORIGINATE?

Terminology in pharmacy and medicine comes from the Latin and Greek languages. Because pharmacy began in Europe, most abbreviations have their origins in a foreign language. Latin and Greek serve as the universal language that all medical personnel can understand. Sometimes knowing the origin of a word or an abbreviation can help a person to remember it.

For example, the *D* and *S* used in abbreviations such as OD and OS, come from the Latin words *dexter* (right) and *sinister* (left). The right side was once associated with skill, as reflected in the word *dexterous*. In contrast, the left side was associated with evil, such as in the word *sinister*. OD is the abbreviation for right eye. OS is the abbreviation for left eye. Remember the "O" is ophthalmic, which is the eye.

INTERPRETING DOCTORS' ORDERS

It is very important for the pharmacy staff to interpret doctors' orders correctly. When writing out the various abbreviations, be sure to write as neatly as possible because other technicians and pharmacists will be reading your handwriting.

In a sense, pharmacy has a language of its own. Abbreviations and acronyms are commonly used to speed up the process of dispensing a drug to the patient. They are also used to help alleviate interpretation errors. For instance, PO is a common pharmacy abbreviation that means by mouth. PO is derived from *per os*; *per* meaning "by" and *os* meaning "mouth" in Latin. A prescriber saves time in writing a script using PO rather than writing out "by mouth." At the pharmacy, there is less chance for error in interpreting the prescriber's handwriting in deciphering PO over the written "by mouth."

A word of caution: some abbreviations may be misinterpreted and actually lead to transcribing errors. QOD is the abbreviation for every other day. QOD has been deciphered as QID, which is four times a day. You can see how it would be easy for the technician to misinterpret a physician's handwriting of QOD versus QID. Be careful when interpreting the abbreviations to make sure the abbreviation makes sense with the rest of the prescribing orders. Read the complete order—in its entirety—before entering information into the computer. Be certain the order makes sense: Does the prescribed strength make sense for the age of the patient? Does the quantity prescribed and length of therapy make sense? How many times a day is the patient ordered to take the medication? Does it coincide with normal prescribing for that medication?

Technicians must learn abbreviations and acronyms to be successful in deciphering prescription orders (see **Tables 6-1** and **6-2**).

Table 6-1 List of Acronyms

ACA	Affordable Care Act
ACD	automated compounding device
ACE	angiotensin converting enzyme
ASA	aspirin
ATC	around the clock
BS	blood sugar
BSC	biological safety cabinet
BSA	body surface area
BUD	beyond use date
CAD	controlled analgesia device
CCB	calcium channel blocker
CEU	continuing education unit
CMS	Centers for Medicare and Medicaid Services
CNS	central nervous system
CSP	compounded sterile product
DAW	dispense as written
DEA	Drug Enforcement Agency
DME	durable medical equipment
DMEPOS	durable medical equipment, prosthetics, orthotics, and supplies
DUR	drug utilization review
EC	enteric coated
EHR	electronic health record
EOB	explanation of benefits
*e*Prescribing	electronic prescriptions
FDA	Food and Drug Administration
GMP	good manufacturing procedure
HCR	health care reform
HCTZ	hydrochlorothiazide
HEPA	high efficiency particulate air
HIPAA	Health Insurance Portability and Accountability Act
HME	home medical equipment

Table 6-1 (Continued)

HRT	hormone replacement therapy
IBU	ibuprofen
ID	intradermal; into the dermal layer of the skin
IM	intramuscular; injection into the muscle tissue
IND	Investigational New Drug
IT	intrathecal; into the space around the spinal cord
IU	international unit
IV	intravenous
IVP	intravenous push
IVPB	intravenous piggy back
LAWB	laminar airflow workbench
LTCF	long-term care facility
LR	lactated ringers
MAC	maximum allowable cost
MAOI	*monoamine oxidase inhibitor*
MDI	metered dose inhaler
MMA	Medicare Modernization Act
MOM	milk of magnesia
MSDS	material safety data sheets
NKA	no known Allergies
NKDA	no known drug allergies
NPI	National Provider Identifier
NTG	nitroglycerin
NSAID	nonsteroidal anti-inflammatory drug
OTC	over the counter
PA	prior authorization
PBM	Pharmacy Benefits Management
PCA	patient controlled analgesia
PDP	prescription drug plan
PHI	protected health information
PPE	personal protective equipment
PPI	patient package insert
RFID	radio frequency identification
RTS	return to stock

(continues)

Table 6-1 (Continued)

SLCPs	scheduled listed chemical products
SNF	skilled nursing facilities
SOP	standard operating procedures
SWI	sterile water for injection
TI	therapeutic index
TCA	tricyclic antidepressant
TPN	total parenteral nutrition
TrOOP	*true out of* pocket (expenses)
U	unit
U&C	usual and customary
UCM	universal claim form
USP	United States Pharmacopeia

Table 6-2 Abbreviations

a	before
$\overline{p}$	after
$\overline{aa}$	of each
$\overline{c}$	with
$\overline{s}$	without
ac	before meals
pc	after meals
pp	after meals (postprandial)
am	morning
pm	afternoon
ad	right ear
as	left ear
au	both ears
APAP	acetaminophen
od	right eye
os	left eye
ou	both eyes
ad	up to
ad lib	as desired
amp	ampule
amt	amount

Table 6-2 (Continued)

bid	twice a day
q	every
QID	four times a day
qd	every day
QOD	every other day—should avoid using; is mixed up with QID
TID	three times a day
bm	bowel movement
C	centigrade
F	Fahrenheit
T	temperature
c	cup
Ca	calcium
Cl	chlorine
Fe	iron
HCl	hydrochloric acid
Mg	magnesium
Na	sodium
NaCl	sodium chloride
K	potassium
KCl	potassium chloride
SO_4	sulfate
$MgSO_4$	magnesium sulfate
MSO_4	morphine sulfate
$FeSO_4$	ferrous sulfate (iron)
PB	phenobarbital
PCN	penicillin
TCN	tetracycline
cc	cubic centimeter
cap	capsule
cm	centimeter
c/o	complaint of
d/c	discharge or discontinue; read the entire order to decipher correct usage
r/o	rule out
comp	compound

(continues)

Table 6-2 (Continued)

D	dextrose (glucose)
D5W	5% dextrose and water
dict	as directed
disp	dispense
dig	digoxin
dx	diagnosis
hx	history
dr	dram; see symbol in **Table 6-3**
ETOH	alcohol
exp	expired
fl	fluid
g	gram
gr	grain
gtt	drop
h	hour
hs	bedtime (hour of sleep)
HA	headache
kcal	kilocalorie
kg	kilogram
L	liter
mL	milliliter
mcg	microgram
mEq	milliequivalent
mg	milligram
mg/kg	milligram of medication needed per kilogram of body weight
lb	pound
gal	gallon
oz	ounce; see symbol in Table 6-3
Tbsp	tablespoonful
tsp	teaspoonful
NS	normal saline (0.9% sodium chloride)
MVI	multivitamin
noc	into the night/darkness; nocturnal
NPO	nothing by mouth; not per os (mouth)
PO	by mouth; per os (mouth)

Table 6-2 (Continued)

oint or ung	ointment
per	by
pr or Ⓡ	rectally; per rectum
PRN	whenever necessary, as needed
pt	patient
pulv	powder
qs	quantity sufficient
qty	quantity
Rx, Script	prescription
Sig, S, Signa	label with directions for use
Susp	suspension
SQ or sc	subcutaneous
sl	sublingual (under the tongue)
STAT	immediately
supp	suppository
syr	syrup
tab	tablet
ud	as directed
vag	vaginal
VO	verbal order
vol	volume
wa	while awake
x	times

Table 6-3 Symbols

♏	minim
ℨ	dram
℈	scruple
Δ	change
℥	ounce
<	less than
>	greater than
= or ::	equal
↑	increase
↓	decrease

This is your checklist to make sure you understand what you need to know for the certification exam. Review chapter content if there is a topic you're uncertain of.
I know:

√	...abbreviations used in pharmacy practice.
	...the importance of correctly interpreting/transcribing prescriber orders.
	...common abbreviation mix-ups.

RESOURCES

1. Hamilton RJ. *Tarascon Pocket Pharmacopoeia*. Burlington, MA: Jones & Bartlett Learning; 2010.
2. Hopper T. *Mosby's Pharmacy Technician: Principles and Practice*. St. Louis, MO: Elsevier Saunders; 2007.
3. Yap D. DEA grants prescriber numbers to certain Massachusetts pharmacists [online article]. Washington, DC: American Pharmacist Association. Available at: http://www.pharmacist.com/AM/Template.cfm?Section=Pharmacy_News&template=/CM/HTMLDisplay.cfm&ContentID=25693. Accessed March 23, 2011.

CHAPTER 6

MULTIPLE CHOICE

Identify the choice that best completes the statement or answers the question.

_____ **1.** The abbreviation for aspirin:

a. ASP

b. A

c. APAP

d. ASA

_____ **2.** The pharmacists asks you to update the patient's EHR. You should update the patient's

a. heart rate readings

b. explanation of health-related items

c. hormone replacement therapy

d. electronic healthcare record

_____ **3.** HIPAA stands for

a. Health Information Portability and Accountability Act

b. Health Insurance Portability and Accountability Act

c. Health Information Privacy and Accountability

d. Health Insurance Payments and Accounts Act

_____ **4.** The patient has no known drug allergies. How is this information abbreviated?

a. KNA

b. No All

c. NKDA

d. NDA

_____ **5.** Transcribe: i tab APAP po qd prn HA

a. Take one tablet of aspirin by mouth every day as needed for headache

b. Take one tablet of acetaminophen by mouth every day as needed for headache

c. Take one tablet of acetaminophen by mouth every day for headache

d. Take one tablet of aspirin by mouth every day after meals for headache

_____ **6.** Translate: ii gtts os bid

a. Place two drops in both eyes twice daily

b. Place two drops in the left ear twice daily

c. Place two drops in the right eye twice daily

d. Place two drops in the left eye twice daily

_____ **7.** The prescription calls for 60 gr. You should fill the prescription for

a. 60 grains

b. 60 grams

c. 60 tablets

d. 60 ounces

_____ **8.** The order is for 10 mg/kg. This means

a. 10 milligrams of medication not to exceed 1 kilogram

b. 10 milligrams of medications needed per kilogram of body weight

c. 10 micrograms of medication per every kilogram the patient weighs

d. 10 milligrams of medication per 10 kilograms of body weight

_____ **9.** Translate: antibiotic ung this noc

a. Take one antibiotic lozenge this evening

b. Apply ointment to affected area

c. Apply antibiotic ointment to affected area this evening

d. Place antibiotic under the tongue in the evening

_____ **10.** Pharmacy abbreviations originate from the _____ and _____ language.

a. Latin and English

b. English and Greek

c. Latin and Greek

d. English and Spanish

ANSWER SECTION

1. D
2. D
3. B
4. C
5. B
6. D
7. A
8. B
9. C
10. C

TASK SHEET

TOPIC TO REVIEW: PHARMACY REGULATIONS

Materials

Pharmacy Technician Exam Review Guide

JB Test Prep: Pharmacy Technician Exam Review Guide

Prepare

1. Read section on federal pharmacy regulations.
2. Take practice test at the end of the chapter.

Study Plan

1. Read pages_____ on _____(date).
2. Take end-of-chapter practice test on_____(date).

Tips

Remembering the dates of the different acts and amendments isn't as important as remembering what changes the new law brought about. Concentrate on how the act or amendment influenced pharmacy rather than on the date.

End of Chapter

List what you need to review.

Federal Pharmacy Regulation and Law

OBJECTIVES/TOPICS TO COVER:

Recall the following regulations pertinent to pharmacy practice:

- ✓ Pure Food and Drug Act
- ✓ Food, Drug, and Cosmetic Act
- ✓ Durham-Humphrey Amendment
- ✓ Kefauver-Harris Amendment
- ✓ OBRA
- ✓ Prescription Drug Marketing Act
- ✓ U.S. Troop Readiness, Veterans' Care, Katrina Recovery, and Iraq Accountability Appropriations Act of 2007
- ✓ FDA Modernization Act
- ✓ HIPAA
- ✓ Controlled Substance Act

- ✓ REMS
- ✓ Poison Prevention Packaging Act (PPPA)
- ✓ Drug Price Competition and Patent-Term Restoration Act
- ✓ Orphan Drug Act
- ✓ Medicare Modernization Act (MMA)
- ✓ Dietary Supplement Health and Education Act (DSHEA)
- ✓ Affordable Care Act
- ✓ Prescribing Authority
- ✓ Respondeat Superior
- ✓ Standard of Care

HISTORY OF PHARMACY LAW

Federal laws relating to the practice of pharmacy were first enacted in the late 1800s. Federal laws were passed to protect the public from unsafe vaccinations and to require vaccinations. The smallpox vaccination, discovered by Edward Jenner in 1796, is the first vaccination on record. With inoculation, a sharp decline in smallpox cases was noted, and the deadly epidemic was gone. However, citizens stopped getting the vaccination, and smallpox attacks returned in different parts of the country. In 1809, Massachusetts was the first state to make it mandatory for citizens to receive the vaccination.

Prior to federal pharmacy laws, each state had its own laws that protected interstate businesses. State Boards of Pharmacy were formed as early as the mid to late 1800s.

A book entitled *The Jungle* by Upton Sinclair actually brought the Food and Drug Administration (FDA) into existence. Sinclair worked undercover in meatpacking plants in Chicago. He wrote about the unhealthy food-handling processes at the plants. In reading Sinclair's findings, the public became concerned and somewhat enraged, which brought about legislation to mandate food processing.

Following legislation brought forth by *The Jungle*, the Scientific Bureau was formed. A group of volunteers called the Poison Squad made up part of the Scientific Bureau. Members of the Poison Squad ingested acids and other poisons to test their effects. In 1906, the Scientific Bureau was transformed into the FDA.

Pharmacy laws exist to protect the public. Most often some type of tragedy preceded the making of these laws, just as Ohio's Emily's Law was preceded by the death of a young girl due to a medication error.

The FDA, the Drug Enforcement Agency (DEA), and State Boards of Pharmacy mandate and regulate pharmacy laws.

This chapter will brief you on the laws affecting pharmacy practice, starting with historical laws up to recent laws.

Pure Food and Drug Act

The Pure Food and Drug Act revolutionized labeling. Up to this point, consumers had no way of knowing the quality of the product. Extravagant and boastful claims were made about medication products: "Fast Growing Hair Tonic," "Cures Sea Sickness." Although the Pure Food and Drug Act did not require labels to list ingredients, the law prohibited misbranded and adulterated drugs. The label could not contain false information about the purity and strength of the product.

- ✓ 1906
- ✓ Sanctioned drug standards
- ✓ Revolutionized drug labeling

Sherley Amendment

While an *act* is a new law, an *amendment* is a change to a current law (act). The Sherley Amendment made an addition to the Pure Food and Drug Act to outlaw labeling medications with fake medical claims meant to trick the buyer.

- ✓ 1912

Food, Drug, and Cosmetic Act

Prior to the Food, Drug, and Cosmetic Act, a medication may have had addictive and dangerous ingredients, but consumers had no way of knowing this. This law brought about premarket safety approval for all new drugs and mandated drug labeling with adequate directions for safe use. The turning point for issuing the Food, Drug, and Cosmetic Act was the elixir sulfanilamide disaster in which the elixir used as an antibiotic contained a poisonous chemical commonly known today as antifreeze and subsequently caused many deaths.

Food, drugs, and cosmetics were also defined in this law. A *drug* was defined as a substance used in diagnosis, cure, treatment, or prevention of disease. A *cosmetic* was defined as a substance applied externally to the human body to cleanse, to beautify, or to affect appearance. A *food* was defined as any substance used for food and drink by man or by animals.

- ✓ 1938
- ✓ Premarket safety approval of all new drugs
- ✓ Drugs labeled with directions for use

Durham-Humphrey Amendment

The Durham-Humphrey Amendment was a change to the Food, Drug, and Cosmetic Act. It amended, or changed, the act to establish two drug classes: nonprescription (over the counter) and prescription drugs. For that reason, the Durham-Humphrey Amendment is also called the Prescription Drug Amendment. The prescription drug class was created for drugs that cannot be used safely without medical supervision.

This amendment also required prescription drugs to bear the phrase, or legend, "Caution: Federal Law Prohibits Dispensing Without Prescription." This is why prescription drugs are also known as *legend drugs*.

Many pharmacy laws are named after either the legislators who worked to pass the law or the individual who suffered the tragedy to make the law possible. The Durham-Humphrey Amendment is named after former vice president Hubert H. Humphrey Jr., who was a pharmacist in South Dakota before beginning his political career. Carl Durham was a pharmacist who represented North Carolina in the House of Representatives.

✓ 1951
✓ Also called Prescription Drug Amendment
✓ Required Rx legend: "Caution: Federal Law Prohibits Dispensing Without Prescription"
✓ Created prescription and nonprescription classes

Kefauver-Harris Amendment

The Kefauver-Harris Amendment was the most significant change to the Food, Drug, and Cosmetic Act. It mandated that drugs must not only be safe but must also be effective. This amendment made new medication approval much stricter in the United States. Before the passage of this amendment, bottled water, a safe product, could be marketed as a medication. Now the manufacturer has to prove that the bottled water is also effective.

The thalidomide tragedy is what brought about the Kefauver-Harris Amendment. Thalidomide was a sedative sold over the counter in Europe. American soldiers returning from World War II active duty in Europe brought home thalidomide. Their pregnant wives took the pill to help ease morning sickness; however, babies were born with severe birth defects.

The Kefauver-Harris Amendment, also called the Drug Efficacy Amendment, emphasized that drugs must be effective. The new law was made retroactive to all drugs marketed between 1938 and 1961. U.S. Senator Estes Kefauver and U.S. Representative Oren Harris were instrumental in passing the law.

✓ 1962
✓ Also called Drug Efficacy Amendment
✓ Drugs must be effective
✓ FDA regulates prescription drug advertising

Fair Packaging and Labeling Act

This act required all consumer products to be honestly and informatively labeled. The label must identify the medication product, the total quantity, and the manufacturer.

✓ 1966

Controlled Substance Act

The Controlled Substance Act (CSA), also known as the Comprehensive Drug Abuse Prevention and Control Act, regulates manufacturing, distributing, and dispensing of controlled medications. This act created a new class of prescription drugs and scheduled the drugs according to potential for abuse.

Whenever a law is created, there must be a way to enforce and regulate the law. The Drug Enforcement Agency (DEA) was formed under the Department of Justice to help regulate the Controlled Substance Act.

✓ 1971
✓ Regulates manufacturing, distributing, and dispensing of controlled medications

✓ DEA formed
✓ Abusable drugs classified according to a schedule

Poison Prevention Packaging Act

The Poison Prevention Packaging Act (PPPA) requires child-resistant and adult-friendly packaging of oral medications. Child-resistant packaging is defined as difficult for 80% of children younger than 5 years of age to open and yet 90% of adults can open the medication packaging. The law is written to protect young children from accidental ingestion and poisoning from medications and household chemicals by creating a barrier to the poisonous product.

Oral medication vials dispensed from the pharmacy directly to the customer must have safety (childproof) lids unless a documented request from the customer for easy-open lids is on file at the pharmacy. There are some exceptions to the child-resistant packaging law. Some medications that are permitted to be dispensed in conventional packaging are sublingual nitroglycerin, sublingual and chewable isosorbide (in limited strength), oral contraceptives in memory-aid packaging, and certain dosage forms and strengths of potassium supplements.

✓ 1970
✓ Child-resistant packaging

Orphan Drug Act

The Orphan Drug Act allowed drug companies to bypass lengthy time requirements for testing new drugs if the drug is intended for a rare disease. This provided an incentive to promote research for rare disease therapy that may have otherwise been overlooked because of budget reasons. Eventual drug sales for a medication used to treat a rare disease may not recoup the high cost of research and development. The Orphan Drug Act helped make rare disease drug research and development more feasible for drug manufacturer companies.

✓ 1983
✓ Manufacturer incentive for medication used to treat rare disease

Drug Price Competition and Patent Term Restoration Act

The Drug Price Competition and Patent Term Restoration Act, also called the Hatch-Waxman Act, was an attempt to resolve a dispute between generic drug and brand-name drug manufacturers. Prior to this act, generic drug manufacturers had to go through the same lengthy approval process as brand-name manufacturers. The act increased the availability of generic drugs by allowing the FDA to approve generic drugs without generic manufacturers repeating safety and effectiveness research that the brand-name drugs had already undergone.

This new law didn't sit well with brand-name manufacturers that were footing the bill for safety and effectiveness research. To be fair to the brand name manufacturers this act allotted the brand-name manufacturers an additional 5-year patent protection for brand-name medications. The extra 5-year patent protection helped manufacturers recoup development costs.

U.S. Senator Orrin Hatch and U.S. Representative Henry A. Waxman were instrumental in passing this act.

✓ 1984
✓ Also called Hatch-Waxman Act
✓ Increased availability of generic drugs

Prescription Drug Marketing Act

The Prescription Drug Marketing Act placed more stringent controls on prescription drug distribution. Retail pharmacies are no longer able to stock drug samples received from a pharmaceutical company's drug representative. Samples cannot be sold or traded. Most often hospitals purchase drugs at a discounted price. According to the act, hospitals cannot sell drugs to other pharmacies. The act was passed to increase buying and selling safety to ensure that drug products purchased by consumers are safe and effective and to avoid the risk of selling counterfeit or expired drugs.

✓ 1987
✓ Increase safety in drug distribution

Omnibus Budget Reconciliation Act

The Omnibus Budget Reconciliation Act is commonly called OBRA. This is important legislation for pharmacy technicians as the passing of this act brought about a higher demand for technicians and increased job opportunities.

President Ronald Reagan wanted to reduce government spending. He looked at ways to reduce astronomical healthcare costs. Through OBRA, the government hoped to save healthcare costs associated with Medicaid patients. To get government reimbursement for Medicaid claims, the pharmacist had to perform a drug utilization review (DUR) on the patient as well as offer counseling to Medicaid patients who receive new medication. Counseling and DUR were believed to save the government money on possible therapeutic duplication, drug–drug interactions, wrong dose of medication, incorrect length of therapy, clinical abuse or misuse, or drug–disease contraindications.

Patient counseling and DUR take up a large chunk of the pharmacists' time, leaving a gap in other pharmacy services. The pharmacy technician is able to perform duties that the pharmacist once did, which allows the pharmacist time to counsel and perform DUR.

✓ 1990
✓ Must offer counseling to patients who receive new medications
✓ DUR

Dietary Supplement Health and Education Act

Under the Dietary Supplement Health and Education Act (DSHEA), the dietary supplement manufacturer, not the FDA, ensures that a dietary supplement is safe before it is marketed. The FDA takes action against any unsafe dietary supplement only after the product reaches the market.

This act defines a dietary supplement as a product taken by mouth that contains a "dietary ingredient" intended to supplement the diet. The ingredient may be vitamins, minerals, herbs, or other botanicals.

✓ 1994
✓ Provides guidelines and definitions of supplements

Health Insurance Portability and Accountability Act

The Health Insurance Portability and Accountability Act (HIPAA) was passed in 1996 and took effect in April 2003. The ruling gave covered entities (pharmacies and other healthcare providers) time to comply with the new privacy regulations. The act was created to ensure the privacy of individuals' protected health information (PHI). Pharmacies and other healthcare providers are now accountable, by law, to keep patient information confidential.

Portability means keeping the electronic interchange of healthcare information secure. In general, the pharmacy must have safeguards in place to ensure the confidentiality, integrity, and availability of all electronic PHI they create, receive, maintain, or transmit. Covered entities had until April 2005 to comply with the security rulings of HIPAA.

The pharmacy must have a HIPAA compliance officer who will help to ensure that individually identifiable health information is protected. Individually identifiable health information includes data:

1. That relates to the individual's past, present, or future physical or mental health or condition
2. That can be used to identify the individual

Examples of common identifiers of an individuals' health information are the patient's name, address, date of birth, and social security number.

All employees must receive HIPAA training.

✓ Signed 1996; compliant 2003 and 2005
✓ Protects confidentiality of patient (PHI)
✓ Patients are given a notice of their individual rights
✓ Security of electronic healthcare information

FDA Modernization Act

The FDA Modernization Act (FDMA) touched every aspect of FDA activities in an attempt to update regulations. Provisions were made for medical devices. The act encouraged drug manufacturers to conduct research for new uses of drugs. Clarifications of extemporaneous compounding were made, and the prescription drug legend that previously read "Caution: Federal Law Prohibits Dispensing Without a Prescription" was replaced with "Rx Only." The act also provided an additional six months of exclusive marketing for manufacturers that develop pediatric medications.

✓ 1997
✓ Improves drug regulations

Drug Addiction Treatment Act

The Drug Addiction Treatment Act authorized office-based treatment for detoxification. Qualifying physicians may prescribe Suboxone and Subutex, which were the first medications approved for office-based treatment of opioid dependence. Prior to the passage of this law, it was illegal for a doctor to prescribe narcotic drugs to treat narcotic dependence. This treatment could only be provided at specially registered clinics. Physicians may also prescribe CIII-CV opioids for detox treatment. Nonqualifying physicians may write detoxification scripts but for no more than a one-day supply of methadone.

✓ 2000
✓ Qualifying physicians may prescribe for office-based treatment:
  ○ buprenorphine (Subutex)
  ○ buprenorphone-naloxone (Suboxone)
✓ Physicians who prescribe detox meds DEA number begins with an "X"

The Best Pharmaceuticals for Children Act

There is inadequate understanding of dosing and safety in most medications used in children, because medications are dosed and labeled for adults. The Best Pharmaceuticals for Children Act gives incentives to study and develop children's medications.

✓ 2002
✓ Study and develop children's medications

Medicare Prescription Drug, Improvement, and Modernization Act

To modernize the Medicare program, prescription drug coverage was made available to Medicare beneficiaries. The Bush administration brought this act forward to help lower healthcare expenses and to improve on the checks-and-balance systems already in place.

✓ 2003
✓ Commonly called the Medicare Modernization Act (MMA)
✓ Makes prescription drug coverage available to patients eligible for Medicare benefits

The Combat Methamphetamine Epidemic Act

This act bans over-the-counter sales of medicines that contain pseudoephedrine and ephedrine, ingredients commonly used to make methamphetamine. The amount of pseudoephedrine and ephedrine that an individual can purchase each day and each month is limited. Purchasers are required to present photo identification, and the pharmacy must maintain purchasing records for at least 2 years.

- ✓ 2005
- ✓ Pharmacies required to keep a logbook of sales (some states require an electronic log book)
- ✓ Products containing ephedrine and pseudoephedrine must be stored either behind the counter or in a locked cabinet
- ✓ Limited quantities may be purchased

U.S. Troop Readiness, Veterans' Care, Katrina Recovery, and Iraq Accountability Appropriations Act of 2007

At a time of national warfare and tragedy, the government looked for a way to funnel money to help war victims and to fund the war. In 2003, Medicare and Medicaid government expenditures were more than $435 billion. In 2002, there were $1.8 billion in judgments and settlements for Medicare fraud. Healthcare costs were, again, at an all-time high, and the government made plans to work to decrease fraudulent activities that lead to high healthcare costs.

Physicians were mandated to use tamper-resistant prescription pads to receive Medicaid reimbursement. Tamper-resistant prescription pads prevent unauthorized copying of a completed or blank prescription pad and prevent the use of counterfeit prescription forms. Tamper-resistant prescription pad requirements include a security watermark on the pad's reverse side, use of tamper-resistant ink, and sequentially numbered blanks or duplicate/triplicate copies.

- ✓ Effective 2008
- ✓ Tamper-resistant prescription pads

Food and Drug Administration Amendments Act

This Food and Drug Administration Amendment Act (FDAAA) changed the Food, Drug, and Cosmetic Act. It requires the FDA to publish a list of all authorized generic drugs on the FDA internet site. The generic listing must include the brand name, the manufacturer of trade name drug, and the date the generic entered the market. The act also requires a Risk Evaluation and Mitigation Strategy (REMS) from manufacturers to ensure that the benefits of a drug outweigh its risks. REMS, in part, is intended to minimize the risk of misuse, abuse, addiction, and overdose of controlled drugs. Some diabetic medications require both the prescribers and the patients to enroll in an REMS program prior to the patient receiving the medications.

- ✓ Signed into public law on 2007
- ✓ REMS

American Recovery and Reinvestment Act

The American Recovery and Reinvestment Act promotes meaningful use of electronic healthcare records technology. Electronic prescriptions, or e-prescribing, is not made mandatory for government reimbursement, but updating health information technology is encouraged. There is a financial incentive through Medicare for physicians who e-prescribe.

- ✓ 2009
- ✓ Commonly referred to as Stimulus Act

Online Pharmacy Consumer Protection Act

The Online Pharmacy Consumer Protection Act, also known as the Ryan Haight Act, addresses problems of online prescription drug trafficking, abuse, and availability. Signed into law by President Bush, this law provides for tough penalties and stronger enforcement against dishonest websites.

The act amends the Controlled Substances Act to prohibit the delivery, distribution, or dispensing of controlled substances over the internet without a valid prescription. The law defines a valid prescription as a prescription issued for a legitimate purpose by a practitioner who has conducted at least one in-person medical evaluation of the patient. The act also requires an online pharmacy:

1. To display on its internet homepage a statement that it complies with the requirements of this act
2. To comply with state laws for the licensure of pharmacies in each state in which it operates or sells controlled substances
3. To post on its internet homepage specified information, including the name, address, and telephone number of the pharmacy, the qualifications of its pharmacist-in-charge, and a certification of its registration under this act
4. To notify the attorney general and applicable State Boards of Pharmacy at least 30 days prior to offering to sell, deliver, distribute, or dispense controlled substances over the internet.

18-year-old Ryan Haight died of an overdose of Vicodin obtained from an internet pharmacy. He told the internet pharmacy that he was a 25-year-old with chronic back pain. His father, a physician, and his mother, a registered nurse, worked to help pass this Act.

✓ 2007
✓ Also called the Ryan Haight Act
✓ Defines valid prescription
✓ Regulations for online pharmacies

Biologics Price Competition and Innovation Act

Part of the Affordable Care Act, the Biologics Price Competition and Innovation Act allows for a quicker approval process for generic copies that are highly similar or interchangeable with biologic medications already approved by the FDA and on the market. Biologics are certain types of medicine such as vaccines and blood components. This act also permits biologic brand manufacturers and innovators 12 years of market exclusivity after FDA approval.

✓ 2009
✓ Improves access to medication therapies

Affordable Care Act

The Affordable Care Act is a healthcare law designed to improve our current healthcare system by increasing access to healthcare coverage. This act is a work in progress with insurance coverage changes scheduled to take place in the future. Some changes that have already been implemented are the ability of Medicare beneficiaries, as well as private insurance participants, to get preventative services at no cost, Medicare Part D donut hole discounts, and insurance coverage for uninsured adults with preexisting conditions. Through this act young adults are able to stay on their parent's insurance plan until they turn 26 years of age.

✓ Increases access to affordable healthcare
✓ 2010

Other Legislation and Achievements

- ✓ Occupational Safety and Health Administration (OSHA) ensures safety of workers in the workplace. Exit signs and personal protective equipment are examples of how OSHA works for the safety and protection of the employee.
- ✓ After seven people died from cyanide-contaminated Tylenol capsules, the government mandated *tamper-resistant packaging* in 1982. Packaging must have an indicator or barrier to entry that, if breached, can provide visible evidence to consumers that tampering has occurred.
- ✓ The Medical Device Amendment of 1976 defined medical devices and classified medical devices based on risk.
- ✓ Compassionate Use Programs help make medications available through accelerated techniques for drug approval and use of investigational drugs.

The FDA continues to offer consumer protection against counterfeit drugs, increased availability of generic drugs, and more informative medication labeling.

PRESCRIBING AUTHORITY

Prescribers are categorized as either top level or midlevel. A top-level prescriber is a physician with the credentialing of a DO or MD, for example. A midlevel prescriber may be a physician assistant (PA) or a nurse practitioner (NP).

Pharmacists generally do not have prescribing authority. However, the DEA has granted registration to pharmacists in seven states: Massachusetts, California, Montana, Washington, North Dakota, North Carolina, and New Mexico. According to the American Pharmacist Association, pharmacists in these seven states who wish to be midlevel prescribers must be part of a program called Collaborative Drug Therapy Management. The midlevel prescribing pharmacist, acting under a physician, may prescribe refills for up to a 30-day supply as well as other prescribing privileges. It is hoped that this movement toward prescribing pharmacists will bridge a gap in medication therapy management (MTM) communications between patient, pharmacist, and physician.

OVERVIEW OF PHARMACY LAWS

Laws are designed to protect the public. *State laws* regulate the practice of pharmacy and dispensing functions while *federal laws* regulate manufacturing and marketing of the drug. States must yield to the federal government if there is a conflicting law between the two. Always follow whichever law (state versus federal) is stricter.

STANDARD OF CARE

The standard of care is the level of performance expected of a healthcare provider in carrying out his or her professional duties. For example, a pharmacy technician who is certified and who has been working in the hospital pharmacy for 25 years will have a higher level of standard of care than a newly hired pharmacy technician with no experience and little education.

A pharmacy technician may be charged with negligence if a patient is injured because the technician failed to perform a reasonable duty. Keep in mind that we are responsible for our actions as well as our failure to act! If in doubt, always remember that our first responsibility is always to provide competent, courteous, and compassionate healthcare to our patients.

RESPONDEAT SUPERIOR

Under this doctrine, pharmacists are liable for employees' acts within the course and scope of employment. *Respondeat superior*, a Latin phrase, translates into "let the master answer."

This is your checklist to make sure you understand what you need to know for the certification exam. Review chapter content if there is a topic you're uncertain of.
I know:

√	...HIPAA rules and regulations regarding patient confidentiality.
	...pharmacy regulations and how to comply.
	...the difference in state and federal pharmacy law and how to comply.
	...which professionals have prescribing authority.

RESOURCES

1. US Department of Health and Human Services. Summary of the HIPPA Privacy Rule. Available at: http://www.hhs.gov/ocr/privacy/hipaa/understanding/summary/. Accessed February 19, 2011.
2. Health Care and You: Understanding the Health Care Law. Available at: http://www.healthcare-andyou.org. Accessed February 2011.
3. Erickson AK. Will medications be safer in the future? *Pharm Today*. 2010;42.
4. US Department of Health and Human Services. US Food and Drug Administration Website. Available at: http://www.fda.gov. Accessed January 2011.

CHAPTER 7

MULTIPLE CHOICE

Identify the choice that best completes the statement or answers the question.

_____ **1.** The act that was the first to revolutionize labeling:

a. Food, Drug, and Cosmetic

b. Pure Food and Drug

c. Durham-Humphrey

d. Fair Packaging and Labeling

_____ **2.** The act that first mandated premarket safety approval:

a. Food, Drug, and Cosmetic

b. Pure Food and Drug

c. Poison Prevention Packaging

d. Durham-Humphrey

_____ **3.** The Prescription Drug Amendment:

a. mandated premarket safety approval for medications

b. mandated easy to read labeling

c. created the IND program

d. created the prescription drug class

_____ **4.** The act that put drug efficacy into place:

a. Food, Drug, and Cosmetic Act

b. Durham-Humphrey Amendment

c. Kefauver-Harris Amendment

d. Fair Packaging and Labeling Act

_____ **5.** The Controlled Substance Act:

a. requires honesty in dispensing medications

b. created the scheduled drug class

c. requires regulation of OTC medications

d. created the prescription drug class

_____ **6.** All medication in vials dispensed directly to the patient must have safety lids unless

a. the patient is older than 65 years of age

c. there is a documented request for easy-open lids on file with the pharmacy

b. the patient has arthritis

d. the medication is a syrup or suspension

_____ **7.** OBRA brought about two important mandates for pharmacists:

a. counseling and DUR

c. adjudication and HIPAA

b. budget restrictions and purchasing options

d. counseling and electronic ordering

_____ **8.** Under HIPAA regulations, pharmacy technicians must

a. offer counseling to patients

c. assist pharmacists in DUR

b. be nationally certified

d. keep patient information confidential

_____ **9.** PHI includes

a. vials and tablet counters

c. personal protective equipment

b. the patient's name and DOB

d. statistical data omitting the patient's name

_____ **10.** The Medicare Modernization Act (MMA) brought about

a. updated pricing for services

c. lower premiums for Medicare beneficiaries

b. prescription drug coverage for Medicare beneficiaries

d. Medicare Part C

_____ **11.** Tamper-resistant prescription pads

a. may help decrease fraud

c. are required for all prescription orders

b. have been replaced with e-Prescribing

d. are mandated through the American Recovery and Reinvestment Act

_____ **12.** Regulations put into place for internet pharmacies selling controlled substances:

a. Ryan Haight Act

c. Controlled Substance Act

b. Emily's Act

d. Compassionate Use Act

ANSWER SECTION

1. B
2. A
3. D
4. C
5. B
6. C
7. A
8. D
9. B
10. B
11. A
12. A

TASK SHEET

TOPIC TO REVIEW: CONTROLLED DRUGS

Materials

Pharmacy Technician Exam Review Guide

JB Test Prep: Pharmacy Technician Exam Review Guide

Prepare

1. Read the section on controlled drugs.
2. Take practice test at the end of the chapter.

Study Plan

1. Read pages_____ on _____(date).
2. Take end of chapter practice test on_____(date).
3. Make flash cards for controlled drugs using http://quizlet.com.
4. Visit the DEA website at http://www.justice.gov/dea.

Tips

1. To help you better understand DEA regulations; find out what filing method your pharmacy uses. Study controlled drugs that you're not familiar with.

End of Chapter

List what you need to review.

Controlled Drugs

OBJECTIVES/TOPICS COVERED:

Name pharmacy procedures required to adhere to the controlled substance laws listed:

- ✓ Controlled Substance Act (CSA)
- ✓ Narcotic Addict Treatment Act
- ✓ Controlled Substance Registrant Protection Act (CSRPA)
- ✓ Valid DEA numbers
- ✓ Security requirements for controlled drugs
- ✓ Theft or loss of controlled drugs
- ✓ Record keeping for controlled drugs
- ✓ Inventory of controlled drugs
- ✓ DEA forms
- ✓ Disposal of controlled drugs
- ✓ Selling pseudoephedrine products

Your role in properly dispensing controlled substances is critical to protecting patient health and safeguarding society against drug abuse and diversion. Diversion of legitimately manufactured controlled substances is a serious problem. Pharmacy technicians can help prevent diversion and control legitimate access to drugs by being aware of various techniques drug abusers and traffickers use to obtain controlled substances.

According to the Drug Enforcement Agency (DEA), look for these warning signs of fraudulent prescription writing:

- ✓ High doses of opioids and benzodiazepines are prescribed for virtually all the patients
- ✓ Drug therapy is not customized for individual patients but instead all patients receive the same therapy
- ✓ Patients live a distance from the pharmacy
- ✓ Most of the patients pay cash rather than use insurance
- ✓ Patients insist on brand-name drugs
- ✓ Prescription is written in different colored inks or different handwriting
- ✓ The patient presents prescriptions written for other people

Pharmacy technicians who are familiar with the regulations of the Controlled Substance Act (CSA) are most successful with compliance.

CONTROLLED SUBSTANCE ACT

The Controlled Substance Act (CSA) came into effect on May 1, 1971. The Controlled Substance Act, also referred to as the Comprehensive Drug Abuse Prevention and Control Act of 1970, was designed to improve the administration and regulation of the manufacture, import or export, and distribution and dispensing of controlled substances. A *closed system* is used to track controlled substances. A closed system enables a controlled drug to be traced from the time it is manufactured to the time it is dispensed.

The DEA was formed to regulate and administer the CSA laws. Before 1970, the DEA was known as the Bureau of Narcotics and Dangerous Drugs.

SUMMARY OF CONTROLLED SUBSTANCES ACT REQUIREMENTS

Every pharmacy that dispenses any controlled substance must be registered with the DEA. Registration is renewed every three years.

Schedule I

These are street drugs. Drugs in this category or schedule have no medicinal value.

Schedule II

- ✓ Pharmacy uses DEA Form 222 to order CII (class II or schedule II) drugs
- ✓ Pharmacy has option to place electronic orders through DEA Controlled Substance Ordering System (CSOS)
- ✓ Drugs are secured in a locked cabinet or dispersed (behind the counter) throughout the pharmacy or another form of secure storage
- ✓ No refills are allowed. A new prescription must be issued
- ✓ Prescriptions must be signed by the prescriber
- ✓ Records of receipt/invoices must be readily retrievable
- ✓ DEA Form 106 is filed to report theft or significant loss
- ✓ Report theft or significant loss immediately to local law enforcement

Schedule III and Schedule IV

- ✓ Records of receipt/invoices must be readily retrievable
- ✓ Prescriptions may be written, electronic, phoned in, or faxed
- ✓ May be refilled up to five times within six months after the date of issue. After five refills or after six months, whichever occurs first, a new prescription is required
- ✓ When refilled the following must be entered on the back of the hard copy:
    - ○ Dispensing pharmacist's initials
    - ○ Date refilled
    - ○ Amount of drug dispensed on refill
- ✓ Fax is considered a hard copy
- ✓ May be called into the pharmacy
- ✓ May be transferred to another pharmacy.
- ✓ Drugs are secured in a locked cabinet or dispersed (behind the counter) throughout the pharmacy or another form of secure storage
- ✓ DEA Form 106 is filed to report theft or significant loss

Schedule V

- ✓ Records of receipt/invoices must be readily retrievable
- ✓ Refills only as authorized by the prescriber (if a prescription is issued)
- ✓ Drugs are secured in a locked cabinet or dispersed (behind the counter) throughout the pharmacy or another form of secure storage

✓ DEA Form 106 is filed to report theft or significant loss
✓ Some schedule V products may be purchased without a prescription by signing a logbook
✓ Fax is considered a hard copy
✓ May be called into the pharmacy
✓ May be transferred to another pharmacy

Note: Certain laws apply to computerized record keeping of controlled drugs.

The 2004 DEA *Pharmacist's Manual* gave three different options for pharmacies to use in filing prescriptions. One option has been excluded from the 2010 revised *Pharmacist's Manual*. Acceptable options for filing prescription records follow:

Option 1—Three separate files, including
  ○ a file for schedule II controlled substances dispensed
  ○ a file for schedules III, IV, and V controlled substances dispensed
  ○ a file for all noncontrolled drugs dispensed

Option 2—Two separate files, including
  ○ a file for all schedule II controlled substances dispensed
  ○ a file for all other drugs dispensed (noncontrolled and schedules III, IV, and V)

Schedule prescriptions must be readily retrievable by using a red "C" stamp.

Note: All records must be maintained for two years, unless state law requires a longer period. Electronic record-keeping systems have the red "C" requirement waived.

PRESCRIPTION REQUIREMENTS

A prescription for a controlled substance must include the following information:

✓ Date issued
✓ Patient's name and address
✓ Prescriber's name, address, and DEA registration number
✓ Drug name
✓ Drug strength
✓ Dosage form
✓ Quantity prescribed
✓ Directions for use
✓ Number of refills (if any) authorized
✓ Manual signature of prescriber

The controlled substance prescription must be written in ink or indelible pencil or typewritten. The pharmacy must not alter the patient's name, prescribed drug, or prescriber's signature on the hard copy. The pharmacist can correct or insert missing dosage form, strength, directions, issue date, and quantity after consulting with the prescriber.

EMERGENCY DISPENSING

At times, a prescriber will phone in a verbal order or fax in an emergency prescription order for a patient needing CII medication. Most often, the emergency order will come in after office hours or on a weekend when the patient needs urgent pain therapy. In these special emergency cases, the CII drug dispensed must be limited to the amount needed to treat the patient during the emergency period, not to exceed a 72-hour time period.

Normally, a written hard copy or an electronic prescription must be received at the pharmacy to dispense a CII drug to the patient. When an emergency CII telephone order comes in, the pharmacist must make a reasonable effort to determine that the prescriber has authority to prescribe the emergency CII drug. And the prescriber must follow up the emergency dispensing request with a written hard-copy prescription within seven days. The hard-copy prescription should have "authorization for emergency dispensing" written on the front.

Exceptions to this rule are that the faxed prescription may serve as the original hard copy if it was issued for home infusion IV to be administered by injection or infusion or if the patient is in a long-term care facility or hospice care.

Another exception to the rule is outlined in the revised 2010 DEA *Pharmacist's Manual* in which a provision was added for emergency dispensing. Emergency prescriptions normally require signed follow-up prescription hard copies. The 2010 revisions allow that, following an emergency oral order of a controlled substance, the prescriber may provide an electronic script in place of a hard-copy prescription as long as the pharmacist documents receiving the emergency oral order and the date of dispensing.

DISPENSING WITHOUT A PRESCRIPTION

Some schedule V drugs may be dispensed without a prescription. A common schedule V drug that can be purchased without a prescription is cough medicine that contains codeine. These medications are kept behind the counter, and certain restrictions apply to purchasing these medications without a prescription. First, only a pharmacist makes distribution. The pharmacist must ensure medical necessity of the need for the product. After the pharmacist has fulfilled his or her professional and legal responsibility, a pharmacy technician may make the actual cash transaction.

A limited quantity of not more than 120 milliliters (4 ounces) of liquid or 24 solid dosage tablets/capsules of schedule V controlled substance may be dispensed to the same purchaser in a 48-hour period. The purchaser must be at least 18 years old, and any customer with whom the pharmacist is unfamiliar should provide identification with proof of age.

The pharmacy must maintain a logbook with the name and address of the purchaser, the name and quantity of the controlled drug dispensed, the date of the sale, and the initials of the pharmacist. Some pharmacies may have an electronic logbook rather than a paperbound book. All records must be kept for at least two years.

SECURITY REQUIREMENTS

The DEA requires pharmacies to keep CII–V substances in a locked cabinet or dispersed within the noncontrolled prescription drug stock to help deter theft. An electronic alarm system is recommended but not required by law.

According to federal law, a pharmacy must not employ anyone who has been convicted of a felony relating to controlled substances in a position that allows access to controlled substances.

ORDERING AND RECEIVING CONTROLLED DRUGS

Pharmacies have the option of ordering CIIs by using the paper DEA Form 222 or by electronically placing an order through the DEA Controlled Substance Ordering System (CSOS). The pharmacist or an authorized person completes and signs official paper order forms. The use of a digital signature is required for electronic ordering. A certification authority issues digital signatures through the DEA.

Pharmacies purchase schedule III–V drugs from the wholesaler in the same manner as other prescription drugs are ordered and purchased.

When CII drugs are received at the pharmacy, the pharmacist must document the actual number of packages received and the date received. CIII–V invoice receipts should also have the date received and a confirmation that the order was accurate. The pharmacist or pharmacy technician who checks in the order should sign the invoice receipt.

Official order forms must be maintained separately from the pharmacy's other business records.

INVENTORY AND RECORD KEEPING

Every pharmacy must maintain complete and accurate records on a current basis for each controlled substance purchased, received, distributed, dispensed, or disposed of. CII inventory records must be kept separate from other controlled drug inventory records. All controlled drug records must be maintained for two years and readily retrievable. This rule applies to both paper and electronic records. Strict and accurate record keeping of controlled drugs includes:

- ✓ Electronic or hard-copy prescription
- ✓ CII order forms
- ✓ Invoices showing receipt of drugs
- ✓ Records of transfers of controlled substances between pharmacies
- ✓ DEA registration certificate
- ✓ Inventory records, including controlled drugs removed from inventory for disposal

Controlled substances must be inventoried every two years (biennial inventory). An actual physical count of CII drugs must be made. Physical count means that the pharmacy technician will actually count each tablet in the stock bottle rather than estimating the amount in stock. CIII–V drugs must have an actual physical count if the bottle holds more than 1000 dosage units and has been opened. Otherwise, an estimated count may be made. Controlled drugs awaiting disposal must be included in the inventory records until actual disposal is made. When a medication not previously listed as a controlled drug is put on the schedule, the drug must be inventoried as of the effective date of scheduling. Pharmacies may hire an outside firm to perform biennial inventory.

DISPOSAL OF CONTROLLED DRUGS

A pharmacy may want to dispose of controlled drugs that are

- ✓ Outdated
- ✓ Returned to the pharmacy from a patient who has expired (passed away)
- ✓ From a partially used vial or ampule of injectable drugs

Hospital or clinic pharmacies or other entities that use injectable controlled drugs will be issued a *blanket authorization* by the DEA for destruction of controlled drugs. The blanket authorization allows the pharmacy to destroy, or to *waste*, injectable drugs without permission each time. Drugs must be *denatured*, or destroyed, in such a manner that they are beyond reclamation. A pharmacy technician is allowed to waste a controlled drug, but a licensed professional, such as a pharmacist or a nurse, must witness the action.

Once a calendar year, retail pharmacies may file DEA Form 41 to request authorization to destroy damaged, outdated, or otherwise unwanted controlled substances. DEA Form 41 will require a list of all drugs to be destroyed, the date and method of destruction, and names of at least two people who will witness destruction. Witnesses should be licensed professionals such as a physician, a pharmacist, a midlevel practitioner, a nurse, or a state/local law enforcement. The DEA office must be notified two weeks before drug disposal.

An outside company or a reverse distributor may be hired by the pharmacy to remove or dispose of controlled drugs. A *reverse distributor* is a company authorized by the DEA to collect outdated and recalled controlled substances from the pharmacy. The company then returns the outdated drugs to drug companies for credit or destroys the drugs at approved incinerators.

Records involving the destruction and removal of drugs must be kept readily available for two years. Information to document when CII drugs are removed from inventory include the date removed, the drug name, strength, dosage form, and quantity removed. Also documented is the lot number and the purpose for removing the drug from inventory. Both the pharmacy technician and the pharmacist will sign the records.

THEFT OR LOSS

Both the DEA and local law enforcement must be contacted if there is theft or significant loss of controlled drugs. Significant loss of controlled drugs may occur over time rather than all at once. Repeatedly coming up a few doses short on your physical count over time may indicate a significant problem that must be reported to the DEA. DEA Form 106 is used to report significant loss or theft. It is *not* used to correct minor inventory shortages. DEA Form 106 can be completed and submitted on paper or online.

If it is determined that the loss is not significant, a record of loss should be placed in the pharmacy's theft/loss file for future reference.

DEA NUMBER

Prescriptions written for a controlled drug must include the prescriber's valid DEA registration number. An example of a DEA number is AB1234567-012. DEA numbers may or may not include the physician's hospital code number (hyphenated numbers). See **Figures 8-1** and **8-2**. The following steps can be taken to determine the number's authenticity.

Step 1: Add the first, third, and fifth number.

Step 2: Then add the second, fourth, and sixth number.

Step 3: Take the total from Step 2 and multiply by 2.

Step 4: Add the numbers you got from steps 1 and 3.

The last numeral in your total should be the same as the last numeral of the DEA number, excluding the hospital code number.

Step 5: Match the last number of your answer in step 4 with the seventh number in the DEA number.

This is not an authentic DEA number, because the numbers don't match.

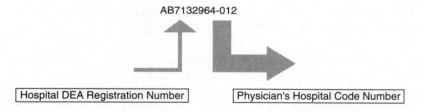

Figure 8-1 DEA Numbers

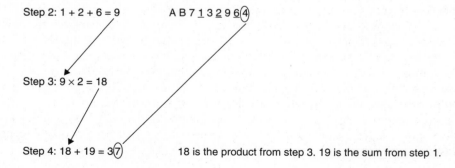

Figure 8-2 DEA Equation

This is not an authentic DEA number, because the numbers don't match.

The first letter in the DEA number signifies the level of prescriber. Letters "A" and "B" are topline prescribers, for instance. The second letter in the DEA number is the first letter of the prescriber's last name. DEA number A *B* 7 1 3 2 9 6 4 may belong to a Dr. *Bennett*.

Military personnel who are prescribers are not required to have a DEA number. Instead of using a DEA number, military prescribers use their service ID number and indicate the branch of service. These prescriptions may be filled off base by any pharmacy.

Midlevel practitioners such as nurse practitioners or physician assistants may have certain prescribing parameters. You should know the state-established parameters where you practice; however, the national certification exam will not ask state-specific questions.

ELECTRONIC PRESCRIPTIONS

Effective June 1, 2010, practitioners have the option of sending electronic prescriptions for controlled substances to pharmacies for dispensing. Pharmacies may now receive, dispense, and archive these electronic prescriptions. Before a prescriber "signs" the electronic prescription, this statement appears: *By completing the two-factor authentication protocol at this time you are legally signing the prescription and authorizing the transmission of the above information to the pharmacy for dispensing. The two-factor authentication protocol may only be completed by the practitioner whose name and DEA registration number appear above.*

Please keep in mind that electronic prescribing is not mandatory; it is an *option*. At this time, prescribers, pharmacies, and institutions voluntarily participate in e-prescribing practices.

Certain rules apply for sending and receiving e-prescriptions:

- ✓ When a controlled substance prescription is received at the pharmacy electronically it must be stored electronically.
- ✓ The electronic health record (EHR) software application that the pharmacy and the prescriber use for e-prescribing must meet DEA requirements.
- ✓ The software program or application is required to run an internal audit for potential security incidents and generate a daily report of such incidents.
- ✓ An independent third party will check the software application and certify that it meets requirements.
- ✓ An electronic prescription must be transmitted from the prescriber to the pharmacy in its electronic form. If transmission of the e-prescription fails, the pharmacy must notify the prescriber.
- ✓ The prescriber has the option to print out a CIII–V e-prescription, sign it, and fax it (rather than sending it electronically).

What Must Controlled Substance e-Prescriptions Contain?

- ✓ Full name and address of patient
- ✓ Drug name
- ✓ Drug strength
- ✓ Drug dosage form
- ✓ Quantity prescribed
- ✓ Directions for use
- ✓ Name, address, DEA number of prescriber
- ✓ Refill information where applicable
- ✓ Prescription date (the day it is signed by prescriber)

PRESCRIPTION MONITORING PROGRAM

As of July 2010, 34 states have established an electronic prescription drug monitoring program for compiling records of CII–IV controlled substances (see **Table 8-1**) dispensed by pharmacies in their state. The prescription monitoring program provides information regarding the prescribing of controlled substances to both prescribers and pharmacies, so they can make informed decisions regarding a patient's need for the substance.

Table 8-1 Controlled Substances Brand/Generic List

Generic Name	Brand Name	Therapeutic Class	Indication/Use	Schedule/Class
1. oxycodone	OxyContin Roxicodone OxyIR Oxyfast	Analgesic Narcotic Opioid	Pain	CII
2. oxycodone/ acetaminophen	Percocet Roxicet Endocet	Analgesic Narcotic Opioid	Pain	CII
3. oxycodone/aspirin	Roxiprin Percodan Endodan	Analgesic Narcotic Opioid	Pain	CII
4. morphine sulfate	MS Contin Roxanol	Analgesic Narcotic Opioid	Pain	CII
5. hydromorphone	Dilaudid	Analgesic Narcotic Opioid	Pain	CII
6. oxymorphone	Opana	Analgesic Narcotic Opioid	Pain	CII
7. meperidine	Demerol Meperitab	Analgesic Narcotic	Pain	CII
8. methylphenidate	Ritalin Concerta	CNS stimulant	ADD ADHD	CII
9. acetaminophen 300 mg/ codeine 30 mg	Tylenol #3	Analgesic Narcotic	Pain	CIII
10. acetaminophen 500 mg/ hydrocodone 5 mg	Vicodin Lortab Lorcet	Analgesic Narcotic	Pain	CIII
11. alprazolam	Xanax	Benzodiazepine	Anxiety	CIV
12. clonazepam	Klonopin	Anticonvulsant Benzodiazepine	Seizures Panic disorder	CIV
13. diazepam	Valium	Benzodiazepine	Agitation Anxiety	CIV
14. lorazepam	Ativan	Benzodiazepine	Anxiety	CIV
15. temazepam	Restoril	Benzodiazepine	Insomnia	CIV
16. promethazine/codeine	Generic only	Narcotic Antihistamine/ cough suppressant	Cold/allergy symptoms	CV

Adverse effects of controlled substances include physical dependence, constipation, sedation, drowsiness, and respiratory distress.

Pharmacies are required to report data twice a month. Although the required controlled substance dispensing data may vary from state to state, general reporting information includes:

✓ Patient name, address, date of birth (DOB), sex
✓ Payment method

- ✓ National Drug Code (NDC) of the dispensed drug
- ✓ Prescriber DEA number
- ✓ Pharmacy identification number
- ✓ Date controlled prescription was filled
- ✓ Prescription number
- ✓ Quantity dispensed
- ✓ Prescription pad serial number (optional)

According to the Substance Abuse and Mental Health Services Administration (SAMHSA), from 1998 to 2008, the number of people seeking treatment for addiction to painkillers jumped 400%. Also reported is misuse or abuse of pharmaceutical pain relievers such as oxycodone and hydrocodone. Prescription drug abuse cases are treated more often than emergency room visits for illicit drugs. And in a growing number of states, deaths from prescription drugs now exceed those from motor-vehicle accidents. According to the DEA, one benefit of a prescription drug monitoring program is to facilitate and encourage the identification, intervention with, and treatment of persons addicted to prescription drugs.

CONTROLLED SUBSTANCES AT LONG-TERM CARE FACILITIES

Many long-term care facilities (LTCF) use an emergency kit that contains a limited amount and type of medications to be administered to residents. The emergency kit, commonly called an e-kit, might contain an emergency supply of heparin flush, epinephrine, Benadryl, and narcotic pain medication. Pharmacy technicians help maintain emergency kits by replacing used and outdated inventory. Complete and accurate inventory records of controlled substances placed in the emergency kit must be maintained.

EPHEDRINE AND PSEUDOEPHEDRINE

The Combat Methamphetamine Epidemic Act of 2005 mandates that training is required to sell non-prescription drug products that contain ephedrine, pseudoephedrine, and phenylpropanolamine. Ephedrine is a naturally occurring drug, and pseudoephedrine is the synthetic or man-made version of ephedrine; *pseudo* meaning false. These drugs are used to make cough, cold, and allergy drug products. Phenylpropanolamine is a veterinarian drug only sold by prescription for animal use. The reason for the combat methamphetamine law is to limit access to ephedrine and pseudoephedrine, which can be used illegally to make methamphetamine. Methamphetamine is a highly addictive drug that is dangerous to use and make. Common street names for methamphetamine are "meth," "crystal," "crank," and "ice." The DEA has put together training materials to ensure that pharmacies understand the requirements and laws for selling ephedrine and pseudoephedrine. Combat methamphetamine laws are nationally recognized; however, some states have tougher laws than the current federal law.

Logbook

The pharmacy must keep a logbook that contains a written or electronic list of sales of drug products that contain ephedrine, pseudoephedrine, and phenylpropanolamine. The pharmacy technician or pharmacist must enter the name of the drug product and the quantity sold in the logbook. The customer will then enter his or her name and address and the date and the time of the sale in the logbook. The customer must also sign the logbook.

Identification and Verification

The customer must show you a photo ID issued by a state or the federal government. You must look at the ID and the logbook to verify that your customer's name on the photo ID matches the name your customer entered in the logbook. Also, verify that the date and time of sale your customer entered in the logbook are correct.

The pharmacy must keep drug products that contain ephedrine, pseudoephedrine, and phenylpropanolamine either behind the counter or in a locked cabinet. After the logbook information has been verified, give the drug product directly to the customer who signed the logbook.

The exception to signing a logbook and showing an ID is if a purchase is made of a single package containing not more than 60 milligrams of pseudoephedrine only. Ephedrine and phenylpropanolamine purchases always require logbook signature no matter what the purchase amount.

Limited Quantities

The pharmacy cannot sell more than 3.6 grams per day to each customer (**Tables 8-2**, **8-3**, and **8-4**). You'll see from the chart that 3.6 grams is a generous quantity and should not limit patients who have a legitimate healthcare need for the product. No matter how many sales you make to a

Table 8-2 Limited Quantities Per Day

Ingredients	Number of Tablets = 3.6 grams
25 mg ephedrine HCl	175 tablets
30 mg pseudoephedrine HCl	146 tablets
60 mg pseudoephedrine HCl	73 tablets
120 mg pseudoephedrine HCl	36 tablets
phenylpropanolamine (PPA)	FDA issued a voluntary recall as being unsafe for human consumption. Veterinary use is by prescription only.
Ingredients	Number of Milliliters (mL) = 3.6 grams
6.25 mg ephedrine HCl / 5 mL liquid	3515 mL
15 mg pseudoephedrine HCl / 1.6 mL liquid	468 mL
7.5 mg pseudoephedrine HCl / 5 mL liquid	2929 mL
15 mg pseudoephedrine HCl / 5 mL liquid	1464 mL
30 mg pseudoephedrine HCl / 5 mL liquid	732 mL
60 mg pseudoephedrine HCl / 5 mL liquid	366 mL

Source: Data from Department of Justice: Drug Enforcement Agency.

Table 8-3 Limited Quantities in a 30-Day Period

Ingredients	Number of Tablets = 9 grams
25 mg ephedrine HCl	439 tablets
30 mg pseudoephedrine HCl	366 tablets
60 mg pseudoephedrine HCl	183 tablets
120 mg pseudoephedrine HCl	91 tablets

The pharmacy cannot sell more than 9 grams in a 30 day period to each customer.
Source: Data from Department of Justice: Drug Enforcement Agency.

Table 8-4 Limited Quantities = 9 grams (mL)

Ingredients	Number of Milliliters (mL) = 9 grams
6.25 mg ephedrine HCl / 5 mL liquid	8788 mL
15 mg pseudoephedrine HCl / 1.6 mL liquid	1171 mL
7.5 mg pseudoephedrine HCl / 5 mL liquid	7323 mL
15 mg pseudoephedrine HCl / 5 mL liquid	3661 mL
30 mg pseudoephedrine HCl / 5 mL liquid	1830 mL
60 mg pseudoephedrine HCl / 5 mL liquid	915 mL

Source: Data from the Department of Justice: Drug Enforcement Agency.

customer, you cannot legally sell more than *3.6 grams per day* of these drug products to the same person.

Keep these rules in mind when selling products that contain ephedrine and pseudoephedrine:

✓ Keep a logbook of sales.
✓ The name on the ID that your customer shows you must match the name your customer entered in the logbook.
✓ These Scheduled Listed Chemical Products (SLCP) must be kept either behind the counter or in a locked cabinet.
✓ The pharmacy can sell only a limited amount (3.6 grams) of these drug products to each customer per day.
✓ Each customer can only buy a limited amount (9 grams) of these drug products in a 30-day period.
✓ Report to local law enforcement and DEA any circumstance that may lead the pharmacy to believe that the purchase of ephedrine or pseudoephedrine will be used to violate the law, for example, a customer purchasing an extraordinarily large quantity or a customer using an uncommon method of payment.

When the new combat methamphetamine laws took effect in 2006, there was an initial decline in meth-related arrests. Studies conducted over the past few years show that, despite the tracking systems, meth-related activity is on the rise. Some states have taken the logbook recording a step further by using an electronic logbook linked to other pharmacies in the state. Linking logbooks allows pharmacies to check instantly whether a buyer has already purchased the legal limits of the ephedrine or pseudoephedrine products. Now, two states—Oregon and Mississippi—require a prescription for pseudoephedrine products.

SUBSEQUENT AMENDMENTS

A number of amendments have been made to the Controlled Substance Act:

✓ Narcotic Addiction Treatment Act of 1974
✓ Controlled Substance Registrant Protection Act of 1984
✓ Domestic Chemical Diversion Control Act of 1993
✓ Comprehensive Methamphetamine Control Act of 1996
✓ Methamphetamine Anti-Proliferation Act of 2000
✓ Drug Addiction Treatment Act of 2000
✓ Combat Methamphetamine Epidemic Act of 2005

Table 8-5 Controlled Substances for Treatment of Addiction

Generic	Use	Brand
buprenorphine	First drug approved for treatment of opioid addiction in physicians' offices	Subutex Butrans Buprenex
naltrexone	Approved for opioid addiction treatment in 1984	Vivitrol Revia
methadone	used to relieve acute opioid withdrawal symptom	Dolophine Methadose

The Domestic Chemical Diversion Control Act of 1993, the Comprehensive Methamphetamine Control Act of 1996, the Methamphetamine Anti-Proliferation Act of 2000, and the Combat Methamphetamine Epidemic Act of 2005 establish a foundation to help the DEA work toward preventing illicit use and abuse of controlled drugs.

Controlled Substance Registrant Protection Act of 1984

Controlled Substance Registrant Protection Act (CSRPA) provides for the federal investigation of pharmaceutical thefts and robberies if replacement cost of the drug taken is $500 or more, if there is a death or a person suffers significant bodily injury during the robbery, or if interstate or foreign commerce is involved in the crime.

Narcotic Addiction Treatment Act of 1974

The Narcotic Addiction Treatment Act and the Drug Addiction Treatment Act amended the Controlled Substance Act (CSA) with respect to the use of controlled substances in the medical treatment of addiction (**Table 8-5**). The acts govern the use of narcotics and the treatment of addiction in the United States.

LEGALIZATION OF MARIJUANA FOR MEDICINAL PURPOSES

As of 2010, 31 states had laws that recognize marijuana's medicinal value. Fourteen states have laws that permit the use of marijuana for medicinal purposes. These states have laws that allow the patient possession and use of marijuana but only with proof of a physician's approval for marijuana use. Most of the states that permit medicinal marijuana allow patients or caregivers to grow marijuana for medical use. Some states list marijuana as a CII medication, which allows for physician prescribing.

Although some state laws permit the use of medicinal marijuana, prescribing and using marijuana violates federal law.

Did you know that marijuana used for medicinal purposes was legal prior to 1970? Let's take a look at the history of medicinal marijuana laws. In 1937, the Federal Marijuana Tax Act made the nonmedical use of marijuana illegal, while medicinal use of marijuana was still legal. The act required physicians who prescribed marijuana and pharmacies that dispensed marijuana to register and pay a substantial tax. The newly required paperwork involved in prescribing and dispensing of medicinal marijuana along with the tax burden led to a reduction in prescribing marijuana.

In 1970, Congress placed marijuana in the CI schedule (no medicinal value) temporarily, pending a report of a national commission. President Richard Nixon supported marijuana as a CI schedule drug, and so it was then placed in the controlled drug class CI with the passage of the Controlled Substance Act in 1970.

This is your checklist to make sure you understand what you need to know for the certification exam. Review chapter content if there is a topic you're uncertain of.

I know:

√	...how to file prescription hard copies.
	...the differences in controlled schedules I–V.
	...top-selling medications in each controlled substance class.
	...regulations in refilling controlled drugs.
	...regulations to follow in transferring prescriptions for controlled drugs.
	...pseudoephedrine and ephedrine laws.
	...procedures to follow when dispensing a CV without a prescription.
	...how to determine a valid DEA number.
	...rules in ordering and storing controlled drugs.
	...inventory and record-keeping procedures for controlled drugs.
	...how to dispose of controlled drugs properly.

RESOURCES

1. Office of Diversion Control. US Department of Justice Drug Enforcement Administration. Available at: www.deadiversion.usdoj.gov. Accessed January 2011.
2. Medical marijuana: Therapeutic Uses and Legal Status. USPharmacist.com. Available at: www.uspharmacist.com. p. 6. Accessed January 2011.

CHAPTER 8

MULTIPLE CHOICE

Identify the choice that best completes the statement or answers the question.

_____ **1.** CII hard copies must be filed by

a. separating CII hard copies from other prescription hard copies

b. the date filled

c. patient name

d. dispersing CII hard copies among other prescription hard copies

_____ **2.** CII prescriptions allow for

a. 5 refills

b. 6 refills

c. no refills

d. 6 months of refills

_____ **3.** Emergency dispensing of CIIs

a. is not permitted

b. allows for a maximum 72-hour supply

c. allows for a maximum 7-day supply

d. is permitted for hospice patients only

_____ **4.** Schedule V logbook includes the

a. name and DOB of purchaser

b. name and quantity of schedule V drug dispensed

c. expiration date of the schedule V drug dispensed

d. pharmacy technician signature

_____ **5.** Inventory for controlled substances must be performed

a. daily

b. monthly

c. once a year

d. every two years

_____ **6.** Determine which DEA number is authentic:

a. AB126536

b. AF2369521

c. BT5623852

d. BF7236253

_____ **7.** What schedule drug is oxycodone?

a. CI

b. CII

c. CIII

d. CIV

_____ **8.** What controlled schedule is Vicodin (acetaminophen/hydrocodone)?

a. CII

b. CIII

c. CIV

d. CV

_____ **9.** Benzodiazepines typically fall into what controlled schedule?

a. CII

b. CIII

c. CIV

d. CV

_____ **10.** Adverse effect of controlled substances:

a. weight gain

b. tinitis

c. delayed development

d. physical dependence

_____ **11.** What is the daily limit per customer of ephedrine or pseudoephedrine purchase?

a. 36 grams

b. 3.6 grams

c. 36 milligrams

d. 9 grams

ANSWER SECTION

1. A

2. C

3. B

4. B

5. D

6. B

7. B

8. B

9. C

10. D

11. B

PRACTICE TEST: CONTROLLED DRUGS

Fill in the letter of the drug type for each drug listed below.

Drug Schedules

a.	CI	d.	CIV
b.	CII	e.	CV
c.	CIII		

_____ **1.** morphine sulfate

_____ **2.** oxycodone

_____ **3.** acetaminophen 300 mg/codeine 30 mg

_____ **4.** promethazine/codeine

_____ **5.** APAP 500 mg/hydrocodone 5 mg

_____ **6.** oxycodone/APAP

_____ **7.** oxycodone/ASA

_____ **8.** temazepam

_____ **9.** lorazepam

_____ **10.** alprazolam

_____ **11.** hydromorphone

_____ **12.** oxymorphone

_____ **13.** meperidine

___ **14.** clonazepam

___ **15.** methylphenidate

___ **16.** diazepam

Brand Name

a.	Restoril	i.	Concerta
b.	Ativan	j.	Roxiprin
c.	Valium	k.	Dilaudid
d.	Klonopin	l.	Opana
e.	Xanax	m.	Demerol
f.	Vicodin	n.	OxyContin
g.	MS Contin	o.	Percocet
h.	Tylenol #3		

___ **17.** oxycodone

___ **18.** oxycodone/ASA

___ **19.** oxycodone/APAP

___ **20.** APAP 300 mg/codeine 30 mg

___ **21.** meperidine

___ **22.** temazepam

___ **23.** alprazolam

___ **24.** morphine sulfate

___ **25.** hydromorphone

___ **26.** methylphenidate

___ **27.** oxymorphone

___ **28.** clonazepam

___ **29.** lorazepam

___ **30.** APAP 500 mg/hydrocodone 5 mg

___ **31.** diazepam

ANSWER SECTION

1. B
2. B
3. C
4. E
5. C
6. B
7. B
8. D
9. D
10. D
11. B
12. B
13. B
14. D
15. B
16. D
17. N
18. J
19. O
20. H
21. M
22. A
23. E
24. G
25. K
26. I
27. L
28. D
29. B
30. F
31. C

TASK SHEET

TOPIC TO REVIEW: ADMINISTRATION AND MANAGEMENT OF PHARMACY PRACTICE

Materials

Pharmacy Technician Exam Review Guide

JB Test Prep: Pharmacy Technician Exam Review Guide

Prepare

1. Read the section on the administration and management of pharmacy practice.
2. Take the practice test at the end of the chapter.

Study Plan

1. Read pages_____ on _____(date).
2. Take end-of-chapter practice test on_____(date).
3. See what a medication error reporting form looks like at www.ismp.org.

Tips

Find out what reference books your pharmacy uses. Look through these books to help you better understand what information to find in each book. For the certification exam, you will want to know which reference book to use to find certain information. Just as we would look up the definition of a word in a dictionary rather than in a phone book, you should know that you would look up AWP in the *Red Book* rather than in the *Physicians' Desk Reference*.

End of Chapter

List what you need to review.

Participating in the Administration and Management of Pharmacy

OBJECTIVES/TOPICS TO COVER:

✓ Identify the regulations in *transferring prescriptions*.
✓ Know safeguards to alleviate *medication errors*.
✓ List the procedures involved in reporting *medication errors*.
✓ Be familiar with common pharmacy *reference materials*.

TRANSFERRING PRESCRIPTIONS

Prescription transfer from pharmacy to pharmacy is communicated directly between pharmacists. By federal law, pharmacy technicians are not allowed to transfer prescriptions. Other rules to transferring prescriptions are as follows:

1. Prescriptions written for noncontrolled drugs may be transferred between pharmacies as long as the number of transfers does not exceed the number of originally authorized refills and the original prescription is still valid.
2. The pharmacist who is transferring the prescription drug order information records the following information:
   ✓ Mark "VOID" on the front of the original hard-copy prescription
   ✓ On the back of the voided hard-copy prescription, document the name, address, and DEA number of the receiving pharmacy and the name of the pharmacist who took the information
   ✓ Document the date of the transfer and the name of the transferring pharmacist
3. Both the hard-copy original and the transferred prescription drug orders are maintained for two years from the date of last refill.
4. Prescriptions written for CII substances may *not* be transferred. There are no refills allowed on a CII prescription and therefore will have no fill amount to transfer to another pharmacy.
5. It is permissible to transfer prescriptions written for controlled substances listed in schedules III, IV, or V on a onetime basis. Pharmacies that share real-time, electronic databases may transfer within the pharmacy network up to the maximum refills permitted by law. Accurate record keeping following a transfer of a controlled drug is important.

The pharmacist who receives the transferred prescription must also document specifics on the transfer, including the date of original dispensing, the pharmacy's name, address, DEA number and prescription number that the prescription was transferred from, date the original prescription was issued, the original number of refills, the number of refills remaining, and other information required by law.

MEDICATION ERRORS

Up to 500,000 preventable injuries occur each year in the United States as a result of medical errors. It is estimated that, for every 3 billion prescriptions filled, 51.5 million errors occur annually. These daunting figures boil down to four medication errors occurring for every 250 prescriptions filled each day in each pharmacy.

According to the Institute for Safe Medication Practices, a medication error is defined as any preventable event that may cause or lead to inappropriate medication use or patient harm while the medication is in the control of the healthcare professional, patient, or consumer. Such events may be related to professional practice, healthcare products, procedures, and systems, including prescribing; written and oral communication; product name, labeling, and packaging; compounding; dispensing; distribution; administration; education; monitoring; and use.

Many pharmacy technicians have a misconception that an error is only when a patient is given the wrong drug. Even if the dispensing mistake is caught by the pharmacist *before* the drug reaches the patient, it is still listed as an error.

When an error occurs the pharmacy technician should report the error to the pharmacy supervisor. The error should also be reported to a national reporting program such as the U.S. Food and Drug Administration's MedWatch or the Institute for Safe Medication Practices Medication Errors Reporting System (see **Exhibit 9-1**).

We are all capable of making mistakes. For this reason, we all need to work together and take the right steps to help prevent errors from happening.

Improving Medication Safety

The Institute of Medicine (IOM) suggests an approach to patient safety that involves identifying medication errors and learning from them through the establishment of a reporting system. There are a few different avenues where medication errors can be reported in confidence and on a voluntary basis; the Institute for Safe Medication Practices (ISMP) has created the Medication Error Reporting Program (MERP).

Exhibit 9-1 Reporting Med Errors

1. MERP at www.ismp.org
2. MedWatch at www.fda.gov. Download a copy of the reporting form and either fax or mail it using the postage-paid, addressed form.

Fax: 1-800-FDA-0178, 1-800-FDA-1080 to report by phone

Examples of medication errors or near errors that may be reported are

✓ Dispensing the wrong drug, such as Topomax instead of Toprol
✓ Dispensing the wrong strength, such as 300mg instead of 30mg
✓ Dispensing the wrong dose of a medication, such as 1 Tablespoonful instead of 1 tsp.
✓ Confusion over look-alike/sound-alike drugs
✓ Incorrect route of administration
✓ Calculation errors
✓ Compounding/preparation errors

It is most important to understand the cause and type of medication errors. The ISMP asks that the following information be included when reporting errors:

1. Describe the error. Tell what went wrong.

2. Tell if the error reached the patient, or if the error reported was discovered before it reached the patient.
3. Document the patient outcome. Did the patient experience an adverse reaction?
4. Indicate the type of practice site the error occurred in (hospital, private office, retail pharmacy, long-term care facility, etc).
5. Give the generic name and brand name of medication involved.
6. Indicate the dosage form, concentration, or strength.
7. Describe how the error was discovered.
8. Share your recommendations for error prevention.

The goal of reporting errors is to reduce medication errors and potential patient harm. Medication error information is collected to see whether there's a trend, and then healthcare professionals are warned of the potential for errors and possible ways to alleviate the error. Drug manufacturers may also be notified of error trends if labeling is a consideration for change.

Pharmacy technicians are able to and should report errors! Without reporting errors, the occurrence may go unrecognized, and the same or a similar error will continue without prevention.

Reporting medication errors is voluntary through MedWatch and MERP; however, you always have the option to include your name as well as your pharmacy name.

As a professional, you never intend to make a mistake when dispensing medications. Being a part of an error that harms a patient can cause emotional distress to the technician and the technician at fault may be characterized as the *second victim*. A non-profit group called National Quality Forum works with healthcare professionals to improve patient safety.

Safe Practices/Improving Patient Safety

The Food and Drug Administration (FDA) has developed programs aimed at improving drug quality and safety. Improving patient safety will come from better drug labeling and more comprehensive postmarketing data. Although the FDA currently performs postmarket surveillance on medications, improvements are needed in collecting postmarket data when a drug is released to the public. Postmarketing is important, because rare adverse events may not have been detected in clinical trial but may only come to light when many more people take the drug. Adverse Event Reporting System (AERS) is a computerized information database designed to support the FDA's postmarketing safety surveillance program for all approved drugs. AERS will be used to track the complete life cycle of the medication.

Another way for the FDA to improve patient safety is through an expanded global presence. The FDA regulatory system was originally built around the concept of drugs manufactured in the United States, as this was the common practice years ago. Today, most products on American pharmacy shelves are either manufactured overseas or contain some ingredients that have been shipped into the United States. Expanded global presence means that the FDA will work to regulate the drugs and drug ingredients manufactured in other countries.

Safe practices to improve patient safety include evaluating pharmacy workflow. Does the workflow promote safety? Areas to evaluate in pharmacy workflow are the dispensing and checking processes and staff workload. Take a look at environmental factors such as pharmacy design, lighting, noise level, and clutter. Staff habits such as work schedules and break times should be logical, with best practices for patient safety in mind. Other ways to improve patient safety:

✓ Use of barcode technology
✓ Electronic prescribing
✓ Communication among pharmacy team members on potential errors. Alert others to potential error.
✓ Clarify prescriptions that are poorly written. Read verbal prescriptions back to the prescriber's office to check for accuracy.

To improve patient safety for pediatric patients, be especially careful when preparing IV medications as well as oral dosing for infants and young children. This group of young patients requires low doses of medications that are often dosed for adults. Make sure syringes are adequate for measuring low-dose volumes, oftentimes less than 0.1 milliliters.

REFERENCE MATERIALS

You will know some drug information about some commonly prescribed medications in your pharmacy setting. With all the medications on the market, it's next to impossible to know everything about every drug. And, really, there is no reason to memorize drug information when a reference book or electronic application is available to look up the information. There are many drug reference books on the market. This section will review well-known reference books, as these are the ones most likely to appear on the certification exam.

Physicians' Desk Reference

Commonly called the PDR, the *Physicians' Desk Reference* is a thick, hardcover book that provides drug information similar to manufacturer's package inserts. Because the drug information contained in a PDR is very detailed, physicians regularly use this reference book for prescribing information. It is also available in electronic format.

Ident-A-Drug Reference

The *Ident-A-Drug Reference* identifies tablets or capsules by the imprint and markings on the tablet/capsule. This reference book gives the National Drug Code (NDC) of the drug along with the generic and brand names and the drug manufacturers. It is also available for a PDA (personal digital assistant) and in electronic format.

Drug Facts and Comparisons

Commonly known as F&C, the *Drug Facts and Comparisons* reference book is a compilation of monographs detailing drug actions, indications, administration and dosage, adverse reactions, warnings, and more. The reference lists both prescription and over-the-counter (OTC) information. It is also available in an online and a CD format.

Orange Book

Published by the FDA, the *Orange Book* is a list of approved drug products and is known for the therapeutic equivalence evaluations that it provides. It is widely accepted as the authoritative source for determining therapeutic equivalence in brand/generic product substitution. The *Orange Book* was originally a bound book with an orange cover. The electronic *Orange Book* drug listings can be accessed free of charge from a link on the FDA website.

United States Pharmacopoeia–NF

The *United States Pharmacopeia–National Formulary* (USP–NF) is a book of standards for medicines, dosage forms, drug substances, excipients, medical devices, and dietary supplements. USP-NF is available in print and in an electronic format.

The well-known *United States Pharmacopoeia–Drug Information* (USP DI), volume 1: *Drug Information for the Health Care Professional* has been discontinued. A similar reference, *DrugPoints*, is available in electronic format.

Drug Topics Red Book

Drug Topics Red Book is the retail pharmacy's guide to average wholesale price (AWP) for prescription and OTC drugs. Commonly called the *Red Book*, it also lists *Orange Book* codes.

Exhibit 9-2 Tips from a Certified Tech

Connie Snyder, CPhT
Fay Pharmacy-Adair, Iowa

I have been employed at the same small independent pharmacy for thirty years. Several years ago I was grandfathered in as a pharmacy technician. I enjoy doing insurance, clerical, long-term care medications, stocking pharmacy shelves, and assisting the pharmacist in his duties.

As the years have passed and laws have changed, so have the pharmacy technician roles. Now, we need to be certified and do continuing education as well as the pharmacist. Today, we can receive prescription requests, count tablets, label bottles, answer phones, and perform administrative functions.

I wanted to become certified to better assist the pharmacist and help serve our customers in a more professional and knowledgeable manner. Good customer service and communication skills are needed because of interaction with patients, coworkers, or others. We, as technicians, help read and verify doses, and that can be a matter of life or death.

Before I became certified I enrolled in a short course offered by a nearby community college to help prepare me for taking the certification test. As soon as I finished the course, within two weeks I applied for the PTCB exam. I went and took the test and passed the first time. The course I had taken prepared me very well and the knowledge of the instructor was most helpful.

I would encourage everyone who intends on working in a pharmacy to become a certified pharmacy technician. Advancement opportunities are sometimes limited; however, you can become a supervisor, do sales, advance to specialty positions, or go on to become a pharmacist. My technician training has helped the pharmacist lighten his duties, and we share most of the duties. I still enjoy working in a small independent pharmacy.

This is your checklist to make sure you understand what you need to know for the certification exam. Review chapter content if there is a topic you're uncertain of.
I know:

√	...safeguards to avoid potential medication errors.
	...steps to take when a medication error occurs.
	...the importance of easy-to-read/understand OTC labeling.
	...common reference sources used in pharmacy practice.

RESOURCES

1. Reprinted with the permission of the National Coordinating Council for Medication Error Reporting and Prevention, © 1998–2011. All Rights Reserved.
2. Courtesy of Ohio Pharmacist's Association. *Ohio Pharm J.* 2010; 59(11): 14–16.
3. Office of Diversion Control. US Department of Justice Drug Enforcement Administration. *Pharmacist's Manual: An Information Outline of the Controlled Substances Act.* Available at: www.deadiversion.usdoj.gov/pubs/manuals/pharm2/pharm_manual.pdf. Accessed January 2011.
4. Institute of Medication of the National Academies (IOM) Committee on Identifying and Preventing Medication Errors; Aspden P, Wolcott JA, Bootman JL, Cronenwett LR, eds. *Preventing Medication Errors.* Quality Chasm Series. Washington, DC: National Academies Press; 2006.
5. Institute of Medication of the National Academies (IOM); Kohn LT, Corrigan JM, Donaldson MS, eds. *To Err Is Human: Building a Safer Heath System.* Washington, DC: National Academy Press; 1999:5
6. Med error reporting. Institute for Safe Medication Practices (ISMP). Available at: http://www.ismp.org. Accessed January 17, 2011.
7. Erickson AK. Will medications be safer in the future? *Pharm Today.* November 2010:40–43.

CHAPTER 9

MULTIPLE CHOICE

Identify the choice that best completes the statement or answers the question.

_____ **1.** Prescription transfer from pharmacy to pharmacy

a. is done by the technicians

b. is against federal law

c. is allowed on a onetime basis

d. is done by the pharmacists

_____ **2.** Prescriptions written for noncontrolled drugs may be transferred between pharmacies

a. one time only

b. as long as the number of transfers does not exceed the number of refills

c. within 1 month of the date on the original prescription

d. with permission from the state board of pharmacy

_____ **3.** Prescriptions written for CII substances

a. may not be transferred

b. may be transferred from pharmacy to pharmacy on an emergency basis

c. may be transferred from pharmacy to pharmacy on a onetime basis

d. may be transferred from pharmacy to pharmacy as long as the original prescription is within date

_____ **4.** A medication error is

a. a nonpreventable event

b. a preventable event that may cause patient harm

c. a nonpreventable event resulting from prescribing error

d. an intentional event that may result in patient harm

_____ **5.** The goal of reporting medication errors is to

a. discipline those responsible for the error

b. track the safest pharmacy setting

c. reduce medication error and potential patient harm

d. alert the public of the safest dispensing pharmacies

_____ **6.** Better drug labeling will help

a. the FDA approve a wider variety of medications

b. pharmacies assess a higher dispensing fee

c. the FDA monitor illegal drug importation

d. improve patient safety

_____ **7.** Pharmacy workflow

a. should promote safe distribution

b. should focus on speed

c. is evaluated every six months

d. evaluates customer satisfaction

_____ **8.** The *Physicians' Desk Reference* (PDR)

a. is used only by physicians when providing dosing instructions for the patient

b. provides drug information similar to a package insert

c. is well-known for providing up-to-date AWP

d. is the most useful reference book for hospital pharmacy

_____ **9.** *Drug Facts and Comparisons*

a. is a compilation of drug monographs

b. is commonly referred to as the DFC

c. gives a general overview of prescription medications

d. is well known for therapeutic equivalence ratings

_____ **10.** The *Orange Book*

a. identifies tablets by the imprint or markings

b. provides information similar to package inserts

c. is known for providing therapeutic equivalence evaluations

d. is a compilation of drug monographs

ANSWER SECTION

1. D
2. B
3. A
4. B
5. C
6. D
7. A
8. B
9. A
10. C

TASK SHEET

TOPIC TO REVIEW: MEDICATION AND INVENTORY CONTROL SYSTEMS

Materials

Pharmacy Technician Exam Review Guide

JB Test Prep: Pharmacy Technician Exam Review Guide

Prepare

1. Read the section on medication and inventory control systems.
2. Take practice test at the end of the chapter.

Study Plan

1. Read pages_____ on _____(date).
2. Take end-of-chapter practice test on_____(date).
3. Memorize pharmacy mandated temperature for room, refrigerator, freezer.

Tips

Look at the NDC numbers on stock bottles in your pharmacy and practice your knowledge of what those numbers stand for.

End of Chapter

List what you need to review.

Maintaining Medication Inventory and Repackaging

OBJECTIVES/TOPICS TO COVER:

After completing this chapter, you will be able to demonstrate an understanding of the topics listed below:

- ✓ Managing inventory
- ✓ Medication storage
- ✓ Inventory concerns for controlled drugs, investigational drugs, and hazardous drugs
- ✓ Recall and returns
- ✓ Emergency ordering
- ✓ Disposal of drugs
- ✓ Repackaging
- ✓ Expiration dating
- ✓ National Drug Code

Managing inventory is a job duty that everyone takes part in. A pharmacy can't serve its patients if medication is not in stock. A pharmacy can't stay in business if products are purchased at too high of a cost for reimbursement equity. Purchasing and stocking too much inventory affects the pharmacy's bottom line. Keeping the right amount of the right inventory products in stock at the right times is a balancing act that pharmacy managers strive to perfect.

INVENTORY TERMS

Inventory are goods the pharmacy stocks. Because pharmacies keep an inventory of products that service their patient needs, ambulatory, or retail, pharmacies will have a different inventory than hospital pharmacies. While different pharmacy settings will carry different types of products, they also have different methods of keeping track of their inventory.

Perpetual inventory is updating or ordering stock on a continuous basis. This method is similar to what many of us do in our homes when we buy groceries. When a gallon of milk is used, we buy a new gallon of milk. When a stock bottle of Lipitor is used, the pharmacy purchases a new bottle of Lipitor. Point-of-service technology makes the process of perpetual inventory relatively easy. The cash register is tied in with the order entry system, so stock is continuously (perpetually) reordered as it leaves the pharmacy with the customer.

Periodic automatic replenishment (PAR) is another method of keeping inventory levels in check. With PAR the pharmacy manager establishes a predetermined optimum stock level for all products in the pharmacy, and when that level is reached, ordering takes place. For instance, the PAR level for 250 milliliters dextrose is 25 bags. When the PAR level is reached, an order is automatically made. PAR levels in the pharmacy can be compared to stocking supplies in our home. Typically there should be at least one dozen eggs on hand at all times. When the egg bucket in the refrigerator gets down to 12 eggs, buy more. To determine the optimum PAR level, the pharmacy manager considers the amount needed on hand to ensure stock doesn't run out before reordering occurs.

Turnover is the rate that inventory is used or sold. A pharmacy that has a quick turnover in stock is managing its inventory well. A quick turnover means that the right products are being purchased and turned over, or sold, to customers. Keys to look for in effective inventory management are minimal outdated products and medication products on hand to fill customer orders.

PURCHASING

Stock is purchased to fulfill the pharmacy's formulary needs. A *formulary* is a list of medications approved for the pharmacy to dispense. An *open formulary* allows the pharmacy to stock any prescribed medication the manager deems necessary. A *closed formulary* limits the medication that can be stocked. The development of a pharmacy formulary is based on cost-effectiveness and meeting the prescribing needs of the community.

Pharmacies may purchase medications from a

- ✓ Wholesaler
- ✓ Manufacturer

Buying from a wholesaler is a one-stop shop. The wholesaler carries prescription medications, over-the-counter (OTC) medications, medical products, and sundries. The wholesaler works as a middleman, buying from the manufacturer and then selling to pharmacies. McKesson, Cardinal Health, and AmerisourceBergen are the "Big Three" drug wholesale companies.

A pharmacy may have a *prime vendor* contract with its wholesaler for a certain dollar amount of business each year, and in turn, the wholesaler gives the pharmacy special pricing.

Commonly, a group of pharmacies unite to form a *purchasing group* to increase their buying power. Purchasing groups enable smaller, independent pharmacies to stay competitive with chain pharmacy pricing by receiving prime vendor pricing for purchasing in bulk.

Instead of purchasing from a wholesaler there are a few instances when the pharmacy may purchase directly from the manufacturer. Nuclear pharmacies commonly purchase directly from the manufacturer, because radiopharmaceuticals have a short half-life and therefore need to be shipped directly to the pharmacy. Additionally, pharmacies that have large buying power may be able to contract with manufacturers to get a lower purchase price for buying direct. When there are special circumstances such as drug shortages, the pharmacy may buy directly from the manufacturer.

RECEIPT OF INVENTORY

When the ordered shipment is received at the pharmacy, a manifest is signed by the technician or other pharmacy staff to indicate delivery and receipt of the supply. Before signing the manifest, the technician will count and verify the number of totes with the delivery driver present. A *manifest* is a listing of the ordered stock that was shipped. The manifest will serve as the pharmacy's receipt of goods, so before signing the manifest, be sure to compare the inventory received against the items listed on the manifest.

When you are unpacking the shipping totes, check the purchase order against the actual stock received. Check for damaged bottles, missing items, miss-picked items, and check to be sure expiration dates are dated well into the future. Miss-picked items are products that are sent in place of products that were ordered, because the warehouse 'picked' the wrong product off the shelf to fill the order.

The technician who checks in the order should be different from the technician who placed the order. Having two different pharmacy personnel perform these important inventory steps is part of the checks-and-balances procedure.

The pharmacy is responsible for the drug shipment as soon as the manifest is signed. The wholesaler is responsible for the shipment from the warehouse to the pharmacy. To discourage drug diversion, manufacturers have started a practice of embedding a computer chip, called a radio frequency identification (RFID), into the medication stock bottle or other product packaging. The computer chip allows that medication product to be tracked from the time it leaves the manufacturer, as it travels to the warehouse, and ends at to the pharmacy site.

DRUG SHORTAGES

A medication that was ordered may not have been shipped due to a drug shortage. Drug shortages may be handled by substituting another drug until the shortage is cleared up. The pharmacist will have to get involved to determine the best therapeutic substitution. Prescribers will also have to be alerted of the drug shortage and the alternative therapy. All pharmacy staff should be notified of drug shortages or back-ordered drugs to provide the best service. Potential results of a drug shortage may involve (1) the pharmacy purchasing the medication from a secondary market of questionable product quality, (2) increased price for the medication that is in short supply, (3) delayed treatment for the patient who is in need of the medication, (4) undue pain and suffering for the patient, and (5) patient death.

At the time of this book printing there are 210 medications in short supply. According to the FDA the reasons for a drug being in short supply is because of production shutdowns due to manufacturing problems, such as contamination in the production facilities; theft from the warehouse or theft during shipment of the medication; and companies that have stopped making certain IV medications because of slim profit margins.

STORAGE AND STOCKING

After the new shipment is checked in, the pharmacy technician will put the stock away. One of the best things a new pharmacy technician can do is to volunteer to put the stock away. This is a great way to become familiar with the layout of the pharmacy. But you must be careful in putting stock away! A misplaced bottle could lead to a medication error. Putting stock away correctly is crucial to workflow. Rotate the stock. This means the new stock is placed on the shelf *behind* the existing stock. The first stock in—with the expiration date closest to today's date—is the first stock that needs to be dispensed to the customer.

Unless otherwise indicated, all medications need to be stored as follows:

✓ In an airtight container
✓ Out of direct sunlight
✓ At room temperature
✓ In low humidity

Lids to stock bottles need to be screwed on tight to keep the bottle as airtight as possible. Vials used to dispense drugs are amber, and stock bottles are blackout plastic to keep direct light and sunlight from penetrating the container and possibly harming the medication. Something you will want to know forever about storing medications is the legal definition of room temperature, refrigerated temperature, and frozen.

Federal law defines   room temperature: 59°–86°F, which is 15°–30°C

refrigerator temperature: 36°–46°F, which is 2°–8°C

freezer temperature: below 32°F, which is 0°C

Purchasing and Storing Controlled Substances

Special considerations are made for purchasing and storing controlled substances. CII drugs are ordered online through the DEA (Drug Enforcement Agency) Controlled Substance Ordering System (CSOS) or ordered on paper using the DEA Form 222. When the CII shipment arrives, the actual shipment received is compared against the pharmacy's copy of DEA Form 222. Document the date received, the drug name, strength, dosage form, and the quantity received. The pharmacist and the pharmacy technician who checked in the order will sign the manifest/purchase order.

The manifest/purchase order for CII drugs is in triplicate. Part three of the manifest is kept on file at the pharmacy for two years.

CII drugs are stored in a secure location to prevent theft and diversion.

Purchasing and Storing Hazardous Drugs and Investigational Drugs

Special considerations are made for ordering, receiving, and storing hazardous substances and investigational drugs. Hazardous drugs such as radiopharmaceuticals, chemotherapy, or antineoplastics may be ordered from the manufacturer and shipped directly to the pharmacy from the manufacturer. As with all drugs, paperwork is filled out to document receipt of the order. Material Safety Data Sheets (MSDS) accompany hazardous drugs. The MSDS lists the chemical properties of the drug and how to provide emergency treatment in the event of accidental exposure to the drug. Pharmacies must have an MSDS on file for each hazardous drug stocked.

The delivery tote that carries hazardous drugs may be orange, red, or yellow and will have the word *hazardous* in bold labeling. Protect yourself by wearing gloves when checking in and stocking hazardous drugs. Males and females of childbearing age should not handle hazardous drugs. This also applies to pregnant or lactating women. All pharmacy personnel should receive training in hazardous drugs prior to handling.

Pharmacy shelves should be labeled to identify hazardous drugs so there is no doubt which drugs are hazardous and where those drugs are stored. In addition, hazardous drugs are to be stored in a separate area of the pharmacy and/or in a safe area where shelving has a lip to help prevent spills. It's good practice to shelve hazardous drugs in breakable containers low to the ground. This will help concentrate spills in the event of accidental breakage.

To eliminate cross-contamination, always use a specially marked counting tray when counting chemotherapy or other hazardous drugs. *Cross-contamination* is when drug residue from one medication is mixed with another drug. Don't count antibiotics on the same tray that hazardous drugs are counted. The antibiotic tablet will collect drug residue powder from the hazardous drug and therefore pose a risk to the patient.

DRUG RECALLS

Drug recalls are classed according to seriousness of the recall. A class 1 recall means that continued use of the product is likely to cause serious adverse effects or death. A class 2 recall means that continued use could cause temporary adverse effects. A class 3 recall is the least serious and means use is unlikely to cause adverse effects.

There are numerous reasons for a drug recall. The drug labeling may be incorrect, there might be a problem with the product packaging, or a certain batch of medication could be contaminated. Most often manufacturers issue voluntary recalls under the direction of the Food and Drug Administration (FDA).

When the pharmacy receives recall notification from the manufacturer or wholesaler, the pharmacy technician will check the product's lot number against the affected lot number on the recall notice. If the lot numbers and/or batch numbers match those indicated on the recall notice, the medication or product is pulled from the pharmacy shelf. The recall notice will provide instructions on how to manage the recalled products. Most of the time, the pharmacy is instructed to send recalled products back to the manufacturer and then reorder a new supply. The technician will have to keep track of paperwork to ensure proper reimbursement credits are issued for the returned, recalled product.

Depending on the seriousness or class of the recall, the pharmacy may need to contact the patient who received the medication or product.

MEDICATION DISPOSAL

According to the U.S. Office of National Drug Control Policy, for young people ages 12–17 years, prescription drugs have become the second most abused drug (behind marijuana). Controlled substances are the prescription drug of choice for abuse and misuse. Prescription drug abuse is at epic proportions in many parts of the country. The Secure and Responsible Drug Disposal Act of 2010 is designed to improve and encourage prescription drug disposal programs. Through the disposal programs, community pharmacies will be allowed to accept all medications from consumers for disposal, including controlled drugs. Consumers will be encouraged to turn in unused and expired medications into the pharmacy. These disposal programs will help to protect our environment from improperly disposed drugs that contaminate our drinking water and threaten our wildlife. Disposal programs will help protect individuals by limiting access to potentially abused drugs.

In 2010, the DEA held a National Take Back Day. Many other "take back" programs for unused medications have been initiated throughout the country as a form of prevention to help keep our communities safe.

It's important to dispose of expired medication appropriately. Flushing unused patient medications down the toilet can contaminate groundwater. Wastewater treatment plants are not designed to remove pharmaceuticals from water supplies. Studies have shown that even small amounts of pharmaceuticals in rivers and streams can have negative effects on the ecosystem. How medication is disposed has an impact on our environment. Common pharmacy practice is to contract with a reverse distributor to manage expired medications. Prior to the passage of the Secure and Responsible Drug Act of 2010, federal law prohibited ambulatory pharmacies from routinely accepting prescription medication returns from customers. Retail pharmacies now have the option to take back unwanted drugs from the public. In the event that the pharmacy does not participate in a drug take back disposal program the pharmacy technician should advise the customer to dispose of their own medication. Current practice is to render the medicine unidentifiable by mixing it with coffee grounds or kitty litter in a sealed plastic baggy.

REPACKAGING

Pharmacies purchase bulk medication at a discounted rate and repackage the drug into unit dose packaging for patient use. Unit dose packaging is used for accurate dosing, distribution, and inventory control.

- ✓ Blister pack
- ✓ Oral syringes
- ✓ Cards
- ✓ OPUS medication cassettes
- ✓ Bubble packs

Each unit dose package must completely identify the medication. The repackaged unit dose must have a National Drug Code barcode, be tamper resistant, and have an assigned expiration date (**Figures 10-1 to 10-6**).

Expiration Dates of Repackaging

Once the manufacturer's stock bottle of bulk medication is opened, the expiration date on the stock bottle is no longer valid. In your home, a can of fruit has a long shelf life, but the minute the can is opened the fruit will spoil sooner than the expiration date on the can. The same concept is true of medications. The manufacturer's expiration date is set to the end of the month. A product with an

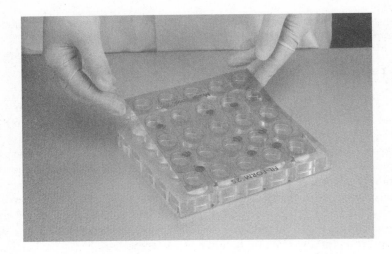

Figure 10-1 Step 1

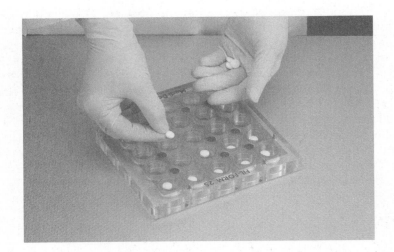

Figure 10-2 Step 2

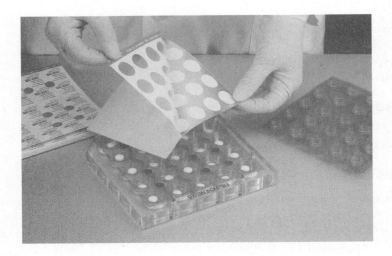

Figure 10-3 Step 3

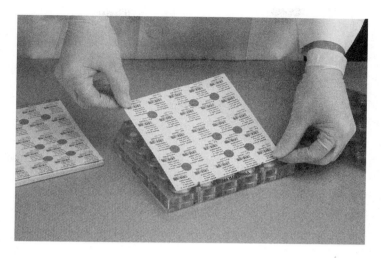

Figure 10-4 Step 4

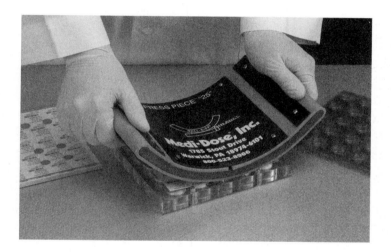

Figure 10-5 Step 5

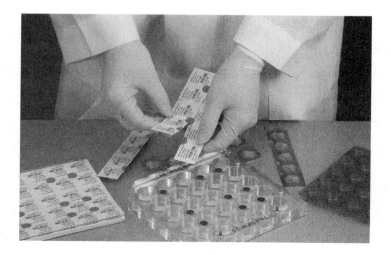

Figure 10-6 Step 6

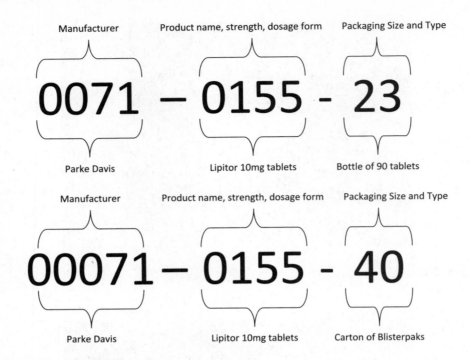

Figure 10-7 National Drug Code

expiration date of October 2015 means the drug is within date through the end of October. Documentation is important when repackaging and setting expiration dates. The pharmacy will use any one of these methods to assign a new expiration date to repackaged medications:

✓ Set the expiration date six months in the future or ¼ the time of the manufacturer's expiration date.
✓ Set the expiration date a maximum of one year into the future, as long as it does not exceed the safety margin given by the drug manufacturer.

Quality assurance (QA) of repackaging involves monitoring routine practices and making various checks throughout the repackaging and distribution process to ensure accuracy of filling and distribution. Pharmacy technicians may contribute to the process by collecting data and suggesting areas for improvement.

NATIONAL DRUG CODE

Every medication and medical product is assigned a National Drug Code (NDC) by the manufacturer. The NDC is a unique 10-digit number that identifies the product. Zeros may be added to the base NDC to allow for electronic configuration (**Figure 10-7**).

This is your checklist to make sure you understand what you need to know for the certification exam. Review chapter content if there is a topic you're uncertain of.
I know:

√	…labeling information found on a stock bottle; identify brand and generic name of drug, expiration date, lot number, drug strength.
	…what the drug NDC number is.
	…how to handle recalled medications.

	…procedures for receiving pharmacy stock.
	…possible reasons for drug shortages and how to respond to shortages and back-ordered drugs.
	…procedures to dispose of medications properly.
	…steps to repackage nonsterile drugs.
	…label requirements when unit dosing.
	…how to calculate expiration dating for repackaged medications.
	…the importance of checking stock bottle expiration dates when receiving and stocking inventory.
	…quality assurance procedures when repackaging.

RESOURCES

1. Congress approves prescription drug disposal legislation to curb abuse, encourage programs like NCPA's Dispose My Meds. September 30, 2010. National Community Pharmacist Association Website. Available at: www.ncpanet.org/index.php/news-releases/764-congress-approves-prescription-drug-disposal-legislation-to-curb-abuse-encourage-programs-like-ncpas-dispose-my-meds. Accessed January 2011.
2. Medi-Dose Inc.
3. US Office of National Drug Control Policy. *Prescription Drug Abuse*. Available at: http://www.whitehouse.gov/ondcp/prescription-drug-abuse. Accessed January 2011.

CHAPTER 10

MULTIPLE CHOICE

Identify the choice that best completes the statement or answers the question.

_____ **1.** A list of goods that the pharmacy stocks is termed

a. protocol

b. want list

c. inventory

d. supply

_____ **2.** Reordering from a predetermined optimum stock level is

a. perpetual inventory

b. periodic automatic replenishment (PAR)

c. turnover

d. formulary purchase

_____ **3.** The rate that inventory is used or sold

a. stock supply

b. purchase point

c. turnover

d. formulary rate

_____ **4.** An open formulary

a. puts limits on medications the pharmacy stocks

b. approves all FDA medications for stock

c. allows all medication dosage forms and strengths for stock supply

d. allows the manager discretion to stock prescribed medications

_____ **5.** Purchasing medications from the manufacturer

a. is common practice for pharmacies

b. occurs in special circumstances

c. is costly and time consuming for the pharmacy

d. is a one-stop shop for the pharmacy

_____ **6.** A listing of ordered stock received at the pharmacy is a

a. manifest

b. billable invoice

c. proven inventory

d. vendor receipt

_____ **7.** Medications should be stored

a. in direct sunlight

b. with no concern to humidity

c. in a cool, dark room

d. in an airtight container

_____ **8.** Federal pharmacy law defines room temperature as

a. 59°–86°F

b. 36°–46°F

c. 59°–66°F

d. 46°–59°F

_____ **9.** Federal pharmacy law defines refrigerator temperature as

a. 0°–32°F

b. 36°–46°F

c. 32°–36°F

d. 36°–59°F

_____ **10.** Special considerations are made for ordering, receiving, and storing

a. OTC medications

b. costly drugs

c. hazardous drugs

d. commonly used medications

ANSWER SECTION

1. C
2. B
3. C
4. D
5. B
6. A
7. D
8. A
9. B
10. C

TASK SHEET

TOPIC TO REVIEW: HAZARDOUS DRUGS

Materials

Pharmacy Technician Exam Review Guide

JB Test Prep: Pharmacy Technician Exam Review Guide

Prepare

1. Read section on hazardous drugs.
2. Take practice test at the end of the chapter.

Study Plan

1. Read pages_____ on _____(date).
2. Take end-of-chapter practice test on_____(date).
3. Make flash cards to help memorize hazardous drugs at quizlet.com.
4. (Add your individualized study plans) _____

Tips

1. Know special procedures and precautions to take when working with hazardous drugs.
2. Find out what hazardous drugs your pharmacy stocks.

End of Chapter

List what you need to review.

Hazardous Drugs

OBJECTIVES/TOPICS COVERED:

✓ List the purpose for proper handling of hazardous drugs.
✓ Summarize exposure guidelines.

Improper exposure to hazardous drugs may cause adverse health conditions to the pharmacy technician. Possible risks associated with hazardous drugs are cancer, organ toxicity, fertility problems, and birth defects. Exposure to hazardous drugs may occur in a number of situations.

✓ During drug compounding and preparation
✓ Transporting the drug to the patient care area
✓ During drug disposal process
✓ Spilling a drug

Exposure to hazardous drugs may occur by inhalation, injection, ingestion, and direct contact. While working with hazardous drugs in the biological safety cabinet, the pharmacy technician may unknowingly inhale toxic fumes either through vapor release due to inappropriate venting of the biological safety cabinet or through improper compounding technique. Inhalation can also occur after compounding when removing gloves or other garb. Ambulatory pharmacy technicians also have inhalation risks with the dust powder from oral tablets.

Injection exposure occurs from accidental needlesticks. Recapping needles used to compound hazardous drugs is an unsafe practice and not recommended. Needless systems or safety needles with self-capping mechanisms are better choices. If a needle must be recapped, use the single-hand sweep method. The single-hand sweep method is done by placing the needle cap on the counter top rather than holding the cap in the opposite hand. Once the needle tip is inside the cap, then use the opposite hand to secure the cap onto the needle and syringe.

Direct contact and ingestion are other routes of possible exposure to hazardous drugs. Direct contact may occur by touching doorknobs, telephones, tables, floors, or other surfaces that have been unknowingly contaminated. When drug contamination on your hand comes in contact with your mouth ingestion may occur. To help avoid ingestion and direct contact, keep gloves clean while in the compounding room. Remove the outer gloves anytime your hands leave the biologic safety cabinet (BSC). Before leaving the compounding room, remove gloves and garb.

SAFETY CONTROLS

Biological Safety Cabinet

Many pharmacies have a class II (type B) BSC for compounding hazardous drugs (**Figure 11-1**). The class II BSC has a vertical laminar airflow. Clean HEPA-filtered air moves from the top of the biological safety cabinet to the work surface area. Rather than "dirty" air blowing at the operator, the safety in laminar vertical airflow is that the intake grills on the work surface collect the air, and most of the air is then exhausted to the outside of the pharmacy. Class II BSCs should always be left running and are certified for quality control every six months by an agency other than the pharmacy.

Class III BSCs are totally enclosed and operate under negative pressure. These cabinets are also called glove boxes and isolators (**Figure 11-2**). The advantage of a totally enclosed cabinet is minimal risk exposure to the technician while compounding activities are performed within the hood. Compounding manipulations are performed through long, heavy-duty rubber gloves attached to the viewing window. When compounding in a glove box, the technician will still don gloves for maximum protection. The class III biological safety cabinet exhaust air is filtered before being released into the outdoor environment.

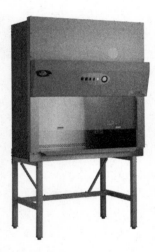

Figure 11-1 Biological Safety Cabinet

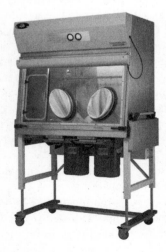

Figure 11-2 Isolator or Glove Box

Personal Protective Equipment

Personal protective equipment (PPE) is commonly called garb. These are the items that the technician wears, or dons, before aseptic compounding. PPE protects both the technician and the drug product.

✓ Powder-free, hazardous-rated nitrile gloves. Must be powder free as the powder may absorb contaminants.
✓ Double glove. The inner glove is placed under the gown sleeve, and the outer glove is placed over the gown cuff.
✓ Change gloves every hour or sooner if there is a puncture or tear or whenever contamination occurs.
✓ Polyethylene gowns of low-permeability fabric.
✓ Eye protection and face mask.
✓ Hair bouffant.
✓ Shoe covers.

Aseptic Technique

Pharmacy technicians must be trained in hazardous drug aseptic compounding. Aseptic technique for hazardous drugs requires extra steps to ensure safety for healthcare workers and the patient. First, all hazardous drugs must be compounded in a biological safety cabinet with airflow vented to the outside environment rather than blown toward the operator and released into the pharmacy. The biological safety cabinet is cleaned with a bleach solution and then disinfected with an alcohol solution.

After garbing and cleaning the biological safety cabinet, gather and stage all compounding supplies and drugs. Check the expiration dating on the drugs and sanitize vials before placing them in the cabinet. Place only necessary items in the BSC, leaving adequate space between each item to allow for airflow. Careful staging allows for fewer times in and out of the cabinet when compounding.

After compounding is completed and checked by the pharmacist, the admixture or final product is wiped down, labeled, and placed for delivery in a zip-lock bag labeled "hazardous."

Remember these key steps when compounding hazardous drugs:

✓ Use luer-lock syringes.
✓ Do not fill a syringe more than ¾ full of a hazardous drug.
✓ IV bags are spiked and primed *before* adding the hazardous drug.
✓ All waste, including wipes used for cleaning the BSC, syringes, needles, and drug vials, are disposed of in hazardous waste bags or containers.
✓ Change gloves every hour or whenever contamination occurs or if there is a suspected puncture or tear.
✓ Wash hands after removing gloves.
✓ Sharps containers and other waste receptacles are labeled as hazardous waste and are not overfilled.

SPILLS

Pharmacies that stock hazardous drugs (**Table 11-1**) will have a spill kit. The spill kit is a box of items used to clean a spill. The kit will have a hand broom and dustpan, wipes, trash bag, chemical deactivator, spill signs, and personal protective equipment, such as goggles, gowns, gloves, and a respirator. The most important thing is to know where the spill kit is kept and to be trained on how to use it! Large spills may require cleanup by a specially trained team.

A small spill is defined as less than 5 milliliters outside of the biological safety cabinet and less than 150 milliliters within the biological safety cabinet. If a hazardous drug spill inside the cabinet contaminates the HEPA (high-efficiency particulate air) filter, the cabinet should be turned off and not used until the filter is changed.

Table 11-1 Listing of Hazardous Drugs

Generic Name	Brand Names	Dosage Form	Classification/Use
tamoxifen	Nolvadex	Tablet	Antineoplastic used to treat breast cancer
methotrexate	Trexall, Rheumatrex	Tablet, injection	Antineoplastic used to treat certain types of cancer, severe psoriasis, rheumatoid arthritis
mitomycin	Mutamycin	Powder for solution of IV or injection	Antineoplastic antibiotic used to treat certain types of cancer
azathioprine	Imuran, Azasan	Tablet, injection	Immunosuppressive used to treat rheumatoid arthritis
bleomycin	Generic only	Powder for solution of injection	Antineoplastic
megestrol	Megace	Oral suspension, tablet	Antineoplastic used to treat certain types of cancer, anorexia, and weight loss in AIDS patients
ganciclovir	Cytovene, Zirgan, Vitrasert	Capsule, ophthalmic implant, powder for solution of injection and IV	Antiviral
vincristine	Vincasar PFS, Oncovin	Powder for solution, solution for IV, injection	Antineoplastic

Complete listing of hazardous drugs found at National Institute for Occupational Safety and Health.

EXPOSURE

Needlestick

It's natural to quickly pull the needle away if there is an accidental stick. However, try to remember to keep the needle in the skin and gently pull back on the plunger to remove any drug that might have penetrated into the skin tissue. Wash the affected area with soap and water and follow up with medical care. Give the Material Safety Data Sheet (MSDS) to the treating physician and remember to complete an incident report noting details of the needlestick.

Other Exposure

For other direct exposure, remove personal protective equipment and other clothing that may have been contaminated. Always wash affected area with soap and water unless otherwise indicated on the MSDS. There is no recommended amount of time to wash the exposed skin, but exposure to eyes recommendations are flushing eyes for 15 minutes with water or eyewash solution of normal saline. Follow up with medical care and always complete an incident report.

Technicians working in all pharmacy settings must be aware of safety measures in dealing with hazardous drugs. Hazardous drugs are not only available in IV form but also available in oral dosage form.

- ✓ Do not crush or split hazardous tablets.
- ✓ Wear hazardous-rated nitrile gloves when stocking and dispensing hazardous drugs.
- ✓ Use a counting tray designated for hazardous drugs.

This is your checklist to make sure you understand what you need to know for the certification exam. Review chapter content if there is a topic you're uncertain of.

I know:

√	...the most common drugs that require special handling procedures.
	...the rules to follow when compounding hazardous drugs.
	...how to respond to hazardous drug spills.

RESOURCES

1. National Institute for Occupational Safety and Health. *NIOSH List of Antineoplastic and Other Hazardous Drugs in Healthcare Settings 2010*. Available at: http://www.cdc.gov/niosh/docs/2010-167/. Accessed March 4, 2011.
2. American Society of Health–System Pharmacists. *Basics of Aseptic Compounding Technique*. Bethesda, MD: Author; 2006.

CHAPTER 11

MULTIPLE CHOICE

Identify the choice that best completes the statement or answers the question.

_____ **1.** Recapping needles

a. should be done quickly

b. is considered an unsafe practice

c. should be done using both hands

d. is a safe practice

_____ **2.** What directional airflow does a biological safety cabinet (BSC) have?

a. universal

b. horizontal

c. vertical

d. tridirectional

_____ **3.** Personal protective equipment includes

a. the biological safety cabinet (BSC)

b. garb

c. OSHA-mandated emergency equipment

d. spill kit

_____ **4.** A safety step when compounding hazardous drugs is to

a. never be in the compounding room alone

b. not fill a syringe more than 3/4 full

c. turn the BSC off immediately after compounding

d. prime IV tubing after adding the hazardous drugs to the bag

_____ **5.** When compounding hazardous drugs,

a. change gloves every hour or whenever contamination occurs

b. change gloves only if there is a suspected puncture or tear

c. change gloves whenever your hands leave the BSC

d. change gloves only if suspected contamination occurs

_____ **6.** A large spill of hazardous drugs is defined as

a. less than 150 mL within the BSC

b. more than 5 mL outside the BSC

c. less than 5 mL inside the BSC

d. more than 150 mL outside the BSC

_____ **7.** In the event of unintended exposure to a hazardous drug,

a. immediately report to the emergency department (ED)

b. flush the area with soapy water for 30 minutes

c. clean the affected area with isopropyl alcohol

d. wash the affected area with soap and water

_____ **8.** A necessary precaution for oral hazardous drugs is to

a. double-count the medication

b. use a separate counting tray designated for hazardous drugs

c. garb up and wear a respirator when counting

d. garb up and wear goggles when counting

_____ **9.** Mutamycin (mitomycin) is used to treat

a. rheumatoid arthritis

b. viral infection

c. certain types of cancer

d. weight loss in AIDS patients

_____ **10.** The generic name for Rheumatrex is

a. Trexall

b. megestrol

c. Megace

d. methotrexate

ANSWER SECTION

1. B

2. C

3. B

4. B

5. A

6. B

7. D

8. B

9. C

10. D

TASK SHEET

TOPIC TO REVIEW: EXTEMPORANEOUS COMPOUNDING

Materials

Pharmacy Technician Exam Review Guide

JB Test Prep: Pharmacy Technician Exam Review Guide

Prepare

1. Read the section on extemporaneous compounding.
2. Take practice test at the end of the chapter.

Study Plan

1. Read pages_____ on _____(date).
2. Take end-of-chapter practice test on_____(date).
3. View extemporaneous compounding equipment at www.gallipot.com.
4. Practice beyond use dating.

Tips

1. Seeing the extemporaneous compounding equipment will help you learn whether this is a topic you're not familiar with. Be sure to take the time to look at the suggested Study Plan websites.
2. Subscribe to a weekly electronic newsletter from *Compounding Today* or visit the website to learn more about extemporaneous compounding at compoundingtoday.com.
3. Another reference website to broaden your learning is the International Journal of Pharmacy Compounding at www.ijpc.com.

End of Chapter

List what you need to review.

Extemporaneous Compounding

OBJECTIVES/TOPICS TO COVER:

✓ Explain the basic concepts of USP Chapter <795>.
✓ Recognize equipment and supplies used in nonsterile compounding.
✓ List steps and procedure followed in nonsterile compounding.

WHAT IS EXTEMPORANEOUS COMPOUNDING?

To understand extemporaneous compounding, it's important to understand the difference between compounding, repackaging, and manufacturing. Repackaging is taking medication from a bulk package and putting that medication into smaller, unit dose packages. Manufacturing is mass producing a medication to be distributed to the public. And compounding is preparing or making a medication in the pharmacy for a patient. Pharmacy compounding is identified as either sterile compounding or nonsterile compounding. This chapter covers nonsterile compounding, which is referred to as *extemporaneous compounding*.

Extemporaneous compounding is the preparation, mixing, assembling, packaging, and labeling of a drug as a result of a licensed practitioner's prescription drug order. Extemporaneous compounding is based on a triangular relationship between the patient who needs the medication, the pharmacist who prepares the medication, and the licensed practitioner who prescribes the medication. This triangular relationship separates compounding in the pharmacy for an individualized patient from bulk manufacturing for wide distribution.

The term *extemporaneous* means to act on the spur of the moment. Nonsterile extemporaneous compounding is done in the pharmacy after the receipt of an unsolicited prescription for an individual patient who is in need of the medication. The U.S. Food and Drug Administration (FDA) views traditional pharmacy compounding as taking an approved drug substance and making a new formulation to meet the medical needs of a specific patient. *United States Pharmacopeia* (USP) chapter <795> outlines pharmacy compounding of nonsterile preparations and is viewed as the authority in the subject matter.

Why Compound?

Nonsterile compounding is individualizing products to meet patient needs.

✓ Children: Many commercial medications are formulated for adult dosages and strength. A medication may be compounded to suit the dosing needs of a child or pediatric patient.
✓ Elderly: A commercially available capsule may be compounded into a suspension dosage form that's easier for the elderly patient to swallow.

✓ Dermatological patients: Some dermatology creams contain dyes, scents, or preservatives that the patient may be allergic to. A preservative-free dermatological cream can be compounded so that the patient responds better to it.

✓ Menopausal patients: Hormone replacement therapy (HRT) is customized to replace the hormones that the body no longer makes. Compounding special orders helps get the right dose and strength of hormone needed.

✓ Hospice patients: Special dosage forms are compounded for patient compliance. For example, medicated lollipops for mouth sores and suppositories for unresponsive patients.

✓ Veterinary patients: Racehorses and dogs receive specially formulated vitamins and nutrition. An antibiotic can be compounded into a biscuit form with chicken flavoring to entice a household pet to swallow the medication. Topical applications are compounded for animals difficult to administer medication to.

Because a compounded medication is individualized for the patient, it may have a type of placebo effect on the patient. The patient sees the physician prescribe something especially for him or her, and the pharmacy makes the medication especially for him or her, so the patient is psychologically beginning to feel better.

Compounding Versus Manufacturing

The FDA Modernization Act of 1997 provides updated definitions and regulations in pharmacy compounding. According to the FDA, a pharmacy is not regulated in the same manner as a drug manufacturer and therefore cannot have a large-scale production of drug products.

Nonsterile compounding…

✓ …is preparing a special medication for a specific patient.
✓ …requires a valid order from a licensed prescriber.
✓ …originates from triangle involvement.
✓ …is making drug products, strengths, dosage forms that are not available from a manufacturer. The pharmacy cannot compound drug products that are copies of commercially available drugs. The pharmacy cannot compound a drug product that has been withdrawn from the market.
✓ …products made by one pharmacy cannot be sold to other pharmacies.

Manufacturing…

✓ …is bulk compounding for nationwide distribution.
✓ …involves advertising.
✓ …involves making generic copies of approved products already on the market.
✓ ….companies will sell their drug product to wholesale companies for distribution.

EXTEMPORANEOUS COMPOUNDING EQUIPMENT

✓ Prescription balance: A class A torsion balance weighs up to 120 grams. Tweezers are used to place the weights on the right pan. Weighing boats are used to hold the substance being weighed in the left pan.

✓ Electronic balance: Electronic balances are more sensitive than a class A balance. An electronic balance will give a more accurate reading for smaller measurements than a class A balance.

✓ Mortar and pestle: The mortar is the bowl, and the pestle is the utensil used to mix or grind. Mortars and pestles come in a variety of sizes and are made of ceramic, glass, and marble **(Figure 12-1).**

✓ Graduated cylinders: Graduated cylinders are used for liquid measure. They are made out of plastic or glass and come in a variety of sizes. For the most accurate measurement, use the graduated size closest to the amount to be measured. Always measure at eye level, bending

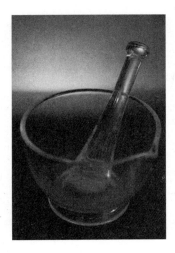

Figure 12-1 Mortar and Pestle

and lowering your eyes to tabletop level for measuring rather than *lifting* the graduate off the table to your eye level. Measure from the bottom of the meniscus.

✓ Spatulas: Spatulas are used to mix ointments and creams and to manipulate dry goods. Spatulas come in different sizes and are made out of hard rubber, stainless steel, or Teflon.

✓ Molds: Molds are used to make tablets, suppositories, lollipops, troches, and lozenges. They may be made out of disposable material or aluminum.

✓ Capsules: Capsules range in size from 000 to 13. Capsule sizing is inversely proportional, which means the size 000 capsules are actually larger and hold a greater quantity of medication than the size 13 capsules. Capsules are made out of gelatin and can be clear or colored. The two parts to the capsule are called the cap and the body.

✓ Pipettes: Pipettes are used for measuring small amounts of liquid. A pipette can be made out of glass or disposable plastic.

✓ Ointment slab: An ointment slab is made out of glass or porcelain and used to mix ointments and other semisolid formulations.

✓ Parchment paper: As in your kitchen at home, parchment paper makes for easier clean up after compounding and is used to help prepare products, such as rolling suppositories.

COMPOUNDING STEPS

Extemporaneous compounding should be performed only by trained individuals in an area of the pharmacy away from mainstream activity, such as a back room. The compounding area should be well lit with temperature and humidity control and sufficient space to allow for organization.

Good manufacturing procedure (GMP) is followed as much as possible by keeping the area as clean as possible. To minimize error, perform compounding steps within the pharmacy's standard operating procedures (SOP).

1. Perform necessary calculations.
2. Gather equipment and supplies such as USP-approved drug ingredients, labels, and final preparation containers.
   a. Routinely calibrate equipment and keep records of calibration.
   b. Clean equipment after each use to avoid cross-contamination and keep records of cleaning.
3. Don garb.
4. Wash hands.

5. Compound only one prescription at a time.

6. Follow the formulation record when compounding.

The pH range is 0–14. 7 is neutral. A pH above 7 is alkaline; lower than 7 is acidic.

Blood = pH 7

Distilled water = pH 7

Orange juice = pH 3

Vinegar = pH 2

Stomach acid = pH 0

---

7. Assess the final product for correct weight, clarity, color, odor, pH, and consistency.

8. Record information about the formulation in the logbook:
  a. Date preparation compounded
  b. Name, strength, dosage form of final preparation
  c. Ingredients used, lot numbers, and amount of ingredients
  d. Equipment used and description of mixing
  e. Beyond use date assigned, storage requirements, and final container used to package the preparation
  f. Quality control procedures such as verification of checking for clarity

9. Package and label the final preparation with:
  a. Name of preparation
  b. Internal lot or batch number assigned to the preparation
  c. Beyond use date
  d. Storage requirements
  e. Initials of certified pharmacy technician or registered pharmacist who compounded the preparation

10. Pharmacist will check the compounded preparation before customer pickup.

11. Pharmacy must properly store the preparation while waiting for customer pickup.

BEYOND USE DATING

Beyond use dates are different from expiration dates. According to USP <795>, the beyond use date is the date after which a compounded preparation is not to be used, and is determined from the date the preparation is compounded.

The manufacturer expiration dates are based on extensive stability testing and are normally set years into the future. Each ingredient used in the final compounded preparation has a different expiration date that was assigned by the manufacturer. The beyond use date set in the pharmacy for the final compounded preparation is no later than 25% of the time remaining until the ingredients used in the formulation expire or six months into the future, whichever date is earlier. The maximum beyond use date is six months.

When water is added to a solid form, the beyond use date is no later than 14 days if the product is refrigerated.

EXTEMPORANEOUS COMPOUNDING TERMS

You should be familiar with common terminology used with extemporaneous compounding.

Preparations will be compounded with the active drug and *inert* or inactive ingredients. An *excipient*, such as flavorings and preservatives, are inert substances added to a preparation to give the desired consistency or form, stability, and effectiveness.

Geometric dilution is a method of adding equal amounts of active and inactive ingredients together to ensure uniformity in mixing.

Trituration and *levigation* are usually done with a mortar and pestle to make a finer powder.

Levigation is also termed wet grinding and involves mixing a solution with the powder to form a paste and then reducing the particle size of the powder by grinding.

Solubilization is dissolving a substance into a solvent. The solvent may be heated to increase the temperature and therefore increase the solubility. An example of solubilization is dissolving a scent into a lotion. The lotion is the *solvent*, and the scent is the *solute*, or the substance being added. To better understand the difference between a solute and a solvent, relate the terms to chocolate milk. The solvent is the milk, and the solute is the chocolate syrup.

This is your checklist to make sure you understand what you need to know for the certification exam. Review chapter content if there is a topic you're uncertain of.
I know:

√	...the importance of calibrating compounding equipment.
	...steps to take when compounding that help ensure accuracy.
	...the difference between beyond use date and expiration date.
	...how to calculate beyond use date.
	...labeling requirements for compounded preparations.

RESOURCES

1. 2010 US Pharmacopeial Convention. Used with permission.

CHAPTER 12

MULTIPLE CHOICE

Identify the choice that best completes the statement or answers the question.

_____ **1.** Extemporaneous compounding is

a. sterile

b. aseptic

c. nonsterile

d. repackaging

_____ **2.** Nonsterile compounding is

a. manufacturing products to extend the role of pharmacy practice

b. individualizing products to meet the needs of the patients

c. repackaging products to ensure safe distribution practices

d. labeling unit dose products to meet federal guidelines

_____ **3.** Extemporaneous compounding is preparing drug products

a. at a more affordable cost than charged by the manufacturer

b. in a sterile environment

c. that are not available from a manufacturer

d. for resale at pharmacy trade shows

_____ **4.** Which graduate size would best suit your needs for measuring 15 mL?

a. 25 mL

b. 50 mL

c. 100 mL

d. 150 mL

_____ **5.** When measuring liquid in a graduated cylinder, measure from the _____ of the meniscus.

a. darkest line

b. bottom

c. top

d. lightest line

_____ **6.** Which capsule size will hold more medication?

a. 13

b. 0000

c. 000

d. 15

_____ **7.** Calibrating equipment means

a. cleaning the equipment

b. performing a test on the equipment to make sure functions are accurate

c. testing the equipment against nonmechanical methods

d. turning the piece of equipment on for operational mode

_____ **8.** The beyond use date (BUD) is

a. the same as the expiration date

b. determined by the date the product is dispensed

c. the date after which a compounded preparation is not to be used

d. the sum of the manufacturers' expiration dates for products used in the preparation

_____ **9.** What is the most accurate BUD for a product compounded on April 3, 2011?

a. October 2011

b. September 2011

c. April 2012

d. April 17, 2011

_____ **10.** What are inert ingredients?

a. active ingredients

b. inactive ingredients

c. passive ingredients

d. unsaturated ingredients

_____ **11.** Flavoring and preservative added to medications are examples of

a. active ingredients

b. excipients

c. binders

d. placebos

_____ **12.** The compounding formulation directs 30 g of derma-bond to be dissolved in 500 mL of gel base. Derma-bond is the

a. inert ingredient

b. solute

c. solvent

d. weighted-solution

ANSWER SECTION

1. C
2. B
3. C
4. A
5. B
6. C
7. B
8. C
9. A
10. B
11. B
12. B

TASK SHEET

TOPIC TO REVIEW: ASEPTIC TECHNIQUE

Materials

Pharmacy Technician Exam Review Guide

JB Test Prep: Pharmacy Technician Exam Review Guide

Prepare

1. Read the section on aseptic technique.
2. Take practice test at the end of the chapter.

Study Plan

1. Read pages_____ on _____(date).
2. Take end-of-chapter practice test on_____(date).

Tips

1. If aseptic compounding is a topic you're not familiar with, call a local hospital pharmacy and ask to visit the pharmacy for a tour. Ask if you could possibly shadow another technician for a few hours. The best way to understand unfamiliar terms, procedures, and equipment is to actually see them in operation!
2. Buddy up with a technician who has experience in aseptic compounding. Professionals are always willing to share their knowledge to help others.

End of Chapter

List what you need to review.

Aseptic Technique

OBJECTIVES/TOPICS TO COVER:

✓ Identify supplies and equipment used in sterile compounding.
✓ Summarize sterile compounding procedures.
✓ Recall USP <797> information.
✓ Understand infection control procedures.
✓ Know what to look for on a vial label.

WHAT IS ASEPTIC TECHNIQUE?

Aseptic technique is sterile compounding procedures used to eliminate the possible contamination of a drug with microbes or particles. Aseptic technique involves the factors of:

✓ Proper manipulation of materials in the laminar airflow workbench (LAWB).
✓ Appropriate garb.
✓ Correct hand washing.
✓ Properly maintained clean room environment and equipment.

A medication that contains microbes can cause a dangerous infection or possibly death for the patient. Parenteral medications and some ophthalmic medications are prepared using aseptic technique. *Parenteral* medications are those that enter the bloodstream directly, such as intravenous (IV) medications.

Proper Manipulation

Hand placement within the LAWB is critical to sterile compounding practices. Proper technique or manipulation is when the technician handles materials without obstructing clean airflow. Depending on the type of LAWB, the airflow in the workbench may flow vertically or horizontally. The key to proper manipulation is that materials within a horizontal LAWB should be handled so that clean air flows over the critical sites unobstructed by the operator's hands. *Critical sites* are the parts of the materials and supplies that come in contact with the medication and will therefore come in contact with the patient. The critical site of the vial is the rubber stopper where medication is withdrawn. The critical site on the syringe is the plunger that touches medication. The entire needle is a critical site. Do not touch the critical sites.

Manipulations within the flow hood should be intentional and well directed. This means no erratic hand movements inside the flow hood that will cause a disruption of airflow. Pharmacy technicians are expected to perform aseptic manipulations meticulously.

Garb

Garb is the personal protective equipment (PPE) worn in the clean room while performing sterile compounding tasks. Shoe covers, gown, hair bouffant, face mask, beard cover, goggles, and gloves are garb. Garb is worn in the clean room to lessen the likelihood of particles falling off the technician's street clothes and shoes as well as skin and hair fibers that would contaminate the medication. Garb is clean, whereas street clothes will have particles. Garb also serves as personal protective equipment for the technician.

Hand Washing

Hands are a large source of contamination, and so strict hand-washing procedures must be followed in the compounding pharmacy. Hands are thoroughly washed and scrubbed and nails are cleaned in the anteroom prior to entering the clean room. An *anteroom* is the preparation room adjacent to the clean room where garbing and hand washing occur and where medications and supplies are kept. Gloves are donned after hand washing.

Once the technician is gowned and gloved and has entered the clean room, gloves are disinfected before performing compounding manipulations within the flow hood. Anytime the technician's hands leave the hood, to reach for a supply off the cart, for instance, the gloves must be re-disinfected with sterile 70% isopropyl alcohol before continuing with work inside the flow hood. Just as we wash our hands often when we cook a meal at home, we must disinfect our gloved hands often when working in the flow hood.

CLEAN ROOM ENVIRONMENT AND EQUIPMENT

The humidity, temperature, and air pressure of the clean room are all factors in sterile compounding and are therefore monitored and regulated. Clean rooms are commonly of positive pressure unless hazardous drugs are being compounded wherein negative room pressure is desired.

According to International Standards Organization (ISO), there are nine levels of clean rooms based on particle counts within 1 cubic meter of room air. A class 1 clean room is the highest level, or the cleanest level, of clean rooms, while a class 8 allows a maximum of 100,000 particles per cubic meter. Clean rooms must be a minimum ISO 7, which is 10,000 particles per square meter.

The clean room, also referred to as the *buffer room*, must meet cleanliness specifications. The floors, walls, ceilings, and shelving must all be kept clean, and documentation of cleaning must be kept.

Large equipment used in the clean room, known as the *primary engineering controls*, consists of laminar airflow workbenches, which are commonly called *hoods*, or *flow hoods*. Laminar airflow means that the airflow is even and constant. The technician must perform aseptic procedures at least 6 inches inside the horizontal airflow hood and place supplies at least 3 inches from the sidewalls of the cabinet (**Figure 13-1**). In a horizontal hood, clean air moves across the workbench from the high-efficiency particulate air (HEPA) filter in the back of the hood to the operator/pharmacy technician standing at the front of the hood.

In a vertical laminar airflow hood, clean air comes from the top of the hood down to the workbench. Glove boxes, biological safety cabinets (BSC), and isolators all have a vertical laminar airflow.

The type of flow hood used in the pharmacy depends on the type of drug being compounded. Hazardous drugs are compounded in a vertical flow hood, because the airflow is vented away from the operator/technician.

Automix compounders and repeater pumps are examples of smaller equipment used in the compounding pharmacy (**Figure 13-2** and **13-3**). All equipment, large and small, must be calibrated, tested for accuracy, cleaned, and maintained. The pharmacy must always keep documentation of equipment maintenance. The rule is, if you do it, document it. If it isn't documented, you didn't do it.

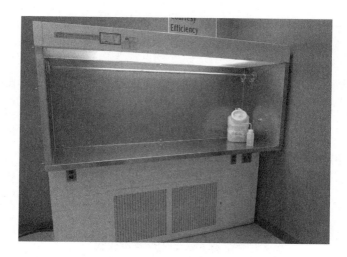

Figure 13-1 Horizontal LAWB

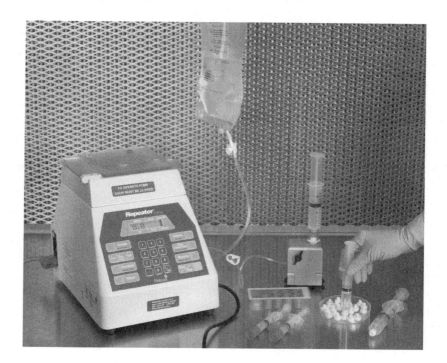

Figure 13-2 Repeater Pump Syringe Filling

Clean room rules to remember:

- ✓ No food or drink. No gum chewing.
- ✓ No pencils.
- ✓ No cardboard.
- ✓ Jewelry removed. No makeup. No artificial nails.
- ✓ No erratic hand movements in the hood.

USP <797>

United States Pharmacopoeia (USP) Chapter <797> was released in January 2004, creating a new national standard for sterile preparations. This standard describes the best practice for quality

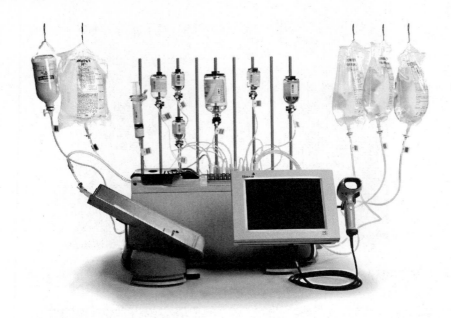

Figure 13-3 Baxa EM2400 Compounder

assurance in sterile compounding. Staff of sterile compounding sites were given time to learn the new rules and to train staff on procedures. The last step in compliance was for pharmacies to have their physical site changes made to comply with anteroom and clean room regulations. Sterile compounding pharmacies were to be fully compliant with <797> regulations by 2008.

USP <797> is looked on as the authority in sterile compounding, and many states model their state rules and regulations after USP <797> guidelines. USP <797> requirements are as follows:

- ✓ There should be a separate area in the pharmacy for sterile compounding. Best controls consist of:
    - ○ an isolated positive or negative pressure clean room; however, the clean room does not have to be a separate room; it can be a separate *area* of the pharmacy
    - ○ a separate anteroom
- ✓ There are basic steps in aseptic compounding technique. Best controls consist of:
    - ○ proper hand-washing
    - ○ gowning or garbing
    - ○ using a LAFW
    - ○ proper manipulations within the LAFW

Supplies

Part of understanding sterile compounding is understanding the supplies and equipment used.

- ✓ *IV solution bags*, or polyvinyl chloride (PVC) flexible bags, come in a variety of sizes with different solutions (**Table 13-1**). The IV bag has two ports: one is the outlet port that the administration set is attached to. The *administration set* is IV tubing used to administer the medication from the IV bag to the patient. The other port on the IV bag is a site for the technician to add medication into the bag. Key points to remember about IV bags are as follows:
    1. *Normal saline* (NS) is commonly referred to as 0.9% *sodium chloride* (NaCl): 9 grams of sodium per 1 liter of water.

2. The *diluent* is the solution used to reconstitute medication. Sterile water (SW) and NS are common diluents.
3. *An isotonic* solution has the same or almost the same concentration of solutes as blood, whereas a *hypertonic* solution is more concentrated (has a higher salt content) than blood. A *hypotonic* solution has a lower salt content than blood.
4. A small volume parenteral (SVP) is less than 250 milliliters. A large volume parenteral (LVP) is 250 milliliters or more.
5. An immediate use compounded sterile product (CSP) has a beyond use date (BUD) of 1 hour. Please refer to **Table 13-1** for types of solutions used in preparing admixtures.

✓ A *piggyback* is a small volume parenteral (SVP) that is added to or *piggybacked* to the main IV therapy that the patient is receiving. Many antibiotics are prepared as piggybacks.

Table 13-1 Types of Solutions Used for Preparing Parenteral Admixtures

Solution Name	Volume Availability	Solution Content	Example of Use
NS	50 mL (mini) 100 mL (mini) 150 mL 250 mL 500 mL 1000 mL	0.9% normal saline or 0.9% sodium chloride	*Isotonic* Dehydration Reconstituting
D5/NS	250 mL 500 mL 1000 mL	5% dextrose in normal saline	*hypertonic* Hydration for patients who are not eating
½ NaCl	500 mL 1000 mL	1/2 normal saline (0.45% sodium chloride) often called ½ normal saline because "full" normal saline is 0.9%; one-half of 0.9 is 0.45. NaCl = salt	*Isotonic* Diluent May be given to patients with low levels of Na or Cl
LR	250 mL 500 mL 1000 mL	Lactated ringers containing Na, K, Ca, Cl	*Isotonic* Large-volume fluid replacement
SW	Vials, bottles, flexible and plastic containers ranges from 50 to 2000 mL	Sterile water Distilled water	*Hypotonic (isotonic when drug is added)* Reconstitute Irrigation, hydration, vehicle for drug distribution
D5W	250 mL 500 mL 1000 mL	5% dextrose in water commonly referred to as "dextrose"	*Isotonic* Used if the patient is at risk for having low blood sugar or high sodium
D10W	250 mL 500 mL 1000 mL	10% dextrose in water	*Hypotonic* Used if the patient is at risk for having low blood sugar or high sodium
D5 ½ NS with 20 mEq KCl	500 mL 1000 mL	20 mEq/L potassium chloride in 5% dextrose and 0.45% sodium chloride	*Hypotonic* Treatment of potassium deficiency

✓ A *port saver* is used to spike IV bags for repeated access. To *spike* an IV bag means that the technician is inserting the spiked or sharp end of the port saver into the medication port of the IV bag. Rule of thumb is that the medication port on the IV bag should not be breached or entered more than three times.

✓ *Vials* are made out of plastic or glass and are single dose or multidose. The medication in the vial is sterile. To withdraw medication, a needle is inserted into the rubber stopper located at the top of the vial. The USP has set forth new labeling standards on vials. Manufacturers will now imprint cautionary statements describing life-threatening risks on the cap overseal of the vial. The beyond use date (BUD) for multidose vials is 28 days. When compounding for a patient with a latex allergy, the rubber stopper of the vial should be completely removed from the vial prior to withdrawing medication.

✓ *Ampules* are made out of glass and are most often used for single-dose purposes (**Figure 13-4**).

✓ An *ampule breaker* is a plastic piece inserted over the neck of the ampule to aid in breaking open the neck of the ampule.

✓ The *syringe* is used for withdrawing medication from a vial or ampule and then instilling medication into the IV bag. Syringes come in a variety of sizes, holding less than 1 milliliter of solution and as much as 60 milliliters of volume. Luer-lock-tension syringes in which the needle is locked into place are most common. The barrel of the syringe has the calibration markings, and the plunger fits inside the barrel. When measuring medication, align the end to the plunger closest to the needle with the correct calibration mark on the barrel (**Figure 13-5**).

✓ Sometimes the pharmacy will pull up medication into the syringe for a nurse to administer it directly to the patient from the syringe. In these cases *syringe caps* are used to cap off the luer-lock end of the syringe.

✓ A *repeating syringe* relates to dose setting and allows for repetitive injection of a prepro-grammed dose amount. Repeating syringes may be used for batch compounding. *Batch compounding* is when many of the same admixtures, or final products, are made at once.

✓ *Needles* are fitted into the syringe and used to draw solutions into the syringe. The hub of the needle is fitted into the syringe by twisting the luer-lock syringe into place while holding the needle in the protective wrapping. The actual needle should never be touched. Needles and syringes transfer liquid medication from one source to another. Needles are distinguished by their length and their gauge. Needles with a larger bore size (*gauge*) are used in pharmacy. The bore of the needle is also called the needle *lumen* and is the hollow part of the needle. The smaller the gauge, the larger the size of the bore. A 1 ½-inch 17-, 18-, or 19-gauge needle is common in the compounding pharmacy, as these larger bore sizes allow for quicker medication draws. Filter needles are used when compounding with medications coming from an

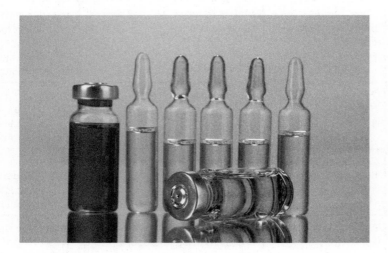

Figure 13-4 Vial and Ampule

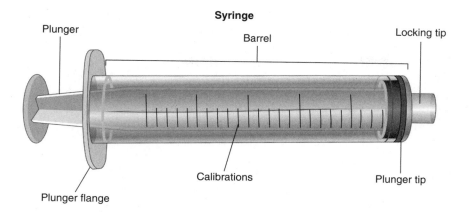

Syringe

Plunger

Barrel

Locking tip

Calibrations

Plunger tip

Plunger flange

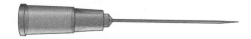

Needle without filter

Needle with filter

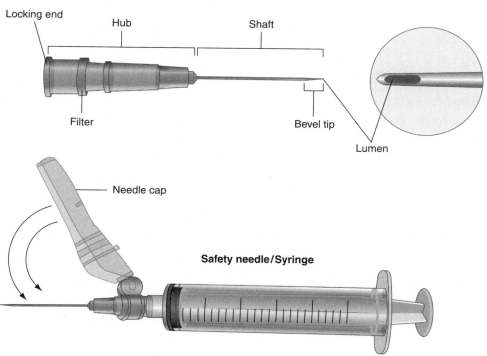

Locking end

Hub

Shaft

Filter

Bevel tip

Lumen

Needle cap

Safety needle/Syringe

Syringe
Barrel - clear part with calibrated measurements
Plunger - the sterile, movable part inside the barrel, measurement is made from the flat rubber end
Locking tip - sterile end where needle is attached or locked into place

Needle
Hub - proximal end of the needle that attaches or locks into the syringe, color-coded according to needle gauge, may or may not contain a filter
Shaft - needle length
Bevel - slanted edge of the needle
Lumen - the opening and hollow barrel inside the needle

Safety needle/syringe
Allows for safe needle re-capping: After using the needle/syringe assembly, press the needle cap over the needle until it locks into place.

Figure 13-5 Needle and Syringe

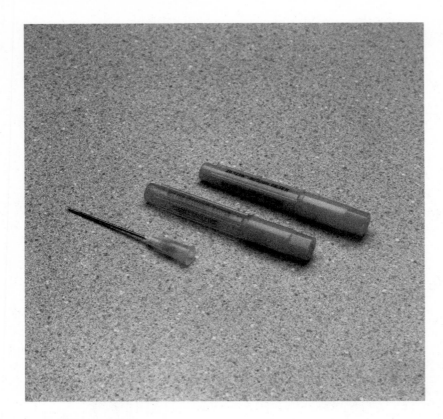

Figure 13-6 Filter Needles

ampule. The filter needle will filter out glass fragments that may have gotten in the medication when the neck of the ampule was snapped off (**Figure 13-6**).

Use	Common Needle Size Used
Subcutaneous (SQ) injection	30 gauge, ½ inch length needle
Intradermal (ID) injection	25 gauge, ⅜ inch length needle
Intramuscular (IM) injection	20 gauge, ½ inch length needle
Intravenous (IV)	20 gauge, 1 ½ inch length needle
Admixture compounding	19 gauge, 1 ½ inch length needle

✓ *Dispensing pins* are used to withdraw medication from vials. When using a multidose vial in which multiple entries will be made into the vial to extract medication, dispensing pins improve aseptic compounding processes by reducing the risk of touch contamination, protecting the medication integrity, and by reducing opportunity for drug loss. Dispensing pins also help to reduce the chance of coring. *Coring* is when small fragments of the vial's rubber stopper may shed into the medication when the needle is inserted into the vial. Coring is not good, and proper needle insertion will help reduce coring. Dispensing pins will also help reduce the chance of coring, because the vial's rubber stopper is penetrated only once by the spike on the dispensing pin rather than multiple times with a needle (**Figure 13-7**).

✓ *Tubing* is a broad term that applies to IV tubing to administer medication to the patient as well as to tubing sets used to transfer medication from one source to another. Accessory items used with tubing include

    ✓ *Male/female adapters* that fit on each end of the tubing to allow for tubing extension.

    ✓ *Clamps* used to close off the tubing so that fluid doesn't run through the tubing while compounding. There are different types of clamps: roller, pinch, and slide.

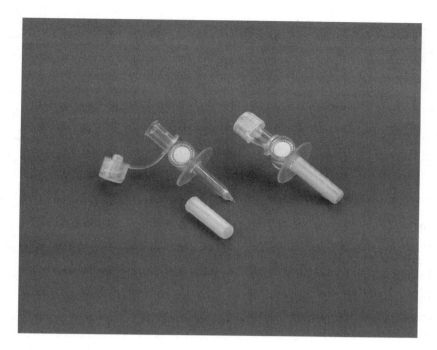

Figure 13-7 Dispensing Pin

✓   A *crimper* used to close off the tubing or to pinch the tubing closed to prevent leaking.

✓   An *evacuated container* is a glass container that has had all of the air vacuumed, or evacuated, out of it to ensure sterility within the container. Evacuated containers range in size from 150 cubic centimeters to 1000 cubic centimeters. The container has a plastic handle that lifts away from the bottle, which allows the bottle to hang from an IV pole. There are graduated markings either embossed in the glass or printed on the label (depending on manufacturer/ maker of the container). The graduated markings allow for reading the container contents while the bottle is inverted (hung from a pole) or sitting upright. Doses of many different medications may be combined into the bulk-evacuated container, such as *pooling* electrolytes for parenteral nutrition.

✓   *Sharps receptacle* is used to dispose of compounding waste, such as needles, syringes, ampules, and alcohol wipes. The sharps container has a fill line and for safety reasons should never be filled above that line. Hazardous waste is disposed of in a separate, specially labeled sharps receptacle.

✓   The most common *antiseptic* is sterile 70% isopropyl alcohol used to disinfect the LAWB. Sterile 70% isopropyl alcohol is used to wipe down ampules and vials and to disinfect gloved hands.

✓   *PCA* and *CAD pumps* are pieces of equipment used to administer IV medication to the patient. Patient-controlled analgesia (PCA) pumps and controlled analgesia device (CAD) pumps have a medication-filled cartridge that locks to prevent patient tampering. The pharmacy will fill the cartridge with pain medication and then program the pump to deliver a set amount of medication according to the prescriber's orders (**Figure 13-8**).

STEPS TO COMPOUND AN IV MEDICATION

1. The pharmacist receives the physician's order.
2. The pharmacist will check over the order for accuracy. Both the pharmacist and the technician should always be sure the order includes all the necessary patient and drug information. Does the ordered medication make sense for the patient's diagnosis? Is the ordered medication strength and quantity reasonable for the patient's age and weight?
3. The technician performs necessary compounding calculations. The pharmacist will check calculations.

Table 13-2 The Following Steps Where Aseptic Practices Begin

4. **Gather equipment** and supplies needed to compound the order.	
5. **Garb** up in the anteroom. Wear shoe covers, hair bouffant, and face mask. Goggles and beard cover may be necessary.	
6. **Hand washing** should include scrubbing and cleaning under nails and washing to the elbows. Hand washing occurs in the anteroom. A nonshedding gown is donned after hand washing.	
7. **Don sterile gloves**. Make sure to have a good glove fit to allow for proper movement with finite objects.	
8. **Stage supplies** before entering the clean room by checking medications for expiration dating and clarity. Check with the order sheet to be sure the right medication was pulled. Wipe down vials and ampules with an alcohol wipe. Enter the clean room with order sheet, medications to be compounded, and supplies.	
9. **Clean and disinfect the LAWB**. Clean and disinfect from the back of the hood (by the HEPA filter) to the front of the hood (where the technician stands). Clean from the top of the hood (ceiling) to the bottom of the hood (workbench). Wipe in broad strokes, being careful not to contaminate an area that has already been wiped clean. Wipe from back to front and top to bottom. The hood is running while cleaning and should run for at least 30 minutes prior to compounding.	
10. **Place the medication and supplies in the flow hood in a logical order of use so that clean air is reaching critical sites**. In a *horizontal air flow hood*, place items close to the clean air coming from the HEPA filter. All items should be placed in a line parallel with the HEPA filter. Work 6 inches inside the hood and 3 inches from the sides. Space items to allow for airflow. Do not place an item behind another item, called *shadowing*, which will obstruct the clean air from reaching the item in the shadow. In a *vertical air flow hood*, place items in a checkerboard pattern to allow HEPA-filtered air coming from the top of the hood to reach each critical site. Avoid placing items in the middle of the workbench, also known as the *zone of confusion*, because of turbulent airflow. The middle of the workbench is the area of *smoke-split*, where the airflow divides and moves to either side of the workbench. It's wrong to place supplies directly in the middle of the vertical airflow hood, because clean air is obstructed.	
11. **Disinfect gloved hands** with sterile isopropyl alcohol and allow hands to dry before compounding. Gloves are redisinfected at regular intervals and each time hands leave and reenter the hood. Gloves are changed if there is a suspected tear.	
12. **Compound** IV medication using correct aseptic technique. Do not obstruct clean airflow to the critical sites. Do not touch critical sites.	
13. **Label** the admixture or the final product.	
14. **Label** multidose vials and opened containers. Seal for **storage**.	
15. **Visual inspection** of the final product. The admixture is clear in color and has no particles.	
16. **Final check** is made by the pharmacist (or technician in *tech check tech* institutions) before delivery to the patient care unit.	
17. Complete compounding **documentation**, including additive lot numbers and expiration dates, calculations, and base solutions used.	
Notes: Garb is removed in the anteroom. Garb should not be worn in the general pharmacy area. When first reporting to work, the pharmacy technician should mop down the clean room. The technician is responsible for periodic cleaning of the anteroom and the clean room.	

HEPA, high-efficiency particulate air; LAWB, laminar airflow workbench.

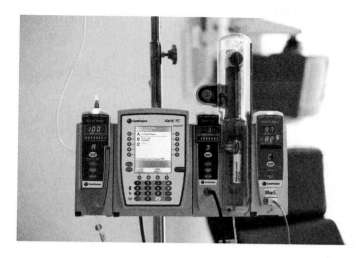

Figure 13-8 Alaris

Patient Name_____ID#_____Rm#_____

BASE SOLUTION:

Drug Additive	Strength	Amount

Start Date_____Start Time_____

Infusion Rate_____

Expiration Date/Time_____
Prepared By_____Date_____Time_____

Figure 13-9 Final Preparation/Admixture Label

Labeling

After compounding is completed, labels are applied to the final preparation admixture. Any vial to be used for more than one dose (multidose vial) must be labeled correctly (**Figure 13-9**). The label on the *final admixture preparation* should include the following:

- **a.** Patient's first and last name
- **b.** Patient room number or location
- **c.** Drug additive name and dose
- **d.** Solution name, strength, and volume
- **e.** Administration instructions:
  - **i** Date and time admixture is to be administered
  - **ii** Route
- **f.** Beyond use date
- **g.** Preparation date
- **h.** Storage instructions
- **i.** Initials of person preparing admixture
- **j.** Initials of person checking admixture

The label on the opened *multidose vial* should include the following:

    a. Date and time of reconstitution
    b. Beyond use date
    c. Diluent name and amount
    d. Final concentration
    e. Initials of the person who reconstituted the vial contents

Know how to read vial labels.

First, look at the name and strength of the drug on the vial label. Does it match your order? The vial label shown in **Figure 13-10** is for Cleocin Phosphate® 150 mg/mL. The generic name of the medication is clindamycin.

    Your checking process may include scanning the barcode on the label or verifying the NDC (National Drug Code) number.

    Next, read the instructions. Does this medication need to be reconstituted? Are there special instructions? The label tells you that the medication in this vial is for IM or IV use. If given intravenously, dilution is required.

    Check the expiration date to make sure the medication is within date. The lot number may need to be recorded in your compounding records.

    The label will also give storage instructions and beyond use date (BUD) information. This label indicates to store at room temperature. This is a multidose vial containing 60 milliliters, and the BUD is 24 hours after opening the vial.

How to Prime Tubing

To prime the tubing means that air is removed from the line, and the medication is brought into the tubing (**Tables 13-3** and **13-4**). Pharmacy personnel will prime the IV tubing for ease of administration on the nursing side.

Reconstituting

Reconstituting a drug is the same in an IV pharmacy as in a retail pharmacy in that a diluent is added to a powdered medication to make that powder into liquid form (**Table 13-5**). The difference is that in an IV pharmacy you are dealing with a sterile, closed-system pressurized vial rather than an open-system stock bottle. Steps are added when reconstituting a vial to maintain the closed-system pressure.

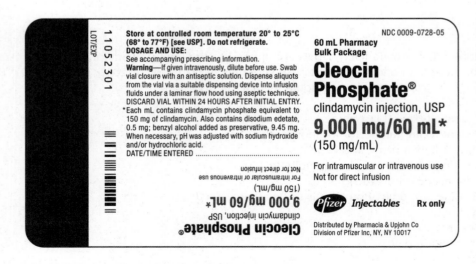

Figure 13-10 Multidose Vial Cleocin 60mL Label

Source: Courtesy of Pfizer

Table 13-3 How to Prime Tubing

Attach administration tubing before medication is added to the IV bag. Do this by:

1. Place the IV bag in first air. Remove plastic cover from administration port.
2. Remove cover from administration tubing set.
3. Close the clamp.
4. Insert the spike from the tubing into the port on the IV bag. Be sure the spike goes through the inner septum of the IV bag.
5. Hang the IV bag on the LAWB rod. Unfold the tubing.
6. **Prime the tubing:**
    7. Place the injection site (end) of the tubing over a cup. Remove the end cover. Remember this is a critical site and should be in first air.
    8. Open the flow regulator and clamps.
    9. Let the drip chamber and tubing fill with fluid. You may need to gently squeeze the IV bag. Prime IV tubing until all air is removed. When fluid drips out of injection end of tubing, clamp.
    10. Squeeze and release drip chamber until fluid level reaches the top of the filter.
    11. Completely close the flow regulator and clamps.
    12. Recap the tubing. Check to make sure the tubing is secure and not leaking by pressing on the IV bag.
    13. Fold the tubing up.

When compounding with hazardous drugs it is necessary to prime the tubing before the hazardous medications are added to the PVC bag.

Table 13-4 Steps to Using a Dispensing Pin

Be sure to perform the following steps in first air:

1. Remove the cap overseal from the top of the vial and swab the rubber stopper. Allow the alcohol to dry from the stopper.
2. Take the dispensing pin out of the protective covering. Remove the cover from the dispensing pin spike.
3. Insert spike firmly into the middle of the rubber stopper of the vial.
4. Add diluent for reconstituting, or withdraw medication from the vial by removing the dispensing pin cap.
5. Place dispensing pin cap face up in first air. This cap will be replaced on the dispensing pin and so must be kept as sterile as possible.
6. Twist the syringe into the dispensing pin hub. (There will not be a needle attached to the syringe.)
7. Remove the syringe after use by twisting off. Replace the dispensing pin cap.
8. Attach a syringe cap or a needle on the end of the syringe.

Note: The dispensing pin is not removed from the vial. The dispensing pin is discarded with the vial.

The *seesaw method* maintains vial pressure by adding air or diluent to the vial then withdrawing vial contents (air or solution) a little at a time, back and forth from syringe to vial.

Sample reconstitution directions for a single-dose vial.

For IM injection or IV infusion. Reconstitute with sterile water for injection according to the following table. SHAKE WELL.

Vial Size	Amount of Diluent	Concentration	Volume
1 g	3.5 mL	350 mg/mL	4 mL

Some medications are reconstituted using a patent-marked drug delivery system. For instance, cefazolin can be reconstituted by using the Duplex delivery system (**Figure 13-11**). The medication

Table 13-5 Reconstituting

Be sure to perform the following steps in first air:

1. Remove cap overseal from the diluent vial.
2. Swab the rubber stopper with an alcohol wipe. Allow the alcohol to dry.
3. Attach the needle to the syringe and pull the plunger to the calibration line a few milliliters less than the amount of diluent needed.
4. Insert the bevel tip of the needle into the rubber stopper at a 90-degree angle. The needle should be bowed as pressure is applied. Once the needle penetrates the rubber stopper, straighten the needle and syringe to a full 180 degrees.
5. Press down on the plunger to instill the air from the syringe into the vial. Do not force air or liquid into the vial against pressure; use the seesaw method instead.
6. Invert the vial; make sure the tip of the needle is in the diluent and pull back on the plunger to withdraw the correct amount of diluent.
7. Final measurements are made before withdrawing the needle from the vial.
8. Use correct technique to add the diluent to the powder vial for reconstitution. Powder is completely dissolved by swirling, shaking, or rolling the vial in the palms of your hands.

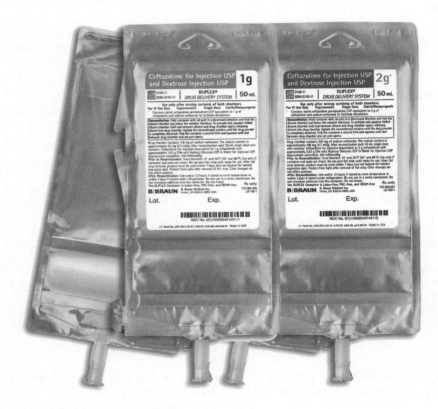

Figure 13-11 Duplex™ Delivery System

and the IV diluent solution are contained within different chambers of the same IV bag. The drug is activated when reconstituted or mixed with the IV diluent solution. The medication is administered to the patient from the same IV bag.

TPN COMPOUNDING

Total parenteral nutrition (TPN) is prepared for a patient who cannot take nutrition orally. Also known as *hyperalimentation*, or "hyperals," these large volume parenteral medications may be prepared for premature babies or patients who have had stomach or intestinal surgery or other conditions that affect the gastrointestinal system.

Each TPN bag is tailor-made for each patient according to the prescriber's orders. Since all TPNs contain dextrose and amino acids with lipids commonly added, the pharmacy may order TPN bags premixed with these ingredients. The technician would then add electrolytes and other medications according to the prescriber's order. Insulin and ranitidine are examples of medications that may be added to the bag.

Electrolyte	Abbreviation
Chloride	Cl
Sodium	Na
Potassium	K
Calcium	Ca
Magnesium	Mg
Bicarbonate	HCO_3

Preparing TPN is a sterile practice performed inside the LAWB. Some pharmacies use the gravity method, in which tubing is connected to the source container and leads to the final solution container (**Table 13-6**). Since gravity rather than a machine allows the transfer of fluid from one container to another, this can be a slow process. An automated TPN compounding machine will be used by pharmacies that frequently prepare a large number of bags. Automated compounding machines must be maintained and calibrated by the technician. *Calibration* steps designed by the manufacturer for the specific automated compounding device (ACD) ensure that the machine is measuring the correct volume.

INFECTION CONTROL

To ensure the health of employees and patients, the compounding pharmacy takes infection control very seriously. Help to keep the pharmacy clean and follow the institution's *policy and procedure* manual to comply with the rules of conduct. Infection control may include hand washing with special soaps to fight resistant bacteria. There may be limitations on prescribing antibiotics to lessen the chance of antibiotic resistance. And pharmacy personnel may need to wear special protective garb before entering an infectious patient's room.

Table 13-6 Steps to Preparing a Total Parenteral Nutrition (TPN) by Gravity Method

Be sure to perform the following steps *aseptically* in first air:	
1. Select an empty polyvinyl chloride (PVC) bag for the final container. (Your pharmacy may carry specialty gravity TPN PVC bags that have the tubing transfer sets preattached.)	
2. Attach the transfer tubing to the final container. You may need to use Y-connectors to add leads to your tubing. Lay the container on the work surface of the hood.	
3. Hang each of the base TPN components from the bar in the hood. Clamp each lead on the tubing. Spike each component bag with the transfer tubing.	
4. Add the base components to the final container one at a time. Do this by unclamping the first lead and measure the volume as it leaves the source container. Clamp the lead/tubing when the desired volume is dispensed. Continue these steps to add each component to the final container.	
5. Add the components in the order as listed on the TPN order sheet. Note: Phosphate must be the first electrolyte and calcium is the last electrolyte added to the admixture.	
6. Remove spikes. Apply a seal to the ports. Crimp tubing as needed.	

QUALITY ASSURANCE

Quality assurance documents that the final product delivered for patient use is the best possible quality. The pharmacy will keep documentation that the technician has been trained in sterile compounding. *Validation testing* is performed to validate, or to prove, that the pharmacy technician is competent in sterile compounding skills and knowledge. Samples are taken from the fingertips of the gloves, from the workbench, and from product preparation to check for possible bacteria growth. Validation testing results of bacteria growth will warrant additional training for the pharmacy technician. This is an opportunity for the pharmacy technician to improve on compounding skills which will help ensure 100% compliance for patient safety.

This is your checklist to make sure you understand what you need to know for the certification exam. Review chapter content if there is a topic you're uncertain of.
I know:

√	...the most common types of sterile compounding solutions.
	...aseptic compounding steps.
	...requirements of a compounded sterile product label.
	...equipment used in sterile compounding.
	...how to maintain a clean environment when aseptically compounding.
	...the importance of checking and calibrating compounding equipment.
	...documentation guidelines for aseptic compounding.
	...sterile compounding quality assurance steps.

Appendix B shows a listing of webinars available through Baxa at www.baxa.com/webinars.

View these webinars to see sterile compounding equipment and procedures.

- ✓ "It's Not Just Food: The Importance of TPN for Patient Outcomes"
- ✓ "Regulatory Challenges to a Hazardous Drug Safety Program"
- ✓ "Improving Sterile Compounding Quality Through Automation"
- ✓ "Implementing a Regional Compounding Program for Compounded Sterile Preparations"

RESOURCES

1. *The United States Pharmacopeia–National Formulary*. USP chapter <797>.
2. CareFusion The Alaris System with Alaris PCA module. Or Alaris® PCA module.
3. Baxa
4. Pfizer

CHAPTER 13

MULTIPLE CHOICE

Identify the choice that best completes the statement or answers the question.

_____ **1.** Aseptic compounding is

a. nonsterile compounding

b. sterile compounding

c. repackaging

d. unit-dosing

_____ **2.** Aseptic technique

a. is required for nonsterile compounding

b. is a natural skill that cannot be learned

c. involves the use of a sterile room

d. involves proper hand manipulations within the LAWB

_____ **3.** According to federal pharmacy law, pharmacy technicians are

a. not permitted to compound IV medications

b. may compound IV medications after completion of a certified college course

c. permitted to compound IV medications

d. able to compound IV medications after completion of 1-year service at the pharmacy

_____ **4.** Medications used for sterile compounding

a. are packaged in vials, ampules, and PVC bags

b. are specially ordered from a compounding distributor

c. are packaged in blister packs and bubble wrap

d. are sterilized in the pharmacy before use

_____ **5.** The key to aseptic compounding is

a. to perform tasks quickly

b. to have the pharmacist observe all steps

c. to align materials in a straight row

d. to keep critical sites in clean air

_____ **6.** Another name for the clean room is the

a. anteroom

b. buffer room

c. sterile room

d. cold room

_____ **7.** Clean room garb is worn

a. to help decrease particle shedding from street clothes and skin

b. to keep the technicians' street clothes clean

c. as an extra precaution and not necessary on a daily basis

d. only when compounding hazardous drugs

_____ **8.** Materials should be placed at least _____ inside the LAWB.

a. 6 inches

b. 6 centimeters

c. 3 inches

d. 3 centimeters

_____ **9.** A multidose vial

a. should be discarded after the first draw

b. is used on a onetime basis

c. should be labeled with the beyond use date

d. can be used up to 1 year after opening

_____ **10.** Immediate use compounded sterile products (CSP)

a. have a 1-hour beyond use date

b. have a 24-hour beyond use date

c. expire in 28 days

d. must be administered within 5 minutes after compounding

ANSWER SECTION

1. B
2. D
3. C
4. A
5. D
6. B
7. A
8. A
9. C
10. A

TASK SHEET

TOPIC TO REVIEW: BASIC MATH REVIEW

Materials

Pharmacy Technician Exam Review Guide

JB Test Prep: Pharmacy Technician Exam Review Guide

Prepare

1. Read section on basic math review.
2. Take practice test at the end of the chapter.

Study Plan

1. Read pages_____ on _____(date).
2. Work sample problems in the chapter.
3. Take end-of-chapter practice test on_____(date).
4. Memorize Roman numerals.
5. Practice math problems and view an online tutorial at www.math.com.

Tips

1. You will be allowed to use a calculator on the exam, but it will be an on-screen calculator or one that is issued by the testing site. Don't be afraid to use a calculator when working the math problems in this chapter. Get used to the functions on the calculator.
2. It's important to have a handle on this basic math before moving on to more advanced pharmacy math. Study in small increments of time throughout the week: 1 hour on Monday, 1 hour on Wednesday, and so forth. Planning a 4-hour study session may become frustrating and may be more than you can retain.

End of Chapter

List what you need to review.

Assess

After completing the problems on the review test, check yourself with the answer key. Then, reread sections of this chapter for suggestions on problem solving. Spend more time reviewing the problems that you had difficulty with on the review test.

Hint: Show your work in solving the problems. This way you can refer to mistakes you may have made in solving the problem.

Hint: Do five problems and then take a break. If one set of problems stumps you, move on to the next set and come back to the difficult problem later.

Basic Math Review

OBJECTIVES/TOPICS TO COVER:

After completion of this chapter, you will be able to solve problems with:

- ✓ Fractions
- ✓ Decimals
- ✓ Roman Numerals
- ✓ Percents
- ✓ Symbols

We all learned math a little bit differently. In our early school years, each of us had a different math teacher who taught math a little bit differently. Many adult students have a fear of math or a strong sense of "not being good at math." It's best to start with a review of basic math concepts. Practice the basic problems until you've reached a level of understanding. Then proceed on to more detailed math problems.

This chapter will start with a review of basic math concepts that you're familiar with. Understanding the fundamentals of math is important for success with more detailed dosage calculation pharmacy math.

TYPES OF FRACTIONS

A proper fraction is when the numerator is less than the denominator, and the fraction is less than 1. Examples of proper fractions follow:

$$\frac{1}{4} \qquad \frac{3}{19} \qquad \frac{5}{7}$$

An improper fraction is when the numerator is greater than or equal to the denominator, and the fraction is greater than or equal to 1. An improper fraction is not the correct way of writing a fraction. An answer to a problem should never be given in the form of an improper fraction. Examples of improper fractions follow:

$$\frac{6}{2} \qquad \frac{15}{11} \qquad \frac{3}{2}$$

A fraction of mixed numbers is when the whole number and proper fraction are combined, and the value is always greater than 1. Examples of mixed number fractions follow:

$$1\tfrac{3}{4} \qquad\qquad 9\tfrac{1}{8} \qquad\qquad 23\tfrac{2}{3}$$

A complex fraction is when the numerator, denominator, or both the numerator and denominator may be a whole number, proper fraction, or mixed number, and the value may be less than, greater than, or equal to 1. Examples of complex fractions follow:

$$\frac{\tfrac{3}{4}}{1\tfrac{2}{3}} \qquad\qquad \frac{5\tfrac{1}{8}}{7} \qquad\qquad \frac{7}{10\tfrac{1}{4}}$$

WORKING WITH FRACTIONS

Reducing Fractions

Fractions must always be reduced to the lowest terms. Always answer problems with a fraction reduced to the lowest or simple terms. To reduce the fraction, find the largest whole number that divides evenly into both the numerator and the denominator of the fraction. Review these examples:

$\dfrac{2}{4}$ Some fractions are easier than others to reduce, because we can guess that 2 will divide evenly into both the numerator and the denominator. The easy math of dividing by 2 can be done in our head.

$$\frac{2}{4} = \frac{1}{2} \qquad\qquad \frac{2 \div 2 = 1}{4 \div 2 = 2} \qquad\qquad \left(\frac{1}{2}\right)$$

$$\frac{11 \div 11 = 1}{22 \div 11 = 2} \qquad \left(\frac{1}{2}\right)$$

$\dfrac{15 \div 5 = 3}{60 \div 5 = 12}$ This fraction is not reduced to simplest terms. $\dfrac{3 \div 3 = 1}{12 \div 3 = 4}$ $\left(\dfrac{1}{4}\right)$

Take it a step further. Both the 3 and the 12 are divisible by 3.

Now you try. Reduce these fractions to simplest terms.

1. $\dfrac{18}{62}$ 2. $\dfrac{12}{90}$ 3. $\dfrac{16}{77}$

Answers are at the end of the chapter.

> Hints that may help you in reducing numbers:
>
> Even numbers are divisible by 2.
>
> A number that ends in 5 or 0 is divisible by 5.
>
> A number that ends in 0 is divisible by 10.

Adding or Subtraction Fractions

To add and subtract fractions, the denominators of the fractions must be the same. Add the numerators. Carry the same denominator across.

$$\frac{1}{15} + \frac{3}{15} = \frac{4}{15}$$

$$\frac{3}{9} + \frac{4}{9} = \frac{7}{9}$$

$$\frac{19}{29} - \frac{17}{29} = \frac{2}{29}$$

If the denominators are not the same, you must first find the least common denominator to add or subtract fractions. Common denominators are numbers that have the same multiple.

$\frac{1}{3} + \frac{3}{5}$ To add these fractions together, find the common denominator. Determine what multiples 3 and 5 have in common. An easy way to determine the common multiple is to multiply $3 \times 5 = 15$.

Whatever you do to the denominator, you have to do the numerator.

For the common fraction $\frac{1}{3}$, the denominator is multiplied by 5 to get the common denominator of 15, so the numerator must also be multiplied by 5:

$$\frac{1}{3} = \frac{1 \times 5}{3 \times 5} = \frac{5}{15}$$

For the common fraction $\frac{3}{15}$, the denominator is multiplied by 3 to get the common denominator of 15, so the numerator must also be multiplied by 3:

$$\frac{3}{5} = \frac{3 \times 3}{5 \times 3} = \frac{9}{15}$$

So

$$\frac{1}{3} + \frac{3}{5} \text{ is the same as } \frac{5}{15} + \frac{9}{15} = \frac{14}{15}$$

$$\frac{7}{9} - \frac{3}{8} \xrightarrow{\text{find the common denominator}} 9 \times 8 = 72$$

$$\xrightarrow{\text{Whatever you do to the denominator, you must do to the numerator}} \frac{7}{9} \times \frac{8}{8} = \boxed{\frac{56}{72}} \quad \frac{3 \times 9}{8 \times 9} = \boxed{\frac{27}{72}}$$

$$\frac{56}{72} - \frac{27}{72} = \frac{29}{72}$$

Now you try. Find the common denominator and add or subtract these fractions.

1. $\frac{3}{7} + \frac{1}{14}$ 2. $\frac{7}{11} - \frac{12}{33}$ 3. $\frac{14}{53} + \frac{2}{3}$

Answers are at the end of the chapter.

> **Need to Know**
>
> You will be allowed to use a calculator on the certification exam. You will use either a handheld calculator furnished by the testing site or an on-screen calculator. You are not allowed to use your personal calculator from home. You will also be given a small dry erase board or scratch paper for calculations.

Multiply Fractions

Multiplying fractions is an easy task. Multiply the numerators and then multiply the denominators. The denominators do not need to be the same to solve a multiplication problem.

$$\frac{3}{5} \times \frac{4}{9} = \frac{12}{45} = \frac{4}{15} \qquad \frac{1}{9} \times \frac{7}{8} = \frac{7}{72} \qquad \frac{5}{6} \times \frac{1}{11} = \frac{5}{66}$$

Now you try. Multiply these fractions. Give your answer in reduced terms.

1. $\frac{3}{8} \times \frac{7}{8}$ \qquad 2. $\frac{4}{7} \times \frac{8}{9}$ \qquad 3. $\frac{1}{14} \times \frac{19}{20}$

Answers are at the end of the chapter.

Dividing Fractions

To divide fractions, invert the second fraction and then multiply.

$$\frac{3}{4} \div \frac{2}{3} = \qquad\qquad \frac{3}{4} \times \frac{3}{2} = \frac{9}{8} = 1\frac{1}{8}$$

$$\frac{7}{12} \div \frac{3}{5} = \frac{7}{12} \times \frac{5}{3} = \frac{35}{36}$$

Now you try. Divide these fractions. Give your answer in reduced terms.

1. $\frac{5}{7} \div \frac{6}{7}$ \qquad 2. $\frac{6}{13} \div \frac{15}{17}$ \qquad 3. $\frac{4}{5} \div \frac{9}{10}$

Answers are at the end of the chapter.

DECIMALS

A quick review of decimals shows that the numbers before the decimal point are whole numbers and the numbers after the decimal point are a fraction of a whole number (**Figure 14-1**). Remember that there is no "ones" place after the decimal. The place values after the decimal point start with the "tenths" place, and the values after the decimal have a "th" on the end of the word: hundredths, thousandths.

Comparing the Value of Decimals

Are you able to look at these decimal values and know which one is the largest or the smallest?

0.125   0.5   0.02

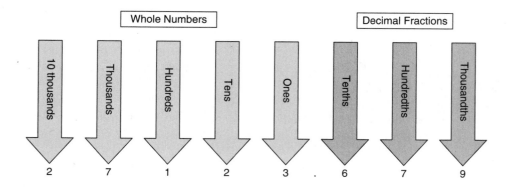

Figure 14-1 Decimals

A trick to determine which decimal value is largest is to align the decimal points and then add zeros to the empty spots (**Figure 14-2**).

First, align the decimal points:
$$0.125$$
$$0.5$$
$$0.02$$

Next, fill zeros in the empty place values:
$$0.125$$
$$0.\mathbf{500}$$
$$0.02\mathbf{0}$$

Now, take off the leading zeros and the decimal point. Look at these as whole numbers:
$$\cancel{0.}125$$
$$\cancel{0.}500$$
$$\cancel{0.0}20$$

You can see that 500 is the largest value, then 125, followed by 20. This helps put the decimal values in the correct order of largest to smallest: 0.5   0.125   0.02
Order these decimal values from largest to smallest: 0.23   0.542   1.71
The correct answer in ordering the decimal values from largest to smallest is 1.71   0.542   0.23
Now you try. Order these decimal values from largest to smallest.

0.003   0.021   0.154   0.158

Answers are at the end of the chapter.

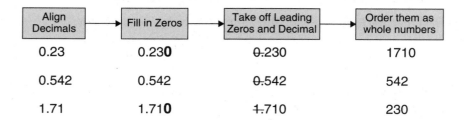

Figure 14-2 Comparing the Value of Decimals

Decimal Values

Keep these points in mind when working with decimals.

1. Zeros added to a decimal fraction before the decimal point or at the end of the decimal fraction *do not* change the value.
   For example,
   .5 is the same value if we add a leading zero 0.5 or if we add a trailing zero .50

   $$.5 = \tfrac{1}{2} \qquad 0.5 = \tfrac{1}{2} \qquad .50 = \tfrac{1}{2}$$

2. In a decimal number, zeros added before or after the decimal point *do change* the value.
   For example,
   1.5 has a zero added after the decimal point 1.05 or a zero added before the decimal 10.5
   Adding these zeros before or after the decimal did change the value,

   $$1.5 \neq 1.05 \qquad 1.5 \neq 10.5$$

3. Possibly the most important point to remember is to **ALWAYS USE LEADING ZEROS**. In pharmacy, the use of leading zeros helps decrease medication errors.

~~.43~~	0.43	1.7	~~1.7~~
NO	YES	YES	NO

ROUNDING NUMBERS

Most often in pharmacy calculations, the figure is rounded to the nearest hundred<u>ths</u> place. For example, 148.0<u>3</u>7 is rounded to 148.04. The 3 is in the hundredths place. The number following the hundredths place or to the right determines whether the 3 will be rounded up or stay the same. Round up if the number to the right is 5 or higher. Keep the number the same if the number to the right is 4 or less.

$$42.3\underline{6}9 = 42.37 \qquad 58.3\underline{4}3 = 58.34 \qquad 184.2\underline{3}654823 = 184.24$$

Knowing how to round numbers is really important, because calculators will give an answer with many figures, such as 85.2366666666666.

Now you try. Round these numbers to the nearest hundredth.

56.321   983.32569   5.42695   7.23335555

Round these numbers to the nearest tenth.

56.3695   78.524   3.256236   692.355698

Answers are at the end of the chapter.

CONVERSION BETWEEN FRACTIONS AND DECIMALS

To convert a fraction to a decimal, divide the numerator by the denominator.

$$\frac{1}{4} = 1 \div 4 = 0.25 \qquad\qquad \frac{1}{8} = 1 \div 8 = 0.125$$

Now you try. Convert these fractions to a decimal. Remember to include a leading zero in your answer. Round the answers to the nearest hundredths place.

$$\frac{5}{9} \qquad\qquad \frac{1}{5} \qquad\qquad \frac{3}{4} \qquad\qquad \frac{4}{25} \qquad\qquad \frac{7}{16}$$

Answers are at the end of the chapter.

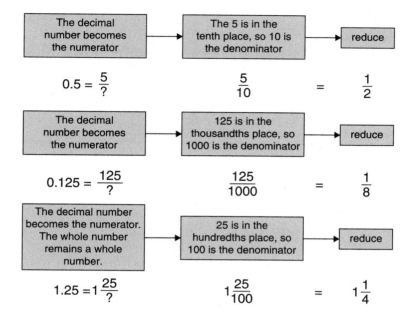

Figure 14-3 Converting Decimals to Fractions

To convert a decimal to a fraction, the decimal number becomes the numerator of the fraction. The denominator is the number 1 followed by as many zeros as there are places to the right of the decimal point. Drop the decimal point and reduce the fraction to the lowest terms.

Now you try. Convert these decimals to fractions. Reduce to the lowest terms.

0.36   0.75   1.5   0.366   2.561

Answers at the end of the chapter.

ADD, SUBTRACT, MULTIPLY, AND DIVIDE DECIMALS

To add or subtract decimals,

- Align the decimal points
- Add zeros to make all decimals of equal length
- Eliminate unnecessary zeros in the final answer

Add   32.6 + 25 + 145.65

1. Align the decimal points

$$\begin{array}{r} 32.6 \\ 25. \\ 145.65 \end{array}$$

2. Add zeros to make all decimals of equal length

$$\begin{array}{r} 32.6\mathbf{0} \\ 25.\mathbf{00} \\ +145.65 \\ \hline 203.25 \end{array}$$

Now you try. Add and subtract these decimals. You *will* be allowed to use a calculator when taking the certification exam. Make sure you key the decimal point into your calculator.

52.36 + 45.21 + 0.4 =   456.35 − 87.70 =

Answers at the end of the chapter.

To multiply decimals,

- Multiply the decimals without concern for decimal point placement
- Put the decimal point in the answer to the *left* as many decimal places as there are in the two decimals multiplied

Multiply 2.36 × 1.4

1. Decimal points do not need to be aligned

$$\begin{array}{r} 2.36 \\ \underline{1.4} \\ 3304 \end{array}$$

2. There are 3 decimal places.

$2.\underline{36}$ 2 decimal places

$1.\underline{4}$ 1 decimal place

3. The answer must have 3 decimal places. 3.304

Now you try. Multiply these decimals. Round to the nearest hundredth. You *will* be allowed to use a calculator when taking the certification exam. Make sure you key the decimal point into your calculator.

25.69 × 453.1 =   0.25 × 1.36 =   7.74 × 0.03 =

Answers are at the end of the chapter.

To divide decimals:

The dividend is the number that will be divided. The divisor is the number that the dividend is divided by.

$1.55 \div 0.2$ is the same as $0.2\overline{)1.55}$ is the same as

(dividend) (divisor)

$\dfrac{1.55}{0.2}$ (dividend) / (divisor)

The divisor should always be a whole number. Move the decimal point to the end of the devisor to make it a whole number.

The decimal point is moved 1 place to the right to make 0.2 a whole number of 2.

Move the decimal point in the dividend the same number of times it was moved in the devisor.

The dividend decimal point is also moved 1 place to the right to turn 1.55 into 15.5

$$0.2\overline{)1.55} = 2\overline{)15.5}$$

Keep the decimal points lined up when completing the division problem. The answer is 7.75

Now you try. Divide these decimals. Round to the nearest hundredth. You *will* be allowed to use a calculator when taking the certification exam. Two points to remember when using the calculator to divide is to make sure to key the decimal point into your calculator. And make sure you enter the dividend and the divisor in the right order. The dividend is entered first, then ÷ the divisor.

$56.2 \div 3.54 =$ $\dfrac{23.6}{1.32} =$ $\dfrac{45}{0.72} =$ $56 \div 3.1 =$

Answers are at the end of the chapter.

PERCENTS

To change a percent (%) to a decimal:

1. Divide by 100 and drop the percent sign $9\% = 9 \div 100 = 0.09$
   -OR-
2. Put in a decimal point two places to the left and drop the percent sign

$$9\% = 9.\% = .0\,9\% = 0.09$$

To change a decimal to a percentage (%):

1. Multiply by 100 and add a percent sign $0.25 \times 100 = 25\%$
   -OR-
2. Move the decimal point two places to the right and put in the percent sign

$$0.25 = 2\,5. = 25\%$$

Now you try. Change these percents to decimals.

55%   3.26%   0.56%   100%

Change these decimals to percents.

0.54   5.8   120   78.3   0.032

Answers are at the end of the chapter.

ROMAN NUMERALS

Roman Numeral	Arabic Numeral
ss	1/2
I or i	1
V or v	5
X or x	10
L or l	50
C or c	100
D or d	500
M or m	1000

You should know these Roman numerals and commit them to memory. You should also know how to translate a series of Roman numerals into Arabic numerals. Do you know what number XXIX is? It is 29. Follow these rules for translating Roman numerals:

1. If a smaller Roman numeral is to the left of a larger Roman numeral, subtract the smaller from the larger. $iv = 5 - 1 = 4$
2. If a smaller Roman numeral is to the right of a larger Roman numeral, add the smaller to the larger. $xi = 10 + 1 = 11$

Now you try. Translate these Roman numerals.

XXIV   XLVII   XIXSS

Translate these Arabic numerals.

52   37   2011

SYMBOLS

< is less than

> is greater than

5 is less than 6   5 < 6

10 is more than 9   10 > 9

Now you try. Compare the value of these fractions, decimals and whole numbers by using the >, < , = symbols.

½ _____ ¼   3 _____ 4.2   ½ _____ 0.5   37 _____ 47

Answers are at the end of the chapter.

Exhibit 14-1 Tips from a Certified Tech

Julia Nichols, CPhT
Colorado Springs, Colorado

As a former stay-at-home mom in Colorado Springs, I decided to attend a pharmacy technician program that would reintroduce me to the workforce. The program was an excellent way to prepare myself for a job as a hospital pharmacy technician. I took interesting classes that gave me a background in pharmacology, physiology, and the business aspect of pharmacies. Even better, the classes provided hands-on training to prepare me for work in either a community or a hospital pharmacy setting.

    Getting ready for the certification exam was not a problem, after the coursework I took at community college. I worked through the exam workbook that was provided with our school textbook. The workbook also came with a practice test CD, but I found that doing old-fashioned pencil and paper practice tests in the workbook was my best strategy. It was also important to memorize the basic metric conversions most often used by pharmacy technicians. The best place for me to study was at our local library, away from the distractions of home and family.

    Now I work part time at a local hospital pharmacy, and it's a great job for me. It's interesting, my coworkers are friendly, and the hours are very flexible. Working in healthcare is a great opportunity; there are always chances to continue your education, and it's a motivating place to improve your own health and well-being.

This is your checklist to make sure you understand what you need to know for the certification exam. Review chapter content if there is a topic you're uncertain of.
I know:

√	...how to convert between fractions and decimals, percent and decimals.
	...how to round.
	...> and < symbols.

PRACTICE TEST ANSWERS

Reducing Fractions

1. $\dfrac{18 \div 2}{62 \div 2}$ $\left(\dfrac{9}{31}\right)$ 2. $\dfrac{12 \div 6}{90 \div 6}$ $\left(\dfrac{2}{15}\right)$ 3.   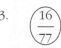

Adding or Subtracting Fractions

1. $\dfrac{3}{7} + \dfrac{1}{14} = \dfrac{3 \times 2}{7 \times 2} = \dfrac{6}{14} + \dfrac{1}{14} = \dfrac{7}{14}$ reduces down to $\boxed{\dfrac{1}{2}}$

2. $\dfrac{7}{11} - \dfrac{12}{33} = \dfrac{7 \times 3}{11 \times 3} = \dfrac{21}{33} = \dfrac{21}{33} - \dfrac{12}{33} = \dfrac{9}{33}$ reduces down to $\boxed{\dfrac{3}{11}}$

$\dfrac{14}{53} + \dfrac{2}{3} = \dfrac{14 \times 3}{53 \times 3} + \dfrac{2 \times 53}{3 \times 53} = \dfrac{42}{159} + \dfrac{106}{159} = \boxed{\dfrac{148}{159}}$

Multiplying Fractions

1. $\dfrac{3}{8} \times \dfrac{7}{8} = \boxed{\dfrac{21}{64}}$
2. $\dfrac{4}{7} \times \dfrac{8}{9} = \boxed{\dfrac{32}{63}}$
3. $\dfrac{1}{14} \times \dfrac{19}{20} = \boxed{\dfrac{19}{280}}$

Dividing Fractions

1. $\dfrac{5}{7} \div \dfrac{6}{7} = \dfrac{5}{7} \times \dfrac{7}{6} = \dfrac{35}{42} = \boxed{\dfrac{5}{6}}$
2. $\dfrac{6}{13} \div \dfrac{15}{17} = \dfrac{6}{13} \times \dfrac{17}{15} = \dfrac{102}{195} = \boxed{\dfrac{34}{65}}$

3. $\dfrac{4}{5} \div \dfrac{9}{10} = \dfrac{4}{5} \times \dfrac{10}{9} = \dfrac{40}{45}$ reduces down to $\boxed{\dfrac{8}{9}}$

Comparing the Values of Decimals
Largest is 0.158, then 0.154, then 0.021, and then 0.003
Rounding to the nearest hundredth

$56.3\underline{2}1 = \boxed{56.32}$ $983.3\underline{2}569 = \boxed{983.33}$ $5.4\underline{2}695 = \boxed{5.43}$ $7.2\underline{3}335555 = \boxed{7.23}$

Round to the nearest tenth

$56.\underline{3}695 = \boxed{56.4}$ $78.\underline{5}24 = \boxed{78.5}$ $3.\underline{2}56236 = \boxed{3.3}$ $692.\underline{3}55698 = \boxed{692.4}$

Converting fractions to decimals

$\dfrac{5}{9} = 5 \div 9 = 0.555 = \boxed{0.56}$ $\dfrac{1}{5} = 1 \div 5 = \boxed{0.2}$

$\dfrac{3}{4} = 3 \div 4 = \boxed{0.75}$ $\dfrac{4}{25} = 4 \div 25 = \boxed{0.16}$

$\dfrac{7}{16} = 7 \div 16 = 0.437 = \boxed{0.44}$

Converting decimals to fractions

$0.36 = \dfrac{36}{100} = \boxed{\dfrac{9}{25}}$ $0.75 = \dfrac{75}{100} = \boxed{\dfrac{3}{4}}$ $1.5 = \boxed{1\dfrac{1}{2}}$

$0.366 = \dfrac{366}{1000} = \boxed{\dfrac{183}{500}}$ $2.561 = \boxed{2\dfrac{561}{1000}}$

Adding and subtracting decimals

$52.36 + 45.21 + 0.4 = $
$$
\begin{array}{r}
52.36 \\
45.21 \\
\underline{00.40} \\
\boxed{97.97}
\end{array}
$$

$456.35 - 87.70 = $
$$
\begin{array}{r}
456.35 \\
\underline{87.70} \\
\boxed{368.65}
\end{array}
$$

Multiplying decimals

$25.69 \times 453.1 = \boxed{11,640.14}$ $\qquad$ $0.25 \times 1.36 = \boxed{0.34}$ $\qquad$ $7.74 \times 0.03 = \boxed{0.23}$

Dividing decimals

$56.2 \div 3.54 = \boxed{15.88}$ $\qquad$ $\dfrac{23.6}{1.32} = \boxed{17.88}$ $\qquad$ $\dfrac{45}{0.72} = \boxed{62.5}$ $\qquad$ $56 \div 3.1 = \boxed{18.06}$

Percent to decimal

$55\% = 55 \div 100 = \boxed{0.55}$ $\qquad$ $3.26\% = 3.26 \div 100 = \boxed{0.0326}$ $\qquad$ $0.56\% = .56 \div 100 = \boxed{0.0056}$

$100\% = 100 \div 100 = \boxed{1}$

Decimal to percent

$0.54 = .54 \times 100 = \boxed{54\%}$ $\qquad$ $5.8 = 5.8 \times 100 = \boxed{580\%}$ $\qquad$ $120 = 120 \times 100 = \boxed{12,000\%}$

$78.3 = 78.3 \times 100 = \boxed{7,830\%}$ $\qquad$ $.032 = .032 \times 100 = \boxed{3.2\%}$

Roman numerals

XXIV is 24 $\qquad$ XLVII is 47 $\qquad$ XIXSS is 19½

Arabic numerals

52 is LII $\qquad$ 37 is XXXVII $\qquad$ 2011 MMXI

Less than/greater than

$\frac{1}{2} > \frac{1}{4}$ $\qquad$ $3 < 4.2$ $\qquad$ $\frac{1}{2} = 0.5$ $\qquad$ $37 < 47$

CHAPTER 14

MULTIPLE CHOICE

Identify the choice that best completes the statement or answers the question.

_____ **1.** $1/8 + 1/2 =$

a. 2/10

b. 1/5

c. 1/10

d. 5/8

_____ **2.** $5/8 + 3 1/12 =$

a. 3 6/20

b. 3 3/10

c. 3 17/24

d. 89/24

_____ **3.** $7/9 - 3/9 =$

a. 4

b. 4/9

c. 10/9

d. 1 1/9

_____ **4.** $57 1/8 - 3 4/5 =$

a. 53 13/40

b. 54 3/8

c. 54 3/5

d. 2133/40

_____ **5.** $1/12 \div 3/5 =$

a. 1/7

b. 3/60

c. 1/20

d. 5/36

_____ **6.** $3/100 \times 75 =$

a. 4/9

b. 2 1/4

c. 235/100

d. 1/10

_____ **7.** What is 2% of 95?

a. 93

b. 93%

c. 1.9

d. 1.9%

_____ **8.** Express 0.4 as a fraction.

a. 4/1

b. 4/100

c. 2/5

d. 0.4/10

_____ **9.** Express 0.23 as a fraction.

a. 0.23/100

b. 23/100

c. 23/10

d. 2 3/10

_____ **10.** What percent (%) is 1/3?

a. 1/3%

b. 0.33%

c. 33.33%

d. 3.3%

___ **11.** What is the decimal of 7 2/3?

a. 7.23

b. 7.2/3

c. 7.67

d. 7.2

___ **12.** How many prescriptions for 30 tablets can be filled with a stock bottle containing a total of 150 tablets?

a. 30

b. 5

c. 3

d. 1

___ **13.** Which of the following is a proper fraction?

a. 3/16

b. 16/3

c. 5/3

d. 2/1

___ **14.** Reduce 15/125 to lowest terms:

a. 3/25

b. 5/41

c. 1/5

d. 5/6

___ **15.** Round 151.23691 to the nearest hundredth place:

a. 151

b. 152

c. 151.24

d. 151.2

___ **16.** Order these decimals from large to small: 0.56, 0.321, 0.9

a. 0.9, 0.321, 0.56

b. 0.56, 0.9, 0.321

c. 0.321, 0.56, 0.9

d. 0.9, 0.56, 0.321

___ **17.** What is the accepted decimal for 7/10?

a. 0.70

b. .7

c. 0.7

d. 7.0

___ **18.** Change 1.3 to a percent:

a. 1.3%

b. 130%

c. 13%

d. 0.013%

___ **19.** IL is:

a. 51

b. 11

c. 49

d. 101

___ **20.** 13 is:

a. XIII

b. IIIX

c. VX

d. XL

ANSWER SECTION

1. D
2. C
3. B
4. A
5. D
6. B
7. C
8. C
9. B
10. C
11. C
12. B
13. A
14. A
15. C
16. D
17. C
18. B
19. C
20. A

TASK SHEET

TOPIC TO REVIEW: MEASUREMENT SYSTEMS AND SYSTEM CONVERSIONS

Materials

Pharmacy Technician Exam Review Guide

JB Test Prep: Pharmacy Exam Review Guide

Prepare

1. Read measurement systems and system conversions.
2. Take practice test at the end of the chapter.

Study Plan

1. Read pages_____ on _____(date).
2. Work sample problems in the chapter.
3. Take end-of-chapter practice test on_____(date).
4. Make flash cards to help memorize system conversions quizlet.com.

Tips

1. You must know the conversion factors to convert between systems: kg to lb, (2.2), oz to mL (30). Commit the conversion factors and formulas to memory.
2. A leading "0" is used in pharmacy. This is a "0" to the left of the decimal point for any decimal that does not include a whole number. The leading zero helps minimize dosing errors by alerting pharmacy to the fact that the dose amount is less than "1."
3. Decimal points must be lined up when adding and subtracting. In multiplication, the decimal places do not need to be lined up but are instead counted when solving the problem. Most decimal errors occur in division. To help avoid errors in division, place the decimal point before calculating.

End of Chapter

List what you need to review.

Measurement Systems and System Conversions

OBJECTIVES/TOPICS TO COVER:

✓ Ratio/proportion problems
✓ Ratio/percentage problems
✓ Measurement systems used in pharmacy practice
✓ Record system conversions
✓ Temperature conversion problems

RATIO AND PROPORTIONS

A *ratio* is a comparison of two like quantities, indicating the relationship of one part of a quantity to the whole. Ratios can be expressed as a fraction, 2/3, or as ratio notation, 2:3.

An example of a ratio is the pharmacist-to-technician ratio of 3 to 1 or 3 technicians to 1 pharmacist or 3:1. There are 4 people working in the pharmacy; 3 are technicians, 1 is a pharmacist.

A *proportion* is when ratios, or fractions, are equal.

$$¾ = 3:4 :: 15:20$$

This proportion reads as ¾ is equal to or the same as 15/20, which is equal to or the same as 3 to 4, which is equal to or the same as 15 to 20.

$$:: \text{ means } =$$

You are able to test two fractions to see whether they're equivalent or equal by multiplying diagonally.

$$\frac{3}{4} = \frac{15}{20} \quad 4 \times 15 = 60$$
$$3 \times 20 = 60$$

Ratio/Percentage

To show a ratio as a percentage, make the first number of the ratio, the numerator, and the second number, the denominator. Then, multiply the fraction by 100 and add the percent sign.

Example: The pharmacist to technician ratio is 1:3. What is the percentage of pharmacists working in a 1:3 ratio? (Answer: 33.33%)

1. Make the first number of the ratio the numerator.	$\dfrac{1}{3}$
2. Make the second number of the ratio the denominator.	
3. Multiply the fraction by 100.	$\dfrac{1}{3} \times 100 = 33.33$
4. Add the percent sign (%).	33.33%

$$1:3 = \frac{1}{3} = 33.33\%$$

You can change this around to show a percentage as a ratio.

Example: 23% of the customers needed allergy medication. How many customers in all needed allergy medication? (Answer: For every 100 customers that came into the pharmacy, 23 of them needed allergy medication.)

1. Change the percent to a decimal by dividing it by 100.	$23\% \div 100 = 0.23$
2. Change the decimal to a fraction and reduce to lowest terms.	$\dfrac{23}{100}$
3. Make the numerator the first number of the ratio.	23:
4. Make the denominator the second number in the ratio.	23:100

$$23\% = 0.23 = \frac{23}{100} = 23 : 100$$

SYSTEMS OF PHARMACEUTICAL MEASUREMENT

The metric system is the most common unit of measure used in pharmacy. Milligrams (mg) and grams (g) are common units of weight used when compounding medications and dosing medications. Kilogram (kg) is another metric unit of weight used most commonly when referring to a patient's weight.

Other systems of measurement used in pharmacy are the apothecary (**Table 15-1**), the avoirdupois, and the household. The avoirdupois system is based on dry weight in which the base unit is

Table 15-1 Apothecary System

Unit	Abbreviation/Symbol
Grain	gr
Scruple	3
Dram	dr
Fluid Dram	fl dr
Ounce	oz
Fluid Ounce	fl oz
Pound	lb
Pint	pt
Quart	qt
Gallon	gal
Minim	♍

a pound. Some of the avoirdupois units of measure are used in the apothecary system, such as the grain (gr), the ounce (oz), and the pound (lb). The apothecary system of measure is an old method first used by early pharmacists. It's important to know the most common apothecary units of measure, because these units are still used in today's pharmacy.

Metric System Base Units

- ✓ Meter (length)
- ✓ Liter (volume)
- ✓ Gram (weight)

Metric Units and Abbreviations

Weight	gram (base unit)—g	
	milligram—mg	
	microgram—mcg (µg)	
	kilogram—kg	
Volume	liter (base unit)—L (ℓ)	A milliliter is the same volume as a cubic centimeter.
	milliliter—mL (mℓ)	1 mL = 1 cc
	cubic centimeter—cc	
Length	meter (base unit)—m	Measurements of length not as commonly used
	centimeter—cm	in pharmacy.
	millimeter—mm	

Apothecary System

- ✓ Fluid measure—minim, fluid dram, fluid ounce, pint, quart, gallon
- ✓ Dry measure—grain, scruple, dram, ounce, pound

Avoirdupois System

- ✓ Grain, ounce, pound

Household System

- ✓ Teaspoonful, tablespoonful, fluid ounce, cup, pint, quart, gallon

The household units of measure are the same in pharmacy as those used in the kitchen with the addition of "ful" on the end of the teaspoon and tablespoon (**Table 15-2**).

SYSTEM CONVERSIONS

Measurements of both weight and volume are constantly used in pharmacy. It's very important that you have a feel for the differences in measurements. It's equally important to understand how to convert metric measurements and how to convert between different measurement systems.
Get a feel for the differences in weights:

A 170-pound patient weighs 77 kg

2.2 pounds = 1 kg

A milligram is a very small unit of measure.

1 teaspoonful of salt weighs about 2300 mg.

1 cup of macaroni and cheese weighs about 228,000 mg.

Table 15-2 Household System

Unit	Abbreviation
Drop	gtt
Teaspoonful	t or tsp
Tablespoonful	T or Tbsp
Ounce as Fluid or Dry Weight	fl oz oz
Gallon	gal
Cup	c
Pint	pt
Quart	qt

Get a feel for the differences in volume:

A milliliter is a lot less than a liter and less than an ounce.

A 12-ounce can of soda pop is about 355 mL

1 ounce = 30 mL

METRIC CONVERSIONS

Converting units within the metric system is easy, because the metric system is based on multiples of 10. The part you may need to practice is which way to move the decimal point. The direction the decimal point is moved depends on whether you're converting to a larger or a smaller unit. You should memorize the measurements in the following tables (**Tables 15-3** and **15-4**). For instance, know that a kilogram is larger than a gram, milligram, and microgram.

Commit to Memory/Know Forever

1 gram = 1000 mg
1 liter = 1000 mL

A milliliter and a cubic centimeter are the same:

1 mL = 1 cc

Table 15-3 Weight Conversions

Weight Unit	Conversion
Kilogram	1 kilogram = 1000 grams
Gram	1 gram = 0.001 kg = 1000 mg
Milligram	1 mg = 0.001 g = 1000 mcg
Microgram	1 mcg = 0.001 mg = 0.000001 grams

Table 15-4 Volume Conversions

Volume Unit	Conversion
Liter	1 liter = 1000 mL
Milliliter	1 milliliter = 0.001 L

Rules to Remember

1. Multiply when going from a larger unit to a smaller unit. Most of the time, you will multiply by 1000. There are 1000 units of measure between a kilogram and a gram, between a gram and a milligram, and between a liter and a milliliter.
   -OR-
2. Move the decimal point to the right. Most of the time, you will move the decimal point three places.
3. Divide when converting a smaller unit to a larger unit. Most of the time, you will divide by 1000.
   -OR-
4. Move the decimal point to the left. Most of the time, you will move the decimal point three places.

Large to small ($\times$)

Small to large ($\div$)

Example: 5 mg = _____ g

1. We are converting from a small unit (mg) to a larger unit (g).
2. We can move the decimal point to the left three spaces.   0   0   5
   -OR-
3. We can divide. $5 \div 1000 = 0.005$
4. The answer is 0.005 grams.   5 mg = 0.005 g

Now you try. Convert these metric measurements.

14 mg = _____ g
1.7 mg = _____ g
0.2 mg = _____ g
130 g = _____ mg
76 g = _____ mg
4567 g = _____ mg
745 L = _____ mL
6 L = _____ mL
909 mL = _____ L

Answers are at the end of the chapter.

CONVERTING BETWEEN SYSTEMS

Sometimes you will need to convert between systems. One of the most common conversions is determining a patient's weight in kilograms when the weight was given in pounds. You will also need to know how to convert between grains and milligrams as well as between milliliters, teaspoonfuls, and ounces.

Converting between systems is not like converting *within* the metric system where you work in multiples of 10. The first step in converting between measurement systems is to know your conversion factors. Conversion factors are approximate, because you're moving from one system to another. You can relate this to using a Walmart brand vacuum cleaner bag in your Hoover vacuum cleaner. The Walmart bag is almost the same as the Hoover brand bag but not an exact fit. You won't get an exact fit, because you're using a bag from a different company. In the same way, there is not an exact conversion factor, because we're moving between two different systems of measure.

Commit to Memory/Know Forever

1 grain (gr) = 60 – 65 mg
1 tsp = 5 mL/cc
1 Tbsp = 3 tsp = 15 mL/cc = ½ fl oz
1 fl oz = 30 mL/cc
1 kg = 2.2 lb
1 in = 2.5 cm

Conversion Factors

Pounds
&
Kilograms } Use conversion factor of 2.2.

Grains
&
Milligrams } Choose to use 60 or 65 as your conversion factor.

Ounces
&
mL/cc } Use conversion factor of 30.

Teaspoonfuls
&
mL/cc } Use conversion factor of 5.

Example:

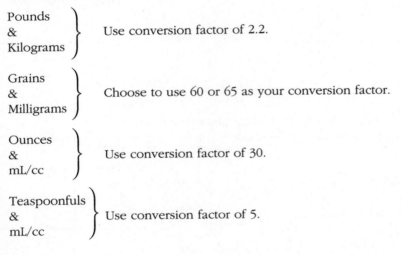

210 pounds = _____ kg

210 ÷ 2.2 = 95.45

Weight in pounds   Conversion factor   Weight in kilograms

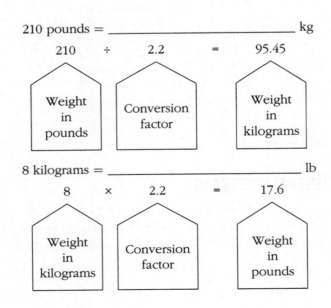

8 kilograms = _____ lb

8 × 2.2 = 17.6

Weight in kilograms   Conversion factor   Weight in pounds

5 gr = _____ mg

| 5 | × | 65 | = | 325 |

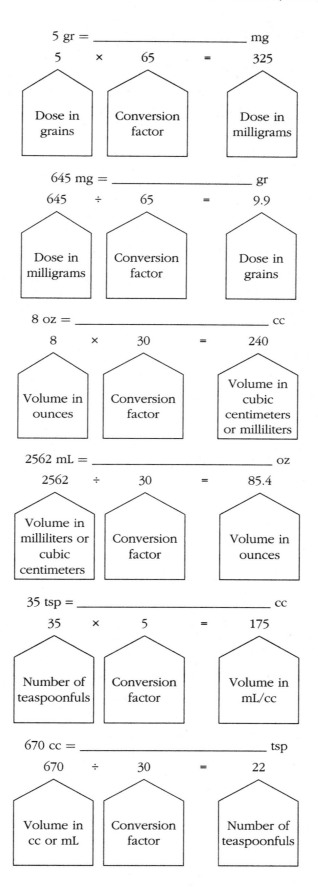

| Dose in grains | Conversion factor | Dose in milligrams |

645 mg = _____ gr

| 645 | ÷ | 65 | = | 9.9 |

| Dose in milligrams | Conversion factor | Dose in grains |

8 oz = _____ cc

| 8 | × | 30 | = | 240 |

| Volume in ounces | Conversion factor | Volume in cubic centimeters or milliliters |

2562 mL = _____ oz

| 2562 | ÷ | 30 | = | 85.4 |

| Volume in milliliters or cubic centimeters | Conversion factor | Volume in ounces |

35 tsp = _____ cc

| 35 | × | 5 | = | 175 |

| Number of teaspoonfuls | Conversion factor | Volume in mL/cc |

670 cc = _____ tsp

| 670 | ÷ | 30 | = | 22 |

| Volume in cc or mL | Conversion factor | Number of teaspoonfuls |

TEMPERATURE CONVERSIONS

It's necessary to know how to make temperature conversions between the Celsius scale and the Fahrenheit scale (**Table 15-5**). You can use a few different formulas to convert the temperatures. Each formula will get you the same answer. Pick the formula that's easiest for you to use and *remember*. You will need to memorize the conversion formulas for your certification exam.

$$C = (F - 32) \div 1.8$$
$$F = (C \times 1.8) + 32$$
$$F = (1.8)\, C + 32$$
$$C = \frac{F - 32}{1.8}$$

Example:
Convert 95°F to its equivalent in Celsius

1. Choose a formula.	$C = (F - 32) \div 1.8$
2. Plug in the numbers you know.	$C = (95 - 32) \div 1.8$
3. Do the math inside the parenthesis first.	$(95 - 32) = 63$
4. Finish the equation.	$C = 63 \div 1.8 = 35$
5. The answer is 35° Celsius.	$C = 35$

Example:
Convert 150°C to Fahrenheit

1. Choose a formula.	$F = (C \times 1.8) + 32$
2. Plug in the numbers you're given.	$F = (150 \times 1.8) + 32$
3. Do the math inside the parenthesis first.	$(150 \times 1.8) = 270$
4. Finish the equation.	$F = 270 + 32 = 302$
5. The answer is 302°F.	$F = 302$

Now you try. Make these temperature conversions.

55°F = _____ C   3°C = _____ F   25°F = _____ C

Answers are at the end of the chapter.

Table 15-5 Boiling and Freezing Point

Celsius	Fahrenheit
Boiling Point	
100°	212°
Freezing Point	
0°	32°

This is your checklist to make sure you understand what you need to know for the certification exam. Review chapter content if there is a topic you're uncertain of.
I know:

√	...how to convert within the metric system.
	...how to convert between measurement systems.
	...common conversion factors.
	...how to express ratios.
	...how to convert between Fahrenheit and Celsius.

PRACTICE TEST ANSWERS

Metric conversions

$$14 \text{ mg} = \underline{\quad 0.014 \quad} \text{ g}$$
$$1.7 \text{ mg} = \underline{\quad 0.0017 \quad} \text{ g}$$
$$0.2 \text{ mg} = \underline{\quad 0.0002 \quad} \text{ g}$$
$$130 \text{ g} = \underline{\quad 130,000 \quad} \text{ mg}$$
$$76 \text{ g} = \underline{\quad 76,000 \quad} \text{ mg}$$
$$4567 \text{ g} = \underline{\quad 4,567,000 \quad} \text{ mg}$$
$$745 \text{ L} = \underline{\quad 745,000 \quad} \text{ mL}$$
$$6 \text{ L} = \underline{\quad 6000 \quad} \text{ mL}$$
$$909 \text{ mL} = \underline{\quad 0.909 \quad} \text{ L}$$

Temperature conversions

$$55°F = \underline{\quad 13 \quad}°C \qquad 3°C = \underline{\quad 37 \quad}°F \qquad 25°F = \underline{\quad -4 \quad}°C$$

CHAPTER 15

MULTIPLE CHOICE

Identify the choice that best completes the statement or answers the question.

_____ **1.** Which equation is correct?

a. 7/10 : : 7/20

b. 3:5 : : 15:25

c. 1/3 : : 3/1

d. 5/16 : : 1:5

_____ **2.** 3:5 is

a. 60%

b. 3/5%

c. 6%

d. 0.6%

____ **3.** Convert 0.35% to a ratio:

a. 35:10,000

b. 35:100

c. 7:20

d. 7:2000

____ **4.** The most common system of measurement in pharmacy:

a. apothecary

b. International Unit (IU)

c. metric

d. household

____ **5.** 50 mL =

a. 5 cc

b. 0.5 cc

c. 50 cc

d. 5000 cc

____ **6.** An order for 65 gr instructs the technician to dispense

a. 65 grams

b. 65 mg

c. 65 grains

d. 65 ounces

____ **7.** What is the conversion factor when converting pounds to kilograms or kilograms to pounds?

a. 22 lbs = 1 kg

b. 22 kg = 1 lb

c. 2.2 lb = 1 kg

d. 2.2 kg = 1 lb

____ **8.** What is the conversion factor used when converting milliliters to ounces?

a. 30 oz = 30 mL

b. 30 oz = 1 mL

c. 30 mL = 1 oz

d. 1 mL = 3 oz

____ **9.** Convert 2000 mg to grams:

a. 200 g

b. 2 g

c. 0.002 g

d. 20 g

____ **10.** 5 liter =

a. 5000 mL

b. 500 mL

c. 0.005 mL

d. 50 mL

____ **11.** How many milligrams are in 1 grain?

a. 6.5

b. 2.5

c. 30

d. 60

____ **12.** Convert 65 grains to milligrams:

a. 1 mg

b. 4225 mg

c. 0.065 mg

d. 1.08 mg

____ **13.** How many milliliters are in 25 teaspoonfuls?

a. 125 mL

b. 5 mL

c. 250 mL

d. 1250 mL

____ **14.** How many kilograms does a 150-pound patient weigh?

a. 330 kg

b. 3.3 kg

c. 6.8 kg

d. 68 kg

____ **15.** Convert 680 mL to ounces:

a. 20,400 oz

b. 22.6 oz

c. 2400 oz

d. 226 oz

____ **16.** Convert 78°F to Celsius:

a. 172°C

b. 46°C

c. 26°C

d. 43°C

____ **17.** What is boiling point on the Celsius scale?

a. 212°

b. 100°

c. 96.8°

d. 120°

____ **18.** What is freezing point on the Fahrenheit scale?

a. 0°

b. −32°

c. 1.8°

d. 32°

____ **19.** Convert 56°C to Fahrenheit:

a. 101°F

b. 133°F

c. 31°F

d. 17°F

____ **20.** How many milliliters are in 1/2 a fluid ounce (fl. oz)?

a. 30 mL

b. 50 mL

c. 15 mL

d. 5 mL

ANSWER SECTION

1. B
2. A
3. D
4. C
5. C
6. C
7. C
8. C
9. B
10. A
11. D
12. B
13. A
14. D
15. B
16. C
17. B
18. D
19. B
20. C

TASK SHEET

TOPIC TO REVIEW: DOSAGE CALCULATIONS

Materials

Pharmacy Technician Exam Review Guide

JB Test Prep: Pharmacy Technician Exam Review Guide

Prepare

1. Read the section on dosage calculations.
2. Take practice test at the end of the chapter.

Study Plan

1. Read pages_____ on _____(date).
2. Work sample problems in the chapter.
3. Take end-of-chapter practice test on_____(date).
4. Find a study buddy to work through problems with.

Tips

1. Make sure you follow the steps. Problems must be set up correctly.
2. Choose one method of working the problems and stick with that method. Use either have/ need or *D/H*.
3. Ask your pharmacist, a co-tech, or a classmate to help you understand problems you may be unsure of.

End of Chapter

List what you need to review.

Dosage Calculations

OBJECTIVES/TOPICS TO COVER

After completion of this chapter, you will be able to exercise the skills in solving these pharmacy calculation problems:

- ✓ Dosage calculations
- ✓ Milligram (mg) of medication per kilogram (kg) of Body Weight
- ✓ Specific gravity
- ✓ IV flow rates
- ✓ Dilutions
- ✓ Alligation
- ✓ Concentrations
- ✓ Powder volume
- ✓ Body surface area (BSA) for children
- ✓ Young's rule
- ✓ Clark's rule

DOSAGE CALCULATIONS: HAVE-NEED EQUATION

Ratios and proportions are commonly used when figuring dosages in pharmacy calculations.

1. A very important step in calculations is to take a look at how you have set the problem up. You must have the problem set up correctly to proceed with the next step.
2. To set the problem up correctly, make sure that the numerators and denominators of both fractions are in the same units. Here is an example of setting the problem up correctly so that units match:

$$\frac{5 \text{ mg}}{1 \text{ mL}} = \frac{8 \text{ mg}}{X \text{ mL}}$$

This problem is set up correctly, because the numerator in both fractions is in the same units (mg) and the denominator in both fractions is the same units (mL).

Example:

The Zofran your pharmacy has in stock is labeled as 5 mg/1 mL. This means that the Zofran contains 5 milligrams of active ingredient for every 1 milliliter of solution. The prescriber orders a dose of 8 mg. How many mL's of the Zofran will need to be drawn up to get the 8 mg ordered?

1. The first fraction that you write down is what you have in stock. Make sure you include the units (mg or mL) with the numbers.

$$\frac{5 \text{ mg}}{1 \text{ mL}}$$

2. The second fraction that you write down is what you need. This is what the prescriber ordered. X is the number you are trying to solve for.

$$\frac{5 \text{ mg}}{1 \text{ mL}} = \frac{8 \text{ mg}}{X}$$

3. Cross off any like labels. The label you're left with is what you're solving for. This is the label that will be carried through to your answer.

$$\frac{5 \text{ mg}}{1 \text{ mL}} = \frac{8 \text{ mg}}{X}$$

4. Cross multiply to solve for X.

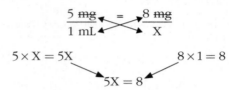

$$5 \times X = 5X \qquad 8 \times 1 = 8$$
$$5X = 8$$

5. Solve for X. X needs to be alone on its side of the equation. To get X to stand alone, divide both sides of the equation by the number that is with the X.

The 5's cancel out

$$\frac{5 \text{ mg}}{1 \text{ mL}} = \frac{8 \text{ mg}}{X} = 5X = 8 = \frac{5X}{5} = \frac{8}{5} = 8 \div 5 = 1.6$$
$$X = 1.6 \text{ mL}$$

6. The last step is to check your answer. Does your answer seem reasonable? If there is 5 mg in 1 mL, does it seem reasonable that there would be 8 mg in 1.6 mL? Yes. This does seem reasonable, and it is the correct dosage.

Try this example:

The label on the stock supply of SoluMedrol is 12 mg/5 mL. The prescriber's order is for 300 mg. How many mL need to be drawn up to get the ordered dosage?

1. Make sure you set your problem up right. Each step in solving hinges on setting up the problem correctly. The left side of the problem—what you write down first—is what you have in stock.

$$\frac{\text{HAVE}}{\underline{\hspace{1.5cm}} \text{ mL}}$$
mg

2. The right side of the equation is what the prescriber ordered.

$$\frac{\text{NEED}}{\underline{\hspace{1.5cm}} \text{ mL}}$$
mg

3. Cross off like labels.
4. Cross multiply to solve for X.
5. Divide each side of the equation by the number with the X. Solve for X. Label your answer.
6. Does your answer make sense?

$$\frac{12 \text{ mg}}{5 \text{ mL}} = \frac{300 \text{ mg}}{X}$$ Set up the problem.

$$\frac{12 \text{ mg}}{5 \text{ mL}} = \frac{300 \text{ mg}}{X}$$ Cross off like labels.

$$12 \times X = 12X \qquad\qquad 5 \times 300 = 1500$$ Cross multiply.

$$12X = 1500$$

$$\frac{12X}{12} = \frac{1500}{12}$$ Divide each side so X stands alone.

$$X = 1500 \div 12 = 125$$

$$X = 125 \text{ mL}$$

DOSAGE CALCULATIONS: $\frac{D}{H}$ EQUATION

The $\frac{D}{H}$ equation can be used to solve dosage calculation problems. You'll get the same answer as you would using the Have-Need equation, but the $\frac{D}{H}$ equation may be easier for you to calculate with. Practice with both of the equations, and use the one that's easier for you to work with.

$$\frac{D}{H} \times Q = X$$

D represents the *Desired Dose*

H represents the dosage the pharmacy has on *hand*

Q is the *Quantity* of the dosage on hand

Same example as we used with the Have-Need equation:
The Zofran your pharmacy has in stock is labeled as 5 mg/1 mL. This means that the Zofran contains 5 milligrams of active ingredient for every 1 milliliter of solution. The prescriber orders a dose of 8 mg. How many mL's of the Zofran will need to be drawn up to get the 8 mg ordered?

1. Plug numbers into the formula that you know. The *D* is the desired dose; the dose the prescriber ordered.

$$\frac{8 \text{ mg}}{H} \times Q = X$$

2. Continue to plug in the numbers that you know. Both *H* and *Q* represent the supply dosage found on the drug label.

$$\frac{8 \text{ mg}}{5 \text{ mg}} \times 1 \text{ mL} = X$$

3. Cross off like labels.

$$\frac{8 \text{ mg}}{5 \text{ mg}} \times 1 \text{ mL} = X$$

4. Divide the *D* and *H* numbers.

$$8 \div 5 = 1.6$$

5. Multiply the *Q* number.

$$1.6 \times 1 = 1.6$$

6. Solve for X and label.

$$X = 1.6 \text{ mL}$$

7. Does the answer seem reasonable?

Please note that when solving problems for drugs supplied in tablets or capsules *Q* is always 1 because the dosage is per 1 tablet or capsule.

Example:

Prescriber's order: furosemide 40 mg po qd
Pharmacy stock supply: Bottle containing furosemide 40 mg per tablet
Dispense: _____ tablet(s)

Answer:

    1. Set up.

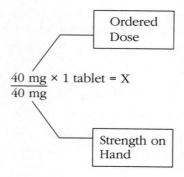

    2. Cross off like labels.

$$\frac{40 \text{ mg}}{40 \text{ mg}} \times 1 \text{ tablet} = X$$

    3. $40 \div 40 = 1$
    4. $1 \times 1 = 1$
    5. X = 1 tablet
    6. Does the answer seem reasonable?

Now you try.

1. Order: nortriptyline 150 mg po qd
    Pharmacy supply: nortriptyline 75 mg per tablet
    Dispense: _____ tablet(s)

Answer at the end of the chapter.

Please note: The *maximum* number of tablets or capsules that will be dispensed for a *single dose* is usually 3. Double-check your calculations if your answer shows a single dose requiring more than 3 tablets/capsules.

2. Order: nortriptyline oral solution 150 mg

  Pharmacy supply: nortriptyline hydrochloride oral solution 10 mg/5 mL

  Dispense: _____ mL

Answer at the end of the chapter.

PARENTERAL DOSAGE CALCULATIONS

IV and other parenteral dosage calculations can be done using the same formulas you just learned for oral medications. Calculate parenteral dosages by using either the Have-Need formula or the $\frac{D}{H} \times Q = X$ formula.

CALCULATION RULES TO REMEMBER

1. Make sure you set your problem up right. Each step in solving hinges on having the problem set up correctly.
2. Make sure the units are labeled. You may have to convert units. Always convert units to what you have in stock.
3. Read the order in its entirety before calculating.
4. Always ask yourself whether the answer you came up with seems reasonable. Is the dosage safe?

Example:

Order: Cleocin 1 g IV

Pharmacy supply: You can see from the label below that the supply on hand is Cleocin Phosphate 150 mg/mL

1. Convert units to what is in stock. The order is for 1 g. The pharmacy is stocked with mg.

$$1 \text{ g} = 1000 \text{ mg}$$

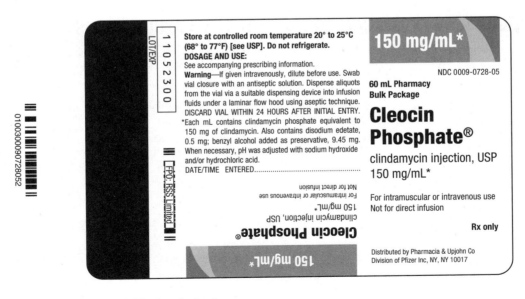

Figure 16-1 Cleocin 150 mg Label

Source: Courtesy of Pfizer

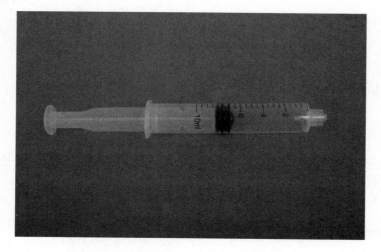

Figure 16-2 10 mL Syringe with Plunger Line at 7 ml

2. Set the problem up. Label the units. Cross off like labels. Solve for X by cross multiplying. Solve for X by dividing to make X stand alone.

$$\frac{150 \; \cancel{mg}}{1 \; mL} = \frac{1000 \; \cancel{mg}}{X}$$

$$150X = 1000$$

$$X = 6.66 \; mL$$

3. Does the answer seem reasonable?

4. Take this calculation problem a step further, and show the calibration line to measure from on this syringe. For this instance $6.66 \approx 7.0$.

MILLIGRAM PER KILOGRAM (MG/KG) DOSAGE CALCULATIONS

Many medications are recommended by mg/kg. This means that a medication is dosed to allow a certain amount of milligrams per kilogram of the patient's body weight.

A prescriber's order will look like this:

Amoxicillin 5 mg/kg po q 12 hours   *pediatric patient weighs 32 pounds*

1. First step is to convert the weight to kg. Recall the conversion factor is 2.2.

$$1 \; kg = 2.2 \; lb$$

You can set up the mg to kg conversion as a ratio equation:

$$\frac{1 \; kg}{2.2 \; lb} = \frac{X}{32 \; lb}$$

$$2.2X = 32$$

$$\frac{\cancel{2.2}X}{\cancel{2.2}} = \frac{32}{2.2}$$

$$X = 14.55 \; kg$$

Or you can simply divide the weight in pounds by the conversion factor.

$$32 \div 2.2 = 14.55$$

Hint: When converting mg to kg, look at kg as approximately 1/2 the weight in pounds.

2. After you have the weight in kg, multiply weight in kg by the prescribed dosage.

$$\frac{14.55 \text{ kg}}{1} \times \frac{5 \text{ mg}}{1 \text{ kg}} = 72.75 \text{ mg}$$

3. Then multiply dose by dosing schedule.
The prescriber's order reads *5 mg/kg p.o. q 12 hours.*
q 12 hours is 2 times a day 72.75 × 2 = 145.5 mg of amoxicillin per day.

Now you try. Solve for this prescriber's order:

Trimox 7.5 mg/kg bid   patient weighs 82 pounds

weight in kg _____

dose _____

daily dose_____

Answer at the end of the chapter.

SPECIFIC GRAVITY

Specific gravity is the ratio of the weight of a substance to the weight of an equal volume of water (the standard) when both have the same temperature and pressure.

The specific gravity for water is 1. This means that 1 mL of water weighs 1 g.

The chart below (**Table 16-1**) gives you an idea of what the specific gravity is for different substances. You should commit to memory that water has a specific gravity of 1. Otherwise, it's not necessary to memorize specific gravity for other substances.

To solve for specific gravity problems,

1. Multiply the volume in mL by the specific gravity (sp gr).
2. Answer is labeled in grams.

Example:
What is the weight of 100 mL of 70% dextrose?
The chart below shows that 70% dextrose has a specific gravity of 1.24.

$$100 \text{ mL} \times 1.24 = 124 \text{ grams}$$

Table 16-1 Specific Gravity

Solution Type	Specific Gravity
Travasol 10%	1.03
70% Dextrose	1.24
5% Dextrose/Lactated Ringers	1.02
SWI (sterile water for injection)	1.00

CALCULATION OF IV RATE AND ADMINISTRATION

Intravenous flow rates are usually described as mL/hr or as drops (gtt) per minute. The best formula to remember for calculating drip rate in mL/hr is the $\frac{V}{T}$ formula:

$$\frac{V}{T} = R$$

$$\frac{\text{Volume (mL)}}{\text{Time (hr)}} = \text{Rate}$$

To use this formula, the volume needs to be in mL and the time in hours.

Example:

A physician orders an *IV fluid of 1 liter D₅W over 10 hours.*

1. Convert units. The volume needs to be in mL.
   Order is for 1 liter.

$$1 \text{ liter} = 1000 \text{ mL}$$

2. Plug numbers into the formula.

$$\frac{V = 1000 \text{ mL}}{T = 10 \text{ hours}} = \text{Rate}$$

3. Work the equation.

$$1000 \div 10 = 100 \text{ mL/hour}$$

To figure drips per minute (gtts/min), we add a component to the $\frac{V}{T}$ formula.

$$\frac{V}{T} \times C = R$$

$$\frac{\text{Volume (mL)}}{\text{Time (min)}} \times \text{Calibration of pump (gtt/mL)} = \text{Rate}$$

The volume needs to be in mL and the time in minutes. The pump calibration or drop factor is in gtt/mL. When you cross off like labels the answer or rate will be labeled in gtt/min.

Example:

Administer a 100-mL SVP over 30 minutes using a 15-drop set. Figure the rate of administration.

1. Convert units if necessary.
2. Plug numbers into the formula. Be sure to label with units.

$$\frac{100 \text{ mL}}{30 \text{ minutes}} \times 15 \text{ gtts/mL} = R$$

3. Cross off like units.

$$\frac{100 \text{ m̶L̶}}{30 \text{ minutes}} \times 15 \text{ gtts/m̶L̶} = R$$

4. Work the equation.

$$100 \div 30 = 3.34 \qquad 3.34 \times 15 = 50$$

5. The rate is 50 gtts/minute.

6. Does this seem reasonable?

Now you try.

1. Your pharmacist asks you to calculate the rate (gtts/min) for a 50-mL infusion to run over 30 minutes, using a 10-drop set.

   Formula_____

   Answer_____gtts/min

2. A 1-liter IV is running at 150 mL/hr. How often will the pharmacy need to have a new bag ready to be administered?

   Formula_____

   Answer_____

Answers at the end of the chapter.

ALLIGATION

Alligations are used to calculate the amount of each solution needed when mixing together solutions with different strengths but the same active ingredient. You will know your problem requires alligation when there are a number of different solutions. Look at this example question. *Prepare 500 mL of dextrose 7% using dextrose 5% (D5W) & dextrose 50% (D50W). How many milliliters of each will be needed?*

You can see that each solution has the same active ingredient of dextrose, and you would not be able to solve this problem using any of the other equations you've learned for dosage calculations. Follow these steps for solving an allegation problem.

1. Draw a tic-tac-toe grid.
2. Put the solution with the highest percent concentration in the upper left corner. Leave off the % sign and write the strength as a whole number.
3. Put the solution with the lowest percent concentration in the bottom left corner.
4. Put the desired concentration strength that the prescriber ordered in the center of the grid. Leave off the % sign and write the strength as a whole number.

$$
\begin{array}{c|c|c}
50 & & \\
\hline
 & 7 & \\
\hline
5 & & \\
\end{array}
$$

5. Subtract the center number from the top left number and put the answer in the bottom right corner. This answer will **always be a positive number**.
6. Subtract the center number from the bottom left number and put the answer in the top right corner. This answer will **always be a positive number**.

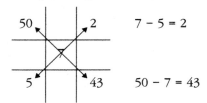

$7 - 5 = 2$

$50 - 7 = 43$

7. Read across the tic-tac-toe grid from right to left.

   To prepare this order, you will need 2 parts of the 50% solution and 43 parts of the 5% solution.

The sum of the numbers in the right column (2 + 43 = 45) is the total number of parts in the 7% solution.

2 parts of the 50% solution is needed

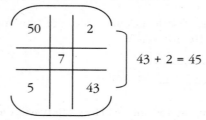

43 + 2 = 45

43 parts of the 5% solution is needed

8. Calculate the actual amount needed to compound the order.

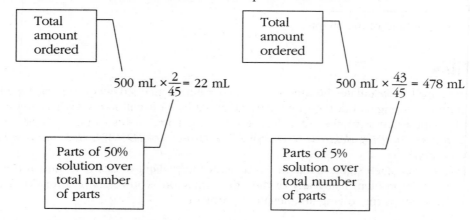

$$500 \text{ mL} \times \frac{2}{45} = 22 \text{ mL}$$

$$500 \text{ mL} \times \frac{43}{45} = 478 \text{ mL}$$

Parts of 50% solution over total number of parts

Parts of 5% solution over total number of parts

The actual amount of 50% strength needed: 22 mL
The actual amount of 5% strength needed: 478 mL

9. Check your calculations. Add the volumes of the two solutions together. The sum should equal the volume ordered by the physician.

$$\begin{array}{r} 22 \text{ mL} \\ +478 \text{ mL} \\ \hline 500 \text{ mL} \end{array}$$

Please make note: Any time sterile water or normal saline (NS) is the diluent, the % strength is zero (0).

Now you try. Solve this alligation problem.

Your pharmacy keeps a stock supply of cortisone cream 20% and cortisone cream 80%. The prescriber's order is for 75 grams of cortisone cream 30%. What quantities of the 20% and 80% concentrations will it take to make the prescribed amount of the 30% cream?

1. Set up the tic-tac-toe grid_____

2. Subtract strengths and find the total parts_____

3. Calculate the actual amount needed of 20% cream_____ 80% cream_____

4. Check your work.

Answer at the end of the chapter.

DILUTIONS

A potent medication would also be referred to as concentrated. Reducing the strength or the concentration of a medication is called dilution. This can be compared to common practices in the home like diluting strong chocolate milk with more milk or diluting strong orange juice with more water.

Concentrated stock medications may be used to compound weaker solutions. You can tell a dilution problem when you're asked to use a higher percent-strength solution to make a lower percent-strength solution.

Example:

How many mL of 20% calcium gluconate are needed to prepare 500 mL of 3% calcium gluconate?
Set up the problem:

$$\frac{\text{volume of stock solution}}{\text{Desired \% strength after dilution}} = \frac{\text{volume needed}}{\text{\% strength of concentration in stock}}$$

Plug in the numbers. Cross off like labels.

$$\frac{X}{3\%} = \frac{500 \text{ mL}}{20\%}$$

Solve for X by cross multiplying:

$$1500 = 20X$$

Solve for X by dividing for X to stand alone:

$$1500 \div 20 = 75$$

X = 75 mL of 20% calcium gluconate 425mL of sterile water (SW) to quantity sufficient (QS)

Does the answer seem reasonable?

Now you try. Solve this dilution problem.

How many mL of 5% magnesium acetate are needed to prepare 100 mL of 1% magnesium acetate?

Answer _____mL

Answer at the end of the chapter.

CONCENTRATIONS

A fraction may be used to express the strength of a solution. Is a ¼-strength solution more concentrated than a ½-strength solution?

✓ The *numerator* of the fraction is the number of parts of *solute*.
✓ The *denominator* of the fraction is the total number of parts of total *solution*.
✓ The *difference* between the denominator (final solution) and the numerator (parts of solute) is the number of parts of *solvent*.

½ strength means $\dfrac{1 \text{ part solute or concentration}}{2 \text{ parts of the total solution}}$

2 − 1 = 1 -----1 part solvent

You should remember the difference between the solute and the solvent. The solute is what is being dissolved. In our kitchen at home, chocolate syrup is the solute in chocolate milk. The powder mix is the solute in Kool-Aid. The solvent is the liquid or semisolid that the solute is dissolved in. Milk is the solvent in chocolate milk. Water is the solvent in Kool-Aid.

Now let's answer the question asked earlier; is a ¼-strength solution more concentrated than a ½-strength solution? No. The ½ strength is more concentrated. It contains 50% medication while the ¼-strength contains 25% medication.

POWDER VOLUME

Parenteral drugs sometimes come in powdered form to be reconstituted. The package insert or label will give directions on what the diluent should be and how much of the diluent should be added to reconstitute. The volume or space that the powder occupies in the vial after reconstitution is called powder volume.

The powder volume equals the final volume minus the amount of diluent added.

$$\text{final volume} - \text{diluent amount} = \text{powder volume}$$

CALCULATING CONCENTRATIONS

A concentration problem will ask you to find the amount of solute needed to make the desired strength or concentration.

Example:

How much medication should be added to the 180 mL solution for a 2/3 strength?
To calculate solutions you may use a ratio-proportion formula to find the amount of solute.

1. Read through the entire order.
2. Convert units if necessary.
3. Set up the equation.

$$\frac{2}{3} = \frac{X \text{ mL}}{180 \text{ mL}}$$

4. Cross off like labels.

$$\frac{2}{3} = \frac{X \cancel{\text{ mL}}}{180 \cancel{\text{ mL}}}$$

5. Cross multiply.

$$2 \times 180 = 360 \qquad 3 \times X = 3X$$

6. Solve for X by dividing so X stands alone.

$$\frac{360}{3} = \frac{\cancel{3}X}{\cancel{3}}$$

$$360 \div 3 = 120$$

$$\left. \frac{120 \text{ mL solute}}{180 \text{ mL solution}} \right\} \qquad \text{reduces to } \frac{2}{3}$$

7. Does the answer seem reasonable?

To calculate solutions, you may also use the $D \times Q = X$ formula. Practice with this formula and decide which formula: $D \times Q = X$ or ratio/proportion is the best formula for you to use.

$$D \times Q = X$$

D (desired solution strength) × Q (quantity of desired solution) = X (amount of solute)
We'll use the same example from the ratio/proportion formula.
How much medication should be added to the 180 mL solution for a 2/3 strength?

1. Read the entire order.
2. Convert units if necessary.
3. Plug numbers into the formula.

$$\frac{2}{3} \times 180 \text{ mL} = X$$

4. Solve for X.

$$120 \text{ mL} = X$$

5. Does the answer seem reasonable?

Now you try. Find out how much solute is needed.

Prepare 1 liter of 3/5 concentration strength.

Conversion 1 liter = _____mL

Equation or Formula_____

Answer_____mL solute

Check Answer_____

DOSING FOR CHILDREN

Most medications are developed and manufactured with the adult patient in mind. The recommended dosing is based on adult patient use. There are ways to determine what the pediatric dose should be for an adult-dosed medication. BSA, Young's rule, and Clark's rule are three formulas used to determine child dosing.

BSA Calculations

Body surface area (BSA) calculations are thought to be the most accurate way to figure patient dosing. While some dosage calculations will rely on either a patient's age or weight, calculating a dosage per body surface area uses the patient's volume. BSA is frequently used to figure dosing for chemotherapy patients where exact dosing is crucial. BSA is also frequently used to figure dosing for young children.

A nomogram is a chart used to find the patient's BSA when determining dosages. The nomogram has a column of height in centimeters and inches and a column of weight in pounds and kilograms. The column in the middle of the nomogram lists BSA.

✓ Use a nomogram
✓ BSA is measured in square meters (m²)

The formula for determining BSA:

$$\text{adult dose} \times \frac{\text{child's BSA}}{1.73 \text{ m}^2} = \text{child's dose}$$

The constant number in the BSA formula is 1.73 m² as this is the surface area of the average adult.

Example:

The order is for an antibiotic with an adult dose of 125 mg per day. What would the dosage for this medication be for a child who has a length of 150 cm and weight of 50 kg?

1. Use the nomogram to find the child's BSA. Put a ruler or straight edge of a paper on the nomogram to align the child's weight and height. The point of intersection is the BSA.
2. Plug the numbers into the formula.

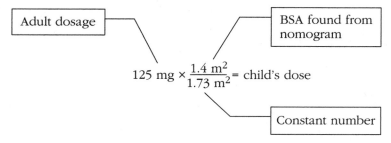

$$125 \text{ mg} \times \frac{1.4 \text{ m}^2}{1.73 \text{ m}^2} = \text{child's dose}$$

3. Cross off like labels and solve.

$$\text{child's dose} = 101 \text{ mg}$$

4. Does the answer seem reasonable?

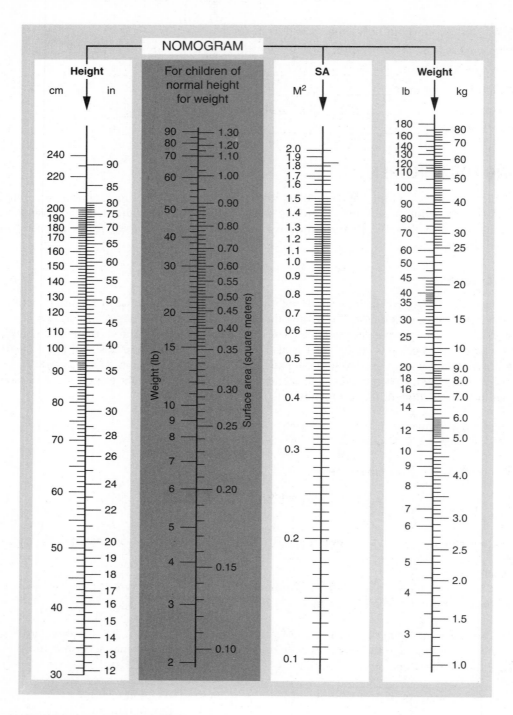

Figure 16-3 Nomogram of ht/wt m²

Reprinted from: Boyd, E. Nelson Textbook of Pediatrics. 1983. Copyright Elsevier

Young's Rule

Young's rule for calculating dosing for children is based on the child's age. The formula has flaws, because it's based strictly on a child's age and sometimes the age of a child doesn't coincide with their size. My 10-year-old daughter, for instance, weighs 110 pounds and is 5'6". Rather than getting a dose based on a 10-year-old, she may be better suited in receiving an adult dose based on her size.

Young's Rule Formula

$$\text{adult dose} \times \frac{\text{child's age in years}}{\text{child's age} + 12} = \text{child's dose}$$

We'll use the same example used for BSA calculations.
The order is for an antibiotic with an adult dose of 125 mg per day. What would the dosage for this medication be for a 13-year-old child who has a length of 150 cm and weight of 50 kg?

1. Plug numbers into the formula.

$$125 \text{ mg} \times \frac{13 \text{ years}}{13 + 12} \quad = \quad 125 \text{ mg} \times \frac{13 \text{ years}}{25 \text{ years}} =$$

2. Cross off like labels.
3. Solve.

$$\text{child's dose} = 65 \text{ mg}$$

Clark's Rule

Clark's rule for calculating dosing for children is based on the child's weight. While this formula will be more accurate than Young's rule, there are still flaws to the formula. The formula is based on an average adult dose and an average adult weight. Anytime averages are used, the accuracy decreases.

$$\text{adult dose} \times \frac{\text{weight of child in lb}}{150 \text{ pounds}} = \text{child's dose}$$

Average adult weight constant number in the formula

We'll use the same example used for BSA and Young's rule calculations.
The order is for an antibiotic with an adult dose of 125 mg per day. What would the dosage for this medication be for a 13-year-old child who has a length of 150 cm and weight of 50 kg?

1. Convert units.

$$50 \text{ kg} \times 2.2 = 110 \text{ pounds}$$

2. Plug numbers into formula.

$$125 \text{ mg} \times \frac{110 \text{ lbs}}{150 \text{ lbs}} = X$$

3. Cross off like labels.
4. Solve for X.

$$\text{child's dose} = 92 \text{ mg}$$

You have worked the same problem using three different formulas, and each formula provided a different answer. You can see that BSA and Clark's rule, the two formulas that deal with the size of the child, provide a more similar answer.

Now you try. Use each formula to figure the appropriate child's dose.

Age: 8   Height: 100 cm   Weight: 20 kg

Average adult dose: 325 mg

BSA answer_____mg

Young's rule answer_____mg

Clark's rule answer_____mg

Answers at the end of the chapter.

This is your checklist to make sure you understand what you need to know for the certification exam. Review chapter content if there is a topic you're uncertain of.

I know:

√	...how to solve dilution problems.
	...the steps to solve a ratio problem.
	...how to use conversions and solve for a weight/weight problem (mg/kg) (lb/kg).
	...how to solve weight/volume equations (specific gravity).
	...formulas to solve for dosage calculations.
	...how to calculate IV drip rates.
	...the meaning of concentration and how to calculate concentration problems.
	...formulas used to figure dosing for children and adults (BSA, Young's rule, Clark's rule).

PRACTICE TEST ANSWERS

Dosage Calculations

Order: nortriptyline 150 mg qd

$$\frac{150 \text{ mg}}{75 \text{ mg}} \times 1 \text{ tablet} =$$

Pharmacy supply: nortriptyline 75 mg per tablet
Dispense_____2_____ tablet(s)

Order: nortriptyline oral solution 150 mg

$$\frac{150 \text{ mg}}{10 \text{ mg}} \times 5 \text{ mL}$$

Pharmacy supply: nortriptyline hydrochloride oral solution 10 mg/5 mL
Dispense_____75_____mL

mg/kg

Trimox 7.5 mg/kg bid   patient weighs 82 pounds

weight in kg____37.27_____ 82 ÷ 2.2
dose _____280 mg_____ 37.27 × 7.5
daily dose___560 mg_____ 280 × 2

IV Administration Rates

Your pharmacist asks you to calculate the rate (gtts/min) for a 50-mL infusion to run over 30 minutes, using a 10-drop set.

$$\frac{V}{T} \times C = R$$

Answer:

$$\frac{50 \text{ mL}}{30 \text{ min}} \times 10 \text{ gtt/mL} = 17 \text{ gtt/min}$$

A 1-liter IV is running at 150 mL/hr. How often will the pharmacy need to have a new bag ready to be administered?

$$\text{Formula} \frac{V}{T} = R$$

1. Convert units. 1 liter = 1000 mL
2. Plug numbers into formula.

$$\frac{\textbf{v}\text{olume is 1000 mL}}{\textbf{t}\text{ime is the unknown (X)}} = \frac{\textbf{r}\text{ate is 150 mL}}{1 \text{ hour}}$$

3. Solve the equation by crossing off like labels and cross multiplying.

$$\frac{1000 \text{ mL}}{X} = \frac{150 \text{ mL}}{1 \text{ hour}}$$

$$1000 = 150X$$

4. Solve the equation by dividing so that X stands alone.

$$\frac{1000}{150} = \frac{15\cancel{0}X}{\cancel{150}}$$

$$1000 \div 150 = 6.67$$

$$6.67 = X$$

Answer: The 1 liter IV bag will need to be changed about every 6½ hours.

Alligation

Answer: 62.5 g of 20% cream and 12.5 g of 80% cream

80		10
	30	
20		50

$10 + 50 = 60$ total parts

$$75 \times \frac{10}{60} = 12.5 \text{ grams } 80\% \text{ cream} \qquad 75 \times \frac{50}{60} = 62.5 \text{ grams } 20\% \text{ cream}$$

Check answer: $62.5 + 12.5 = 75$

Dilution

X = 20 mL magnesium acetate

Concentration

Prepare 1 liter of 3/5 concentration strength.
Conversion: 1 liter = 1000 mL

Equation or formula: $\frac{3}{5} \times 1000 = X$

Answer: 600 mL solute

Check answer: $\frac{600}{1000}$ reduces to $\frac{3}{5}$

Children's Dosing

Age: 8   Height: 100 cm   Weight: 20 kg
Average adult dose: 325 mg
BSA answer: Nomogram BSA 0.75   141 mg
Young's rule answer: 130 mg
Clark's rule answer: Conversion from 20 kg to pounds is 44 pounds   95 mg

DRUG CALCULATION PRACTICE TEST – BEGINNER

MULTIPLE CHOICE

Identify the choice that best completes the statement or answers the question.

_____ **1.** Order: Lasix 80 mg
Pharmacy stock: 20 mg/mL
How much will the pharmacy dispense?

a. 20 mL
b. 4 mL

c. 40 mL
d. 2 mL

_____ **2.** Order: Ancef 560 mg IV qd
Pharmacy stock: cefazolin (Ancef) 1 g/5 mL
How much will the pharmacy dispense?

a. 2800 mL
b. 28 mL

c. 2.8 mL
d. 5 mL

_____ **3.** Order: Rocephin 287 mg IV qd
Pharmacy supply: 1 g/5 mL
How much will the pharmacy dispense?

a. 14 mL
b. 5 mL

c. 140 mL
d. 1.4 mL

_____ **4.** Order: Camptosar 35 mg IV
Pharmacy stock: Camptosar 40 mg/2 mL
How much will the pharmacy dispense?

a. 1.75 mL
b. 175 mL

c. 17.5 mL
d. 2 mL

_____ **5.** What is the powder volume of a medication that is reconstituted with 4 mL of sterile water and has a final concentration of 250 mg/5 mL and final volume of 8 mL?

a. 1 mL
b. 8 mL

c. 5 mL
d. 4 mL

_____ **6.** Order: 1500 mL over 12 hr
What is the infusion rate?

a. 125 mL/hr
b. 12.5 mL/hr

c. 1500 mL/hr
d. 100 mL/hr

_____ **7.** Order: 400 mL over 8 hours with an IV tubing set drip rate of 10 gtt/mL
What is the infusion rate?

a. 8 gtts/min
b. 480 gtts/min

c. 10 gtts/min
d. 40 gtts/min

_____ **8.** Order: 0.04 mg/kg IM q2hr prn
Pharmacy supply: 10 mg/5 mL
Patient weight: 25 lb

What amount is dispensed for one dose?

a. 0.04 mg

b. 11.4 mg

c. 0.46 mg

d. 4.6 mg

____ **9.** Order: 0.04 mg/kg IM q2hr prn
Pharmacy supply: 10 mg/5 mL
Patient weight: 25 lb
How much will the pharmacy dispense?

a. 23 mL

b. 0.23 mL

c. 5 mL

d. 0.46 mL

___ **10.** Order: 120 g 45% hydroxycream
Pharmacy supply: hydroxycream 80% and hydroxycream 5%
What strengths are needed of each cream to compound the order?

a. 40 g of 80% and 80 g of 5%

b. 63.6 g of 80% and 56.4 g of 5%

c. 37 g of 80% and 83 g of 5%

d. 56.4 g of 80% and 63.6 g of 5%

___ **11.** Use Clark's rule to calculate the pediatric dose.
Recommended adult dose: 520 mg po TID
Child's weight: 62 lb

a. 173 mg

b. 215 mg

c. 57 mg

d. 21.5 mg

ANSWER SECTION – BEGINNER

1. B

You can use either $\frac{D}{H} \times Q = X$

or the have:need ratio-proportion method

Have in stock $\frac{20\ mg}{1\ mL}$ Need (Dr. order) $\frac{80\ mg}{X}$

Cross off like labels (mg)

Cross multiply: $20 \times X = 20X$ $1 \times 80 = 80$

Divide each side of the equation by 20 to solve for X

$$\frac{20X}{20} = 1X \qquad\qquad \frac{80}{20} = 4$$

X = 4mL

2. C

Always convert to what you have in stock

Convert mg to g   560 mg = 0.56 g

Set up the problem in ratio-proportion (Have-Need) or use formula $\frac{D}{H} \times Q = X$

$$\frac{1\ g}{5\ mL} = \frac{0.56\ g}{X}$$

Cross off like labels (g) and solve for X

Cross multiply: $1 \times X = 1X$ $5 \times 0.56 = 2.8$

Divide each side of the equation by 1 to solve for X

$$\frac{1X}{1} = \frac{2.8}{1}$$

X = 2.8mL

3. D

Always convert to stock supply

287 mg = 0.287 g

$$\frac{D}{H} \times Q = X$$

$$\frac{0.287\ g}{1\ g} \times 5\ mL =$$

Cross off like labels and solve

X = 1.435 round to 1.4 mL

4. A

$$\frac{D}{H} \times Q = X$$

$$\frac{35\ mg}{40\ mg} \times 2\ mL = X$$

Cross off like labels and solve

5. D

Final volume minus diluent added

$8 - 4 = 4$

6. A

$$\frac{V}{T} = R$$

$$\frac{1500\ mL}{12\ hr} = 125\ mL/hr$$

7. A

$\frac{V}{T} \times C = R$ volume divided by time, times the calibration equals the rate (time must be in minutes)

Convert hours to minutes: 8 hours × 60 minutes = 480 min

$$\frac{400 \text{ mL}}{480 \text{ min}} \times 10 \text{ gtts/mL} =$$

400 mL/480 minutes × 10 gtts/1 mL =

Cross off like labels (mL) and you are left with gtts/minutes
Multiply to solve: 400 × 10 = 4000   480 × 1 = 480
4000/480 reduces to 8.33 or 8 gtts/min

8. C
Convert lb to kg   25 lb ÷ 2.2 = 11.36 round to 11.4 kg
11.4 kg × 0.04 mg = 0.456 round to 0.46 mg

9. B
Use the answer from problem #8 of 0.46 mg/dose
Set the problem up
$$\frac{10 \text{ mg}}{5 \text{ mL}} = \frac{0.46 \text{ mg}}{X}$$

10 mg/5 mL = 0.46 mg/X
Cross off like labels and cross multiply
10 × X = 10X   5 × 0.46 = 2.3
Divide both sides by 10 to solve for X
10 ÷ 10 = 1   2.3 ÷ 10 = 0.23
X = 0.23 mL

10. B
Alligation
Make a tic tac toe grid:
Desired strength in the middle, higher strength in top left, lower strength in bottom left
Subtract strengths

```
80 |     | 40
   | 45  |
5  |     | 35
```

80 − 45 = 35
45 − 5 = 40
Add the two parts 35 + 40 = 75
40 ÷ 75 = 0.53   0.53 × total amount needed 120 g = 63.6 g needed of 80% cream
35 ÷ 75 = 0.47   0.47 × total amount needed 120 g = 56.4 g needed of the 5% cream
Check your answer by adding 63.6 + 56.4 = 120

11. B

adult dose 520 mg × $\dfrac{\text{weight of child 62 lb}}{150 \text{ lb}}$ = 214.9   Round to 215 mg

DRUG CALCULATION PRACTICE TEST – INTERMEDIATE

MULTIPLE CHOICE

Identify the choice that best completes the statement or answers the question.

_____ **1.** The pharmacy stocks Zofran 5 mg/1 mL. The patient is prescribed 17 mg. How many mLs will be dispensed to fill the order?

a. 17 mL

b. 3.4 mL

c. 5 mL

d. 0.29 mL

_____ **2.** Pharmacy stock: Lipitor 20 mg tablets
Order: Lipitor 40 mg po qd
Dispense _____ for a 30 day supply

a. 60 tablets

b. 20 tablets

c. 30 tablets

d. 40 tablets

_____ **3.** Pharmacy stock: metoprolol 50 mg tablets
Order: metoprolol 150 mg po BID x 10 d
Dispense _____

a. 300 tablets

b. 20 tablets

c. 60 tablets

d. 30 tablets

_____ **4.** Pharmacy stock: calcium gluconate 10%
Order: calcium gluconate 4% 100 mL
How much of the calcium gluconate 10% is needed to prepare the order?

a. 100 mL

b. 40 mL

c. 400 mL

d. 10 mL

_____ **5.** Which solution is the most concentrated?

a. 0.9% NaCl

b. ½ NS

c. 5% Dextrose

d. 0.25% KCl

_____ **6.** The pharmacy technician prepares 500 mL of 1/3 strength dextrose. How much dextrose is added to gain the 1/3 strength?

a. 0.33 mL

b. 33 mL

c. 167 mL

d. 333 mL

_____ **7.** Nifedipine: Adult dose 120mg/day
Figure the dosing for a 25 kg child who is 120 cm tall with a BSA of 1.3m^2

a. 120 mg

b. 100 mg

c. 90 mg

d. 95 mg

_____ **8.** Use Clark's rule to determine a 10-year-old child's dose who weights 45 kg. The adult dose is 75 mg/day.

a. 50 mg

b. 74 mg

c. 45 mg

d. 5 mg

_____ **9.** What is the percent (%) strength of 500 mL of a 12% solution that is diluted to 1500 mL?

a. .04%

b. 45%

c. 4%

d. 0.4%

_____ **10.** How much time will it take a 1L IV bag to empty with an administration rate of 100 mL/hour?

a. 1 hour

b. 100 minutes

c. 8 hours

d. 10 hours

ANSWER SECTION – INTERMEDIATE

1. B

2. A

3. C
150 mg × 2 = 300 mg per day × 10 days = 3000 mg needed
3000 mg needed ÷ 50 mg tablets in stock = 60 tablets needed

4. B

5. B
0.9% NaCl contains 0.9% medication and 99.1% solvent
1/2 NS contains 50% medication in 50% solvent
5% Dextrose contains 5% medication and 95% solvent
0.25% KCl contains 0.25% medication in 99.75% solvent

6. C

7. C

8. A
Convert 45 kg to lb: 45 kg = 99 lb
75 mg/day × 99 lb = 7425
7425 ÷ 150 lb = 49.5 = 50 mg

9. C

10. D

DRUG CALCULATION PRACTICE TEST—ADVANCED

Use the label information to answer the following questions.

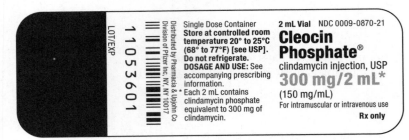

Figure 16-4 Cleocin 2mL label

Source: Courtesy of Pfizer

1. **Physician's Order:** Cleocin 400 mg IV
   What amount is dispensed to fill the order?

   How many vials will be used?

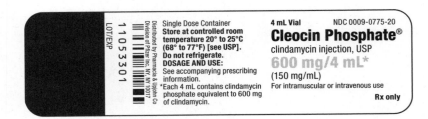

Figure 16-5 Cleocin 4mL label

Source: Courtesy of Pfizer

2. **Physician's Order:** Cleocin 300 mg IV TID
   What amount will be dispensed to fill the order for a 24-hour period?

   How many vials will be used?

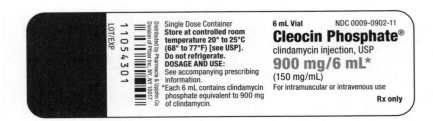

Figure 16-6 Cleocin 6mL label

Source: Courtesy of Pfizer

3. **Physician's Order:** Cleocin 850 mg IV
   What amount will be dispensed to fill the order?

   How many vials will be used?

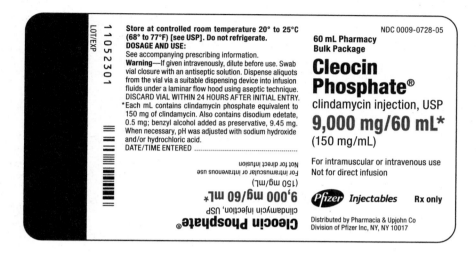

Figure 16-7 Cleocin 60mL label

Source: Courtesy of Pfizer

4. **Physician's Order:** Cleocin 250 mg IV
   What amount will be dispensed to fill the order?

   How many orders for 250 mg will this vial provide?

ANSWER SECTION – ADVANCED

1. The label reads 150 mg/mL. There are 2 mL in the vial.
Have in stock: $\frac{150 \text{ mg}}{1 \text{ mL}}$
Need: 400 mg
Set up the problem with *Have* on one side and *Need* on the other side.

$$\frac{150 \text{ mg}}{1 \text{ mL}} = \frac{400 \text{ mg}}{X}$$

Cross off like labels.

$$\frac{150 \text{ m̶g̶}}{1 \text{ mL}} = \frac{400 \text{ m̶g̶}}{X}$$

Cross multiply.

$$150 \times X = 150X \qquad\qquad 400 \times 1 = 400$$

Divide each side of the problem by the number with the X.

$$\frac{150X}{150} = \frac{400}{150}$$

$$150X \div 150 = X \qquad\qquad 400 \div 150 = 2.67$$

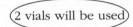

X = 2.67mL dispensed to fill the order   2 vials will be used

2. The label reads 150 mg/mL. The vial contains 4 mL.
The order is for 300 mg TID or 3 times a day. $300 \times 3 = 900$ mg needed for a 24-hour period.
Set up the problem with *Have* on one side and *Need* on the other side.

$$\frac{150 \text{ mg}}{1 \text{ mL}} = \frac{900 \text{ mg}}{X}$$

Cross off like labels.

$$\frac{150 \text{ m̶g̶}}{1 \text{ mL}} = \frac{900 \text{ m̶g̶}}{X}$$

Cross multiply.

$$150 \times X = 150X \qquad\qquad 900 \times 1 = 900$$

Divide each side of the problem by the number with the X.

$$\frac{150X}{150} = \frac{900}{150}$$

$$150X \div 150 = X \qquad\qquad 900 \div 150 = 6$$

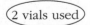

X = 6 mL dispensed to fill the order for 24 hours   2 vials used

3. The label reads 150 mg/mL. The vial contains 6 mL.
Set up the problem with *Have* on one side and *Need* on the other side.

$$\frac{150 \text{ mg}}{1 \text{ mL}} = \frac{850 \text{ mg}}{X}$$

Cross off like labels.

$$\frac{150 \text{ mg}}{1 \text{ mL}} = \frac{850 \text{ mg}}{X}$$

Cross multiply.

$150 \times X = 150X$ $\qquad\qquad$ $850 \times 1 = 850$

Divide each side of the problem by the number with the X.

$$\frac{150X}{150} = \frac{850}{150}$$

$150X \div 150 = X$ $\qquad\qquad$ $850 \div 150 = 5.67$

$\boxed{X = 5.67 \text{ mL dispensed to fill the order}}$ $\qquad$ (1 vial is needed)

4. The label reads 150 mg/mL. This is a bulk, multidose vial containing 60 mL. Set up the problem with *Have* on one side and *Need* on the other side.

$$\frac{150 \text{ mg}}{1 \text{ mL}} = \frac{250 \text{ mg}}{X}$$

Cross off like labels.

$$\frac{150 \text{ mg}}{1 \text{ mL}} = \frac{250 \text{ mg}}{X}$$

Cross multiply.

$150 \times X = 150X$ $\qquad\qquad$ $250 \times 1 = 250$

Divide each side of the problem by the number with the X.

$$\frac{150X}{150} = \frac{250}{150}$$

$150X \div 150 = X$ $\qquad\qquad$ $250 \div 150 = 1.67$

$\boxed{X = 1.67 \text{ mL dispensed to fill the order}}$

The vial holds 60 mL. Divide the volume of the vial by the dosage volume to find out how many doses can be pulled from this bulk vial.

$60 \div 1.67 = 35.93$ $\qquad$ (35 doses of 1.67 mL can be pulled from this 60-mL vial)

TASK SHEET

TOPIC TO REVIEW: BUSINESS CALCULATIONS

Materials

Pharmacy Technician Exam Review Guide

JB Test Prep: Pharmacy Technician Exam Review Guide

Prepare

1. Read the section on business calculations.
2. Take practice test at the end of the chapter.

Study Plan

1. Read pages_____ on _____(date).
2. Work sample problems in the chapter.
3. Take end of chapter practice test on_____(date).

Tips

Relate the business math problems to real-life situations. Does your answer make sense?

End of Chapter

List what you need to review.

Business Calculations

OBJECTIVES/TOPICS TO COVER:

✓ Perform pharmacy business calculations.

MARKUP AND DISCOUNT

The pharmacy sells medications at a higher price than they are purchased. The difference is called gross profit, and it is also referred to as markup.

$$\text{selling price} - \text{purchase price} = \text{markup or gross profit}$$

Example
A supply of a medication sells for $105 and costs the pharmacy $30. What is the markup?

$$\$105 - \$30 = \$75$$

The mark up rate is computed as:

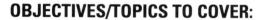

$$\frac{\text{markup}}{\cos t} \times 100 = \text{markup rate (\%)}$$

$$\frac{\$75}{\$30} \times 100 = 250\%$$

Discount
To figure discount, multiply the purchase price by the discount rate.

$$\text{purchase price} \times \text{discount rate} = \text{discount}$$

Take that a step further to figure the discounted price.

$$\text{purchase price} - \text{discount} = \text{discounted price}$$

Example
The pharmacy purchases 10 cases of vitamins at $100 per case. The vitamins were purchased at the annual trade show and therefore receive a 10% discount. What is the discounted purchase price?

$$\text{Full purchase price: } \$100 \times 10 \text{ cases} = \$1000$$
$$\text{Discount: } \$1000 \times 10\% = \$100$$
$$\text{Discounted price: } \$1000 - \$100 = \$900$$

AVERAGE WHOLESALE PRICE

Third-party insurance companies typically reimburse a pharmacy based on the average whole-sale price (AWP) of the medication. Therefore, there is an incentive for a pharmacy to purchase a medication below its AWP. The lower the AWP of the drug, the more profitable the pharmacy can be.

To figure pharmacy reimbursement from the third-party payer, add the AWP to the allotted dispensing fee.

$$prescription\ reimbursement = AWP + dispensing\ fee$$

Example
Lipitor tablets come in a quantity of 90 and have an AWP of $100. The pharmacy has an agreement with McKesson (the supplier) to purchase the drug at the AWP minus 5%. The third-party insurer will reimburse AWP plus 5% plus a $2 dispensing fee. How much profit does the pharmacy make on this prescription of 90 tablets?

Amount of discount from the supplier: $100 × 5% = $5.00

Purchase price of drug: $100 − $5 = $95

Third-party payment: $100 × 5% = $5

$100 + $5 = $105

Third-party payment: $105 + $2 dispensing fee = $107

Pharmacy profit: $107 − $95 = $12

INVENTORY MANAGEMENT

A common inventory goal is to move the dollar amount of inventory stock every 30 days. This means that, if the pharmacy inventory is $425,000, the pharmacy has sales equal to or greater than $425,000 every 30 days. This inventory goal is referred to as 30 *days' supply*, not to be confused with days supply for dispensing medication prescriptions.

Use this formula to determine inventory usage and days' supply:

$$\frac{value\ of\ inventory}{average\ daily\ cost\ of\ products\ sold} = number\ of\ days'\ supply$$

Example
Pharmacy total inventory: $189,990

Sales last week: $37,980

Pharmacy costs last week: $33,147

What is the pharmacy's days' supply?

1. Determine the pharmacy's average daily costs:

$$\$33,147 ÷ 7 = \$4735$$

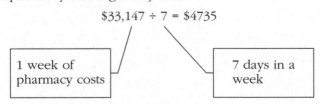

1 week of pharmacy costs   7 days in a week

2. Divide the value of the inventory by the average daily costs to determine the number of days' supply:

$$\frac{\$189,990}{\$4735} = 40\ days$$

This means it takes approximately 40 days for the pharmacy to move or to sell the value of its inventory. To reach a 30 days' supply the pharmacy may need to reduce inventory.

This is your checklist to make sure you understand what you need to know for the certification exam. Review chapter content if there is a topic you're uncertain of.
I know:

√	...how to figure markup.
	...how to use information to find inventory goals and days' supply.

CHAPTER 17

MULTIPLE CHOICE

Identify the choice that best completes the statement or answers the question.

_____ **1.** Horn Pharmacy has total overhead expenses of $570,000. How much money must be made in sales to have an 18% profit?

a. $102,600

b. $672,600

c. $467,400

d. $31,666

_____ **2.** Ms. Emsteve has prescription drug coverage insurance that gives the pharmacy a capitation fee of $300 a month. During allergy season, she had prescriptions for $70.25, $55, $37.50, $87, and $63.49. Who came out ahead, Ms. Emsteve's insurance company or the pharmacy?

a. Ms. Emsteve's insurance company came out ahead. The drugs totaled $313.24.

b. Neither came out ahead. The capitation fee allows for overages.

c. The pharmacy came out ahead.

d. Neither came out ahead. Ms. Emsteve pays the difference out of pocket.

_____ **3.** Jen ordinarily pays a purchase price of $4 a bottle for a generic brand of vitamins, but if she buys the vitamins by the case (24), she will get a 10% discount. How much will Jen pay for a case of vitamins?

a. $96.00

b. $105.60

c. $9.60

d. $86.40

_____ **4.** An 8 oz bottle of antibiotic has an AWP of $35. Feel Good Pharmacy can get the antibiotic from McKesson wholesaler for AWP minus 10%. How much will Feel Good Pharmacy pay?

a. $3.50

b. $25.00

c. $38.50

d. $31.50

_____ **5.** Furosemide has an AWP of $35. The pharmacy will purchase furosemide for AWP minus 10%. Catelynn's insurance company will reimburse the pharmacy AWP + 6%, whereas Emma's insurance company will reimburse the pharmacy AWP + 5% plus pay a $2 dispensing fee. How much will the pharmacy make from each of the prescriptions, and which provides a higher profit?

a. Emma's prescription yields a higher profit of $7.25

b. Catelynn's prescription yields a higher profit of $5.60

c. Emma's prescription yields a higher profit of $37.10

d. Catelynn's prescription yields a higher profit of $38.75

_____ **6.** The pharmacy is running a promotion of 25% off the purchase of the second bottle of vitamins. Ms. Muhr buys two bottles of vitamin C at $5/bottle and one bottle of vitamin E for $4. What is the total cost before tax?

a. $10.50

b. $12.75

c. $14.00

d. $1.25

_____ **7.** What is the markup on stock for which the pharmacy paid $456 and billed patients $792.87?

a. $1248.87

b. $456.00

c. $792.87

d. $336.87

_____ **8.** What is the markup percentage rate for stock that the pharmacy paid $717.54 for and charges patients $998.02 for?

a. 280%

b. 2.8%

c. 39%

d. 139%

_____ **9.** The pharmacy has a total inventory value of $98,500. The average daily cost of inventory is $4159.00. The pharmacy sold $21,560 last week. What is the pharmacy's days' supply?

a. 24 days' supply

b. 308 days' supply

c. 9 days' supply

d. 41 days' supply

_____ **10.** Determine the average daily costs.

Inventory total: $2,265,190   Average weekly costs: $245,009

a. $323,598

b. $35,001

c. $350.01

d. $3235.98

ANSWER SECTION

1. B

$570,000 \times 0.18$ (18%) $= $102,600

$102,600 + $570,000 = $672,600

2. A

3. D

4. D

5. A

6. B

7. D

8. D

9. A

10. B

TASK SHEET

TOPIC TO REVIEW: PRACTICE TESTS

Materials

Pharmacy Technician Exam Review Guide
JB Test Prep: Pharmacy Technician Exam Review Guide
Calculator

Prepare

Take certification practice tests.

Study Plan

Each practice test has 50 questions. Take these tests one at a time. Take the test in its entirety.

Tips

1. Take the practice tests as a final step in reviewing before sitting for your certification exam. Go over questions you miss and make sure you understand why your answer was wrong and how the correct answer was chosen. Review any information you're unsure of after taking the practice tests.
2. Both the ExCPT and PTCE websites have online practice tests. There is a fee to take the practice tests.
3. www.TestPrepReview.com is a free online source for practice tests. Access this web page and then click on the PTCB Exam Practice choice found on the left column of the home page. It's a great advantage to practice your knowledge using a computer, as this will be the format for your actual certification exam.

End of Chapter

List what you need to review.

Assess

1. You should take the time to check over all missed questions to find out why your answer was wrong and how the correct answer was found.
2. Missing 5 questions on a 50-question practice test would put you at a 90%.

Certification Practice Tests

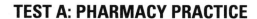

CHAPTER 18

TEST A: PHARMACY PRACTICE

MULTIPLE CHOICE

Identify the choice that best completes the statement or answers the question.

_____ **1.** A prescription hard copy is filed by

a. patient's last name
b. date filled

c. prescription number
d. date written

_____ **2.** An acute care medication order includes the patient's

a. DOB, room number, diet
b. room number, allergies, weight

c. allergies, diagnosis, address
d. diagnosis, prescriber's name, insurance information

_____ **3.** To triage orders in the pharmacy,

a. categorize orders for the next shift
b. determine the level of care for the patient

c. act on the first order received
d. act on the most urgent order first

_____ **4.** Unit dose medications

a. are an outdated medication delivery system
b. are individually packaged and labeled

c. are high risk for med errors
d. are an unrecoverable expense for the pharmacy

_____ **5.** Routine medication orders are filled for a(n) _____time period in the hospital pharmacy.

a. 8-hour
b. 1-week

c. 12-hour
d. 24-hour

_____ **6.** In all cases, which medications are permitted to be delivered via pneumatic tube?

a. CII's

b. STAT orders

c. medications in glass bottles

d. routine unit dose medications

_____ **7.** One reason for having an accurate and up-to-date patient profile is

a. to ensure proper third-party billing

b. to share patient information with the prescriber

c. to check for possible drug–drug interactions

d. to ensure the patient is living a healthy lifestyle

_____ **8.** The patient profile is a building block

a. to MTM

b. to pay-for-service healthcare

c. to patient-centered self-care

d. to OBRA

_____ **9.** The pharmacy technician assists in medication therapy management (MTM) by

a. counseling the patients

b. collecting and recording patient data

c. dispensing the correct medication

d. handling calls from third-party insurance

_____ **10.** Nonadherence refers to

a. nonpayment of an insurance claim

b. a patient refusing counseling by the pharmacist

c. nonpayment of a medication copay

d. a patient not taking his or her medication as prescribed

_____ **11.** Pharmacy automation

a. is uncommon in retail pharmacy

b. is designed to reduce medication error

c. is designed to take the place of the technician

d. will decrease productivity in the pharmacy

_____ **12.** Certain prescription packaging must contain the medication name and dose in a scannable format referred to as

a. unit dose

b. UPC symbol

c. barcode

d. labeling

_____ **13.** What part of Medicare insurance provides hospitalization coverage?

a. Part A

b. Part B

c. Part C

d. Part D

_____ **14.** What part of Medicare insurance provides coverage for DMEPOS?

a. Part A

b. Part B

c. Part C

d. Part D

_____ **15.** What part of Medicare insurance provides prescription drug coverage?

a. Part A

b. Part B

c. Part C

d. Part D

____ **16.** Medicaid is primarily available to

a. patients 65 years and older

b. patients 65 years and younger

c. patients who can't afford medical care

d. young patients covered under their guardian's healthcare

____ **17.** Individuals eligible for both Medicare and Medicaid are termed

a. dual eligible

b. double eligible

c. dual benefit earners

d. double beneficiaries

____ **18.** Which of the following is a military health plan?

a. workers' compensation

b. TRICARE

c. Medicaid

d. TROOP

____ **19.** A flat monthly reimbursement fee paid by the insurance company to the pharmacy is termed a

a. copay

b. deductible

c. capitation fee

d. adjudication

____ **20.** The transmission of insurance claims online is termed

a. online approval

b. acceptance

c. adjudication

d. approval

____ **21.** Which of the following is a common reason for a rejected insurance claim?

a. invalid person code

b. invalid patient address

c. refill quantity not matched

d. pharmacy not covered

____ **22.** The procedure of asking the insurance carrier for a nonformulary medication to be dispensed is termed

a. approval

b. postapproval

c. prior grant

d. prior authorization

____ **23.** The National Provider Identifier (NPI) number is

a. optional for retail pharmacies

b. optional for acute pharmacies

c. mandatory for pharmacies that transmit electronically

d. optional for pharmacies that transmit electronically

____ **24.** A Universal Claim Form (UCF) is

a. a paper claim used to bill for certain pharmacy supplies and services

b. an electronic form used to bill for certain pharmacy supplies and services

c. required for adjudication

d. completed by the third-party payer and mailed to the pharmacy for approval

____ **25.** A preferred list of drugs is termed a

a. protocol

b. formulary

c. handbook

d. utilization guide

___ **26.** Transcribe: i tab po bid ac

a. Take one tablet by mouth three times a day

b. Take one tablet by mouth twice daily

c. Take one tablet by mouth twice daily before meals

d. Take one tablet by mouth twice daily after meals

___ **27.** Transcribe: ii caps tid pp prn po

a. Take two capsules by mouth three times a day after meals as needed

b. Take two capsules by mouth twice a day after meals as needed

c. Take two capsules by mouth three times a day per physician as needed

d. Take two capsules by mouth twice daily per physician as needed

___ **28.** Transcribe: ii gtts AD QID

a. Instill two drops in the right eye every other day

b. Instill two drops in the left ear four times a day

c. Instill two drops in the left eye four times a day

d. Instill two drops in the right ear four times a day

___ **29.** The drug class for PCN:

a. calcium channel blocker (CCB)

b. antibiotic

c. analgesic

d. proton pump inhibitor (PPI)

___ **30.** Prescription transfer from pharmacy to pharmacy

a. is done by the pharmacists

b. is done by the patient

c. is done by the pharmacy technicians

d. is not permitted by federal law

___ **31.** Prescriptions written for a controlled substance III–IV

a. may not be transferred

b. may be transferred on a onetime basis

c. may be transferred from pharmacy to pharmacy up to 2 years from the dated hard copy

d. may be transferred on an emergency basis

___ **32.** Reporting of medication errors

a. is done only by the pharmacist in charge

b. is voluntary

c. is done only by the healthcare worker who had the error

d. is mandatory

___ **33.** The Orange Book is

a. a compiling of monographs detailing drug actions and indications

b. a book of standards

c. the authority for determining therapeutic equivalence in product substitution

d. a guide to AWP

___ **34.** The Red Book is

a. a set of standards for pharmacy practice

b. used to identify tablets and capsules by their unique markings

c. used in retail pharmacy to find detailed drug information

d. a guide to AWP for prescription and OTC drugs

___ **35.** Who is responsible for inventory?

a. the pharmacy manager

b. the pharmacy technician

c. central supply

d. everyone on the pharmacy team

___ **36.** Updating or ordering stock on a continuous basis is termed

a. inventory purchase

b. perpetual inventory

c. turnover

d. periodic automatic replenishment (PAR)

___ **37.** The technician who checks in the shipment of stock

a. should be the first on shift for the day

b. should remove radio frequency identification (RFID) from the packaging

c. should be different from the technician who placed the order

d. should be the same technician who placed the order

___ **38.** Rotating stock means that

a. new stock is shelved in front of existing stock

b. new stock is shelved behind existing stock

c. stock is returned to the manufacturer for fresh stock

d. stock is routinely checked for outdates

___ **39.** Pharmacy-mandated room temperature is

a.   36°–46°F

b.   15°–30°F

c. 56°–69°F

d. 59°–86°F

___ **40.** Pharmacy-mandated refrigerated temperature is

a. 36°–46°F

b. 2°–8°F

c. 15°–30°F

d. 59°–86°F

___ **41.** A listing on how to provide emergency treatment in the event of accidental exposure to a drug is listed

a.   in the Red Book

b.   on the manifest

c. on the MSDS

d. in the Orange Book

___ **42.** Cross-contamination occurs when

a. the manufacturer recalls a drug because of contamination

b. drug residue from one medication is mixed with another medication

c. drugs are mixed up during the shipping process

d. hazardous medications are shelved incorrectly

___ **43.** The most serious drug recall:

a. class 1

b. class 2

c. class 3

d. class 4

___ **44.** Which step should the pharmacy technician make when receiving a drug recall notice?

a. forward the notice to the pharmacist

b. contact the drug manufacturer to determine whether the affected product was shipped to your pharmacy

c. check the pharmacy stock lot number against the affected lot number on the recall notice

d. immediately contact patients to inform them of the recall and potential adverse effects

___ **45.** Medication disposal programs

a. help limit unauthorized access to unused pharmaceuticals

b. are voluntary in all states

c. help the pharmacy manage inventory

d. are time consuming and have not been statistically proven to help our environment

___ **46.** A company hired by the pharmacy to manage outdated medications is a

a. reverse distributor

b. distributor

c. manufacturer

d. prime vendor

___ **47.** Use the 1/4 method to determine the expiration date of a medication repackaged on March 10, 2011. The stock bottle expiration date is 3/2014.

a. 3/2012

b. 9/2011

c. 12/2011

d. 3/2014

___ **48.** A 10-digit number that identifies the drug product is termed:

a. National Drug Code (NDC)

b. National Provider Identifier (NPI)

c. Current Procedure Terminology (CPT)

d. Drug Enforcement Agency (DEA)

___ **49.** Unintended exposure to hazardous drugs

a. should be reported to MedWatch

b. will not occur when the pharmacy technician is properly trained

c. is a risk to pregnant women only

d. may be a risk to the health of the pharmacy technician

___ **50.** The pharmacy technician may risk unintended exposure to a hazardous drug

a. when administering the drug to the patient

b. during shipment of the drug from the supplier to the pharmacy

c. during drug compounding and preparation

d. when disposing of patient urine

ANSWER SECTION

1. C
2. B
3. D
4. B
5. D
6. D
7. C
8. A
9. B
10. D
11. B
12. C
13. A
14. B
15. D
16. C
17. A
18. B
19. C
20. C
21. A
22. D
23. C
24. A
25. B
26. C
27. A
28. D
29. B
30. A
31. B
32. B
33. C
34. D
35. D

36. B

37. C

38. B

39. D

40. A

41. C

42. B

43. A

44. C

45. A

46. A

47. C

48. A

49. D

50. C

TEST B: ASEPTIC COMPOUNDING

MULTIPLE CHOICE

Identify the choice that best completes the statement or answers the question.

_____ **1.** Aseptic technique is

a. sterile compounding procedures

b. nonsterile compounding procedures

c. repackaging oral unit dose

d. compounding creams, lotions, and troches

_____ **2.** Aseptic technique involves

a. proper manipulation of materials on the countertop

b. proper hand washing

c. a particle-free clean room

d. government-mandated training

_____ **3.** Proper aseptic technique is when the technician

a. handles materials without obstructing clean airflow

b. completes hand washing requirements every 15 minutes

c. facilitates airflow from the clean room into the LAFB

d. keeps an airtight seal on all critical sites

_____ **4.** The critical site of the needle is

a. the bevel tip

b. the hub

c. the shaft

d. the entire needle

_____ **5.** An example of aseptic compounding personal protective equipment (PPE):

a. LAWB

b. anteroom

c. garb

d. clean room

_____ **6.** An example of garb:

a. hair scarf

b. face mask

c. specially fitted shoes

d. overcoat

_____ **7.** Hand washing takes place in

a. the LAWB

b. the clean room

c. the buffer room

d. the anteroom

_____ **8.** Gloves are disinfected

a. before entering the buffer room

b. upon reentry into the hood to perform compounding

c. once an hour

d. after each syringe draw

_____ **9.** Clean rooms are _____ _____ for standard compounding.

a. positive pressure

b. negative pressure

c. not regulated

d. high humidity

_____ **10.** Hazardous drug compounding requires a clean room of:

a. positive pressure

b. negative pressure

c. high humidity

d. refrigerator temperature

_____ **11.** Clean rooms must be a minimum International Standards Organization (ISO):

a. 1

b. 8

c. 7

d. 10

_____ **12.** Clean rooms are also referred to as

a. buffer rooms

b. anterooms

c. hood rooms

d. pressurized rooms

_____ **13.** Aseptic compounding must be performed at least _____ inside the LAWB.

a. 3 inches

b. 1 inch

c. 3 feet

d. 6 inches

_____ **14.** Erratic hand movements within the hood should be avoided, because

a. clean air currents may be disrupted

b. vials and ampules may be broken

c. compounding errors may occur

d. viruses may spread to the compounded products

_____ **15.** The standard for aseptic compounding:

a. USP <795>

b. USP <797>

c. FDA rules and regulations

d. DEA rules and regulations

___ **16.** Normal saline:

a. D5W

c. Na

b. 0.9% NaCl

d. 9% NaCl

___ **17.** Term used for a solution used to reconstitute medication:

a. solute

c. admixture

b. diluent

d. CSP

___ **18.** The pharmacist asked Jennifer to reorder LVP D_5W. What size bags should Jennifer order?

a. 100 mL

c. 25 mL

b. 1000 mL

d. premixed quick grab

___ **19.** A piggyback is

a. LVP

c. SVP

b. commonly used for fluid replacement

d. commonly used for TPN

___ **20.** What is the term for inserting a needle-tipped apparatus into the medication port of an IV bag?

a. port saving

c. insertion

b. spiking

d. entering

___ **21.** Used for withdrawing and instilling medications:

a. syringe

c. ampule

b. port saver

d. vial

___ **22.** The pharmacist asked Emma to compound 10 SVP of ampicillin. Emma will

a. create a unit dose

c. create a repeat compound

b. create a batch compound

d. repackage the compound

___ **23.** What type of needle is used when withdrawing medication from an ampule?

a. luer-lock

c. filter

b. tension

d. large gauge

___ **24.** Which needle has the largest bore size?

a. 20 gauge

c. 19 gauge, 1 1/2 inch

b. 12 gauge

d. filter

___ **25.** The term used when fragments of the vial's rubber stopper are found in the medicine:

a. coring

c. fragmented

b. shedding

d. contaminated

___ **26.** Combining doses of many different medications is termed:

a. spiking

c. pooling

b. coring

d. mixing

___ **27.** How long should the compounding hood run prior to use?

a. 3 minutes

b. 30 minutes

c. 1 hour

d. 15 minutes

___ **28.** When cleaning the horizontal flow hood, wipe from _____ to _____.

a. bottom to top

b. rod to top

c. top to bottom

d. base to rod

___ **29.** What is the term for placing one item behind another, obstructing first air?

a. zoning

b. backwash

c. filtering

d. shadowing

___ **30.** How should items be placed in the vertical airflow hood?

a. checkerboard pattern

b. parallel with the front of the hood

c. directly in the middle of the workbench

d. parallel with the back of the hood

___ **31.** In the vertical airflow hood, the airflow divides at the middle of the workbench creating

a. backwash

b. a zone of confusion

c. shadowing

d. an aseptic field

___ **32.** What is desired of the final compounded sterile preparation (CSP) when conducting the visual inspection?

a. clear in color and no particles

b. amber in color with few particles

c. clear and concise labeling

d. clear in color with less than 2 particles

___ **33.** A vial used for more than one dose:

a. single dose vial

b. variable vial

c. multidose vial

d. disposable vial

___ **34.** Removing the air from IV administration tubing is termed

a. bleeding the tubing

b. folding the tubing

c. preparing the tubing

d. priming the tubing

___ **35.** Reconstituting is adding

a. powder to a liquid medication

b. diluent to a powder medication

c. medication to an IV bag

d. sterile water to a liquid medication for dilution

___ **36.** When working with a vial,

a. force air into the vial before withdrawing medication

b. withdraw medication and then add air to maintain vial pressure

c. add to and withdraw from the vial in a seesaw method

d. withdraw from the vial before adding medication

___ **37.** TPN may be compounded for a patient

a. who cannot eat or drink

b. training for a sporting event

c. who is on a solid-food diet

d. dieting to lose weight

___ **38.** All TPNs contain

a. lipids

b. dextrose

c. potassium

d. insulin

___ **39.** When compounding, what electrolyte should be added last to the TPN?

a. potassium

b. phosphate

c. calcium

d. magnesium

___ **40.** Methods to show the final compounded sterile preparation is of good quality:

a. infection control

b. quality assurance

c. infection assurance

d. quality checklist

___ **41.** What steps will pharmacy technicians who perform sterile compounding go through?

a. validation testing

b. infection screening

c. safe-handling assurance

d. control testing

___ **42.** Another name for TPN:

a. hyperalimentation

b. feeders

c. fluids

d. hypoalimentation

___ **43.** A glove box or isolator is

a. used to sterilize equipment

b. used for hazardous drug compounding

c. not as safe as a horizontal airflow hood

d. located in the pharmacy anteroom

___ **44.** Personal protective equipment (PPE)

a. protects the technician and the product

b. covers the technician's eyes to eliminate drug sprays

c. can be reworn from shift to shift

d. should be worn home at the end of the work shift

___ **45.** Clean the vertical airflow hood from _____ to _____.

a. top to bottom

b. bottom to top

c. outside to inside

d. inside to outside

___ **46.** How often should the LAWBs be cleaned?

a. once a week

b. at the beginning of the work shift

c. once a day

d. at the beginning and the end of the work shift, and periodically in-between times

___ **47.** What type of syringe is most often used with sterile compounding?

a. slip

b. luer-lock

c. glass

d. 50 mL

___ **48.** Rule to follow while compounding in the clean room:

a. no gum chewing or eating

c. work at a slow pace

b. no paper or pens

d. frequent hand washing

___ **49.** A common needle size used in sterile compounding:

a. 25 gauge, 1 inch

c. 19 gauge, 1 1/2 inch

b. 30 gauge, 1 inch

d. 13 gauge, 1/2 inch

___ **50.** Medication that requires sterile compounding:

a. oral medications

c. otic and IV

b. ophthalmic and IV

d. parenteral and otic

ANSWER SECTION

1. A
2. B
3. A
4. D
5. C
6. B
7. D
8. B
9. A
10. B
11. C
12. A
13. D
14. A
15. B
16. B
17. B
18. B
19. C
20. B
21. A
22. B
23. C
24. B
25. A
26. C
27. B
28. C
29. D
30. A
31. B
32. A
33. C
34. D
35. B

36. C

37. A

38. B

39. C

40. B

41. A

42. A

43. B

44. A

45. A

46. D

47. B

48. A

49. C

50. B

TEST C: MATH

MULTIPLE CHOICE

Identify the choice that best completes the statement or answers the question.

_____ **1.** Round to the hundredth place: 57.03269

a. 57

b. 57.03

c. 57.033

d. 57.0327

_____ **2.** Round to a whole number: 63.589

a. 63

b. 64

c. 63.6

d. 63.59

_____ **3.** Round to the tenth place: 89.0923

a. 90

b. 89.09

c. 89.1

d. 89

_____ **4.** In the fraction 1/4, 4 is the

a. numerator

b. denominator

c. equivalent

d. remainder

_____ **5.** What fraction is equivalent to 1/4?

a. 4/16

b. 1/2

c. 3/8

d. 25%

_____ **6.** Which one is a mixed number?

a. 13/24

b. 0.236

c. 4 2/3

d. 22%

_____ **7.** Reduce to lowest terms: 8/16

a. 1/8

b. 1/2

c. 4/8

d. 2/4

_____ **8.** Reduce to lowest terms: 74/100

a. 74/100

b. 4/30

c. 2/15

d. 37/50

_____ **9.** Reduce to lowest terms: 8 9/27

a. 8 3/9

b. 8 1/9

c. 8 1/3

d. 9/27

_____ **10.** 1/2 + 3/4 =

a. 6/4

b. 4/6

c. 1 1/4

d. 2/3

_____ **11.** 12/15 + 1/15 =

a. 13/15

b. 13/30

c. 3/10

d. 3/5

_____ **12.** 10 1/4 + 6 2/3 =

a. 17

b. 16 11/12

c. 16 3/7

d. 16/17

_____ **13.** 12/34 − 8/34 =

a. 5/34

b. 2/17

c. 4

d. 1/8

_____ **14.** 3/5 − 1/10 =

a. 4/10

b. 2/5

c. 1/2

d. 1/5

_____ **15.** 10 7/8 − 4 3/5 =

a. 6 11/40

b. 6 4/8

c. 6 1/4

d. 6 1/5

_____ **16.** 3/5 × 1/4 =

a. 1/3

b. 4/9

c. 3/20

d. 1/6

___ **17.** 13/22 × 4/5 = (lowest terms)

a. 52/110

b. 13/55

c. 26/55

d. 1/12

___ **18.** 5 2/5 × 3 1/4 =

a. 17 11/20

b. 351/20

c. 15 3/9

d. 15 3/20

___ **19.** 5/30 ÷ 11/20 =

a. 55/60

b. 11/12

c. 1/3

d. 10/33

___ **20.** 3 5/8 ÷ 1 1/4 =

a. 29/10

b. 4 5/10

c. 2 9/10

d. 2 1/10

___ **21.** Align these numbers in order of greatest to smallest: 0.235, 1.35, 0.569

a. 1.35, 0.235, 0.569

b. 0.235, 0.569, 1.35

c. 1.35, 0.569, 0.235

d. 0.569, 0.235, 1.35

___ **22.** Convert 5/16 to a decimal:

a. 5.16

b. 0.3125

c. 0.4

d. .516

___ **23.** Convert 0.651 to a fraction:

a. 651/1000

b. 651/100

c. 0.651/1000

d. 6 51/100

___ **24.** Convert 2.33 to a mixed number:

a. 2 33/10

b. 3 3/10

c. 2 1/10

d. 2 33/100

___ **25.** Find the answer and round to the nearest hundredth: 36.5 ÷ 3.2 =

a. 11.40

b. 11.406

c. 11.4

d. 11.41

___ **26.** 9% is the same as:

a. 9

b. 90

c. 0.9

d. 0.09

___ **27.** 52% is the same as:

a. 52

b. 0.052

c. 5.2

d. 0.52

___ **28.** What percent (%) is 3.25?

a. 325%

b. 3.25%

c. 0.0325%

d. 0.325%

___ **29.** What is the Arabic numeral for XXIX?

a. 31

b. 29

c. 1920

d. 21

___ **30.** What is the Roman numeral for 2011?

a. MMVI

b. MXXIX

c. MMXI

d. MMIX

___ **31.** Order these fractions from largest to smallest: 1/2, 1/4, 3/5, 2/9

a. 1/2 > 1/4 < 3/5 > 2/9

b. 1/2 > 1/4 > 3/5 > 2/9

c. 1/2 < 1/4 > 3/5 > 2/9

d. 1/2 > 1/4 < 3/5 = 2/9

___ **32.** Convert 25°F to Celsius:

a. −2°C

b. 46°C

c. −4° C

d. 77°C

___ **33.** Convert 77°C to Fahrenheit:

a. 25°F

b. 271°F

c. 52°F

d. 171°F

___ **34.** Convert 110°F to Celsius:

a. 43°C

b. 230°C

c. 34°

d. 57°

___ **35.** What is 32% of 150?

a. 48

b. 468

c. 4800

d. 4.68

___ **36.** What is 0.9% of 100?

a. 9000

b. 0.9

c. 9

d. 90

___ **37.** 1 liter is the same as:

a. 1 mL

b. 1000 mL

c. 0.0001 mL

d. 0.001 mL

___ **38.** Convert 10 mg to grams:

a. 10,000 g

b. 0.1 g

c. 1000 g

d. 0.01 g

___ **39.** Convert 2.6 liter to mL:

a. 2600 mL

b. 0.026 mL

c. 260 mL

d. 0.26 mL

___ **40.** 63 mL is the same as:

a. 6.3 L

b. 63 cc

c. 0.63 L

d. 0.63 cc

___ **41.** The pharmacy has a 52 kg bulk supply of compounding powder. 72% of the compounding powder has been used. How many kilograms have been used?

a. 15 kg

b. 72 kg

c. 0.72 kg

d. 37 kg

___ **42.** One vial of medication contains 6 doses. How many doses are in 3 1/2 vials?

a. 18 doses

b. 2 1/2 doses

c. 21 doses

d. 21 1/2 doses

___ **43.** One tablet contains 125 mg of active medication. How many milligrams of medication is in 7 1/2 tablets?

a. 16.6 mg

b. 875 mg

c. 937.5 mg

d. 166 mg

___ **44.** How many 25 mL doses can you get from a 1-liter bottle?

a. 40 doses

b. 4 doses

c. 25 doses

d. 250 doses

___ **45.** The prescription calls for a 0.235 mg tablet. The pharmacy carries 0.355 mg tablets. Which tablet is a higher dose?

a. 0.235 mg

b. 0.355 mg

c. both round up to 1.0 mg; same dose

d. both round up to 0.3 mg; same dose

___ **46.** The pharmacy tech mixed a cleaning solution using 15 2/3 mL of isopropyl alcohol and 230 1/2 mL of distilled water. What is the total volume of the cleaning solution?

a. 245 7/6 mL

b. 246 1/6 mL

c. 245 3/5 mL

d. 245 1/3 mL

___ **47.** The pharmacy stock supply of D_5W 250-mL bags is 26 1/4 boxes. There are 20 D_5W bags in each box. How may D_5W bags are in stock?

a. 525 bags

b. 520 1/4 bags

c. 46 1/4 bags

d. 650 bags

___ **48.** The pharmacy had 53 new customers in 2010. 17 new customers were male. What percentage (%) of new customers were male?

a. 9%

b. 3%

c. 36%

d. 32%

___ **49.** One stock bottle holds 2000 mL. How many milliliters are in this bottle if it is 3/4 full?

a. 1500 mL

b. 150 mL

c. 15 mL

d. 26 mL

___ **50.** The pharmacy filled 380 prescriptions on Monday. 36% of those prescriptions were for antibiotics. How many antibiotic prescriptions were filled on Monday?

a. 105 prescriptions

b. 344 prescriptions

c. 137 prescriptions

d. 320 prescriptions

ANSWER SECTION

1. B
2. B
3. C
4. B
5. A
6. C
7. B
8. D
9. C
10. C
11. A
12. B
13. B
14. C
15. A
16. C
17. C
18. A
19. D
20. C
21. C
22. B
23. A
24. D
25. D
26. D
27. D
28. A
29. B
30. C
31. A
32. C
33. D
34. A
35. A

36. B

37. B

38. D

39. A

40. B

41. D

42. C

43. C

44. A

45. B

46. B

47. A

48. D

49. A

50. C

TEST D: PHARMACY CONVERSIONS

MULTIPLE CHOICE

Identify the choice that best completes the statement or answers the question.

_____ **1.** Choose the true equation:

a. 1:9 : : 9:1

b. 3/5 : : 9/15

c. 7:8 : : 8:16

d. 9/10 : : 18/25

_____ **2.** Choose the correct percentage (%) for 7:20:

a. 0.35%

b. 7/20%

c. 0.725%

d. 35%

_____ **3.** 0.9% NaCl is

a. 9 grams per 1000 mL

b. 0.009/100

c. 0.009 grams per 1000 mL

d. 9/10

_____ **4.** 75 cubic centimeters (cc) =

a. 0.75 mL

b. 7.5 mL

c. 750 mL

d. 75 mL

_____ **5.** Show 57% as a ratio:

a. 0.57:100

b. 0.57:10

c. 57:100

d. 5.7:10

_____ **6.** An order for 77 gr instructs the technician to dispense

a. 77 grams

b. 77 grains

c. 77 mg

d. 77 gallons

_____ **7.** What is the conversion factor when converting kilograms to pounds?

a. 1 kg = 2.2 lbs

b. 1 lb = 2.2 kg

c. 1 lb = 22 kg

d. 22 kg = 1 lb

_____ **8.** Convert 90 mL to ounces:

a. 9 oz.

b. 3 oz.

c. 270 oz.

d. 2700 oz.

_____ **9.** 9000 mg =

a. 9 g

b. 90 g

c. 0.009 g

d. 900 g

_____ **10.** 20 gram =

a. 200 mg

b. 0.02 mg

c. 20,000 mg

d. 2,000 mg

_____ **11.** Convert 5.7 liters to milliliters:

a. 0.0057 mL

b. 570 mL

c. 5700 mL

d. 57 mL

_____ **12.** How many grains are in 325 mg?

a. 5 gr

b. 21,125 gr

c. 0.325 gr

d. 2113 gr

_____ **13.** Arrange the fractions in order from largest to smallest: 1/2, 3/15, 9/10:

a. 3/15, 9/10, 1/2

b. 1/2, 3/15, 9/10

c. 9/10, 1/2, 3/15

d. 1/2, 9/10, 3/15

_____ **14.** Solve for x in this proportion 30:50 = x:10

a. 5

b. 9

c. 3

d. 6

_____ **15.** Solve for x in the proportion 0.25:5 = x:10

a. 25

b. 0.5

c. 5

d. 2.5

_____ **16.** 850 mg = _____ g

a. 0.85

b. 850,000

c. 8.5

d. 85

___ **17.** 693 mg = _____ kg

a. 693,000

b. 693,000,000

c. 0.000693

d. 0.693

___ **18.** The prescription dose ordered is 0.0825 g. The pharmacy stocks 7.5 mg tablets. How many tablets are needed to fill the prescription?

a. 110 tablets

b. 11 tablets

c. 1 tablet

d. 7 1/2 tablets

___ **19.** 1 tsp = ____ mL

a. 15 mL

b. 30 mL

c. 5 mL

d. 50 mL

___ **20.** How many 1 tbsp doses in a 4 fl oz bottle?

a. 4 doses

b. 120 doses

c. 24 doses

d. 8 doses

___ **21.** 500 mL = _____ L

a. 5 liters

b. 1/2 liter

c. 500,000 liters

d. 50 liters

___ **22.** You are to fill an order for #25, 10 gr tablets of pain medication. Pharmacy stock supply: 100 mg, 150 mg, 250 mg, and 325 mg tablets. To fill this order, how many tablets will you need and of what strength?

a. #1 250 mg tablet

b. #7 100 mg tablets

c. #17 325 mg tablets

d. #50 325 mg tablets

___ **23.** A child weighing 54 lb is to take Tylenol. The physician orders 1 mg/kg tid. What is the child's dose?

a. 24.5 mg TID

b. 118.8 mg TID

c. 54 mg TID

d. 73.5 TID

___ **24.** A child with an ear infection weighs 45 lb. The prescriber ordered Trimox 15 mg/kg po bid. What daily dose will the child receive?

a. 306 mg po BID

b. 300 mg po qd

c. 1485 mg po BID

d. 1485 mg po qd

___ **25.** 1/4 gr = _____ mg

a. 2.4 mg

b. 240 mg

c. .015 mg

d. 15 mg

___ **26.** How many teaspoonfuls are in 1 tablespoonful?

a. 15

b. 3

c. 5

d. 30

___ **27.** 5°C = _____F

a. 9°

b. 41°

c. −48.6°

d. 48.6°

___ **28.** 113°F = _____°C

a. 45

b. 203

c. 81

d. 235

___ **29.** Solve for x in this equation 2:11 = x:77:

a. 7

b. 2

c. 22

d. 14

___ **30.** How many milliliters are in an 8-ounce bottle?

a. 8 mL

b. 240 mL

c. 400 mL

d. 120 mL

___ **31.** One capsule of medication contains 350 mg. How many milligrams are in #30 capsules?

a. 10,500 mg

b. 11.67 mg

c. 1050 mg

d. 3000 mg

___ **32.** 100 mL of the suspension contains 15 mg of active drug. How many milligrams (mg) are in 300 mL of suspension?

a. 150 mg

b. 45 mg

c. 130 mg

d. 200 mg

___ **33.** Order: i tsp bid × 10 days. What amount should be dispensed to fill the order?

a. 20 mL

b. 200 mL

c. 100 mL

d. 2 mL

___ **34.** What ratio is D_5W (5% dextrose)?

a. 1 mg of dextrose to 20 mL water

b. 5 g of dextrose to 100 mL water

c. 5 g dextrose to 1000 mL water

d. 1 g dextrose to 200 mL water

___ **35.** What ratio is $D_{10}W$ (10% dextrose)?

a. 1:100

b. 10:25

c. 1:1000

d. 10:100

___ **36.** 1255 mL = _____L

a. 1255.000 L

b. 0.0001255 L

c. 1.255 L

d. 125.5 L

___ **37.** 55.7 g = _____mg

a. 0.0557 mg

b. 55,700 mg

c. 0.557 mg

d. 5570 mg

___ **38.** 35 mg = _____gr

a. 0.035 gr

b. 0.54 gr

c. 2275 gr

d. 227 gr

___ **39.** The pharmacy has X gr tablets in stock. The order is for #4 300 mg tablets. How many X gr tablets should be dispensed to fill the order?

a. 4

b. 8

c. 30

d. 2

___ **40.** Order: 200 cc q 4hr. How many ounces should be dispensed for a one-day supply?

a. 40 fl oz

b. 7 fl oz

c. 1200 fl oz

d. 12 fl oz

___ **41.** Order: 25 mg BID. How many grams are dispensed for a 30-day supply?

a. 1500 g

b. 1.5 g

c. .075 g

d. 7.5 g

___ **42.** 2 L = _____cc

a. 2

b. 200

c. 0.002

d. 2000

___ **43.** Convert 67°C to Fahrenheit:

a. 121°

b. 37°

c. 5°

d. 153°

___ **44.** Using 200 mL, you are to prepare a 1/4-strength solution. What will the ratio of solvent to solute be?

a. 5:150

b. 50:200

c. 50:150

d. 4:200

___ **45.** The family doctor ordered 50 mg/kg/day divided every 12 hours. The child weighs 50 lb. How many milligrams (mg) will the patient receive per dose?

a. 2750 mg/dose

b. 23 mg/dose

c. 1150 mg/dose

d. 568 mg/dose

___ **46.** Order: 9 oz. phenergan with codeine syrup. Pharmacy stock supply: 500 cc bottle 1/4 full and a 400 cc bottle 1/3 full. Do you have enough supply on hand to fill the order?

a. yes; with 200 cc left over

b. no; have less than 6 oz in stock

c. no; have 258 cc in stock

d. yes; with no supply left over

___ **47.** A patient must take 1 tsp of medication every day until gone. How many days will a 6 oz bottle last the patient?

a. 1 day

b. 36 days

c. 5 days

d. 30 days

___ **48.** 0.36 L = _____mL

a. 0.00036

b. 0.0036

c. 3.6

d. 360

___ **49.** 560 mg = _____g

a. 0.56

b. 0.056

c. 560,000

d. 5.6

___ **50.** 552 mL = _____cc

a. 0.552

b. 552

c. 552,000

d. 0.00552

ANSWER SECTION

1. B
2. D
3. A
4. D
5. C
6. B
7. A
8. B
9. A
10. C
11. C
12. A
13. C
14. D
15. B
16. A
17. C
18. B
19. C
20. D
21. B
22. D
23. A
24. A
25. D
26. B
27. B
28. A
29. D
30. B
31. A
32. B
33. C
34. B
35. D

36. C

37. B

38. B

39. D

40. A

41. B

42. D

43. D

44. B

45. D

46. C
needed 270 cc
500 cc bottle has 125 cc left in it
400 cc bottle has 133 cc left in it

47. B

48. D

49. A

50. B

TEST E: DOSAGE CALCULATIONS

MULTIPLE CHOICE

Identify the choice that best completes the statement or answers the question.

_____ **1.** 1/2 normal saline (NS) is

a. 0.5% NS

b. 50% NS

c. 45 grams of sodium chloride in 100 mL of solution

d. 0.45 grams of sodium chloride in 100 mL of solution

_____ **2.** 2 L D_5W IV to infuse in 24 hours by infusion pump. What is the drip rate?

a. 0.8 mL/hr

b. 12 mL/hr

c. 83 mL/hr

d. 8.3 mL/hr

_____ **3.** Order: IVF: 100 mL NS with antibiotic to infuse in 25 minutes. The drop factor is 20 gtt/mL. What is the flow rate?

a. 4 gtts/minute

b. 80 gtts/minute

c. 20 gtts/minute

d. 5 gtts/minute

____ **4.** The BSA of the child is 1.17 m²
The recommended adult dose is 15 mg
What will be the dose given for this child?

a. 1.7 mg

c. 10.1 mg

b. 17 mg

d. 1.8 mg

____ **5.** 1/4-strength medication will have:

a. 1 part solute
   4 parts solvent
   5 parts solution

c. 1 part solute
   1 part solvent
   4 parts solution

b. 1 part solute
   3 parts solvent
   4 parts solution

d. 0 part solute
   1 part solvent
   4 parts solution

____ **6.** 200 mL of 1/4-strength peroxide solution for irrigation is best described as:

a. 25 mL peroxide 175 mL water

c. 150 mL peroxide 50 mL water

b. 50 mL peroxide 150 mL water

d. 175 mL peroxide 25 mL water

____ **7.** *Use this order to answer questions 7–11.*
Order penicillin 15 mg/kg/day po give q 6h for a child who weighs 40 lb.
How much does the child weigh in kilograms?

a. 88 kg

c. 1.8 kg

b. 8.8 kg

d. 18 kg

____ **8.** Order penicillin 15 mg/kg/day po give q 6h for a child who weighs 40 lb.
Using your answer from question 7: How many milligrams (mg) should the child receive per dose?

a. 67.5 mg

c. 45 mg

b. 675 mg

d. 450 mg

____ **9.** Order penicillin 15 mg/kg/day po give q 6h for a child who weighs 40 lb.
Using information from questions 7 and 8: How many milligrams (mg) will the child receive per day?

a. 600 mg

c. 720 mg

b. 270 mg

d. 450 mg

___ **10.** Order penicillin 15 mg/kg/day po give q 6h for a child who weighs 40 lb.
Using information from questions 7–9, pharmacy stock supply—penicillin 100 mg/5 mL. How many
   milliliters should be given per dose?

a. 337.5 mL

c. 15 mL

b. 67.5 mL

d. 3.4 mL

___ **11.** Order penicillin 15 mg/kg/day po give q 6h for a child who weighs 40 lb.
Pharmacy stock supply—penicillin 100 mg/5mL
Using information from question10, how many teaspoonfuls (tsp) will be administered per dose?

a. 3 tsp

c. 5 tsp

b. 3 1/2 tsp

d. less than 1 tsp

___ **12.** A 1-liter IV bag is running at 150 cc/hr. When will the fluid be done running?

a. 1 hour

b. a little less than 6 hours

c. 3 hours

d. between 6 and 7 hours

___ **13.** Order: 500 mg Cefzil in 100 mL of $D_{10}W$—infuse over 2 hours with a 10 drop set
What is the rate of infusion?

a. 10 mL/hr

b. 20 mL/hr

c. 50 mL/hr

d. 5 mL/hr

___ **14.** Order: Effexor XR 300 mg po bid × 5 days
Stock supply: 150 mg tablets
How many tablets will be dispensed to the patient?

a. 20 tablets

b. 5 tablets

c. 3000 tablets

d. 600 tablets

___ **15.** Order: Lipitor 40 mg po qd × 90 day supply
Stock supply: Lipitor 20 mg
How many tablets will be dispensed to the patient?

a. 2 tablets

b. 90 tablets

c. 180 tablets

d. 40 tablets

___ **16.** Order: Trimox 0.275 g po q 12h × 7 days
Stock supply: Trimox 150 mg/5 mL
How many milliliters(mL) will be dispensed to the patient?

a. 3850 mL

b. 385 mL

c. 128.3 mL

d. 12.8 mL

___ **17.** Order: Trimox 0.275 g po q 12h × 7 days
Stock supply: Trimox 150 mg/5 mL
How much Trimox will be administered per dose?

a. 9 mL

b. 5 mL

c. 1375 mL

d. 275 mL

___ **18.** Order: Trimox 0.275 g po q 12h × 7 days
Stock supply: Trimox 150 mg/5 mL
Using your answer from problem 17, how many teaspoonfuls (tsp) will the patient be administered
   per dose?

a. 1 tsp

b. 2 tsp

c. 3 tsp

d. 4 tsp

___ **19.** Order: Cleocin 2 g IV q 8h
Stock supply: Cleocin 4 g/200 mL
What amount will be prepared for the first dose?

a. 200 mL

b. 250 mL

c. 100 mL

d. 4 mL

___ **20.** Order: Cleocin 2 g IV q 8h
Stock supply: Cleocin 4 g/200 mL
What amount will be administered to the patient for the day?

a. 800 mL

c. 300 mL

b. 200 mL

d. 500 mL

___ **21.** Order: Levaquin 0.2 g q 8 h
Stock supply: Levaquin 50 mg/5 mL
How much will need to be dispensed for one dose?

a. 20 mL

c. 5 mL

b. 1000 mL

d. 50 mL

___ **22.** Order: Levaquin 0.2 g q 8 h
Stock supply: Levaquin 50 mg/5 mL
How much will the pharmacy need to prepare for a 24-hour time frame?

a. 20 mL

c. 60 mL

b. 3000 mL

d. 50 mL

___ **23.** Order: Ranitidine 150 mg po qid × 20 days
Stock supply: 150 mg scored tablets
Stock supply: 300 mg scored tablets
Which stock supply should be used to fill this order?

a. #80 300 mg

c. #40 150 mg

b. #80 300 mg split

d. #40 300 mg split

___ **24.** Order: propofol 2.5 mg/kg
Stock supply: propofol 10 mg/mL
Patient weight: 205 lb
How many milliliters (mL) of propofol will be administered?

a. 23.25 mL

c. 10 mL

b. 232.5 mL

d. 0.23 mL

___ **25.** Order: Zofran 8 mg po bid × 2 days
Stock supply: Zofran 4 mg tablets
How many tablets should be dispensed?

a. 16

c. 4

b. 32

d. 8

___ **26.** Order: Gleevec 400 mg po TID × 5 days
Stock supply: Gleevec 100 mg tablets
How many tablets should be dispensed for a 5-day supply?

a. 60

c. 24

b. 12

d. 1200

___ **27.** Order: metronidazole 30 mg/kg/day IV in divided doses q 6h
Stock supply: metronidazole reconstituted suspension 500 mg/100 mL
Patient weight: 162lb
How many milliliters (mL) will the patient receive per dose?

a. 2220 mL

b. 111 mL

c. 100 mL

d. 555 mL

___ **28.** Order: metronidazole 30 mg/kg/day IV in divided doses q 6h
Stock supply: metronidazole reconstituted suspension 500 mg/100 mL
Patient weight: 162 lb
What amount must the pharmacy have ready for a 24-hour time period?

a. 444 mL

b. 400 mL

c. 555 mL

d. 2220 mL

___ **29.** Order: Cleocin 200 mg IV q 4h
Stock supply: Cleocin Phosphate 600 mg/4 mL
What amount is needed for one dose?

a. 12 mL

b. 4 mL

c. 1.3 mL

d. 3.1 mL

___ **30.** Order: Cleocin 200mg IV q 4h in NS
Stock supply: Cleocin Phosphate 600 mg/4 mL
What amount of Cleocin will the pharmacy need to prepare for a 24-hour time period?

a. 1.3 mL

b. 3.6 mL

c. 7.8 mL

d. 78 mL

___ **31.** Order: Penicillin G 1 million U IM today
Stock supply: Penicillin G Sodium 5,000,000 Units/mL
How many milliliters are needed to fill the order?

a. 1 mL

b. 2 mL

c. 20 mL

d. 0.2 mL

___ **32.** Order: Zithromax 500 mg po qd × 4 days
Supply stock: 100 mg/5 mL in a 50-mL bottle
Supply stock: 200 mg/5 mL in a 100-mL bottle
Supply stock: 100 mg/5 mL in a 100-mL bottle
Supply stock: 100 mg/5 mL in a 300-mL bottle
What is the best choice for supply stock?

a. 100 mg/5 mL in a 50-mL bottle

b. 200 mg/5 mL in a 100-mL bottle

c. 100 mg/5 mL in a 100-mL bottle

d. 100 mg/5 mL in a 300-mL bottle

___ **33.** Order: Zithromax 500 mg po qd × 4 days
Supply stock: 100 mg/5 mL
What quantity will be dispensed to the patient for the full order?

a. 25 mL

b. 100 mL

c. 5 mL

d. 500 mL

___ **34.** Product Label

> *Parenteral drug product should be SHAKEN WELL when reconstituted and inspected visually for particulate matter prior to administration. If particulate matter is present, discard.*
> *Single Dose Vial IM injection*
> recommended 50 mg/kg/day divided into 3 doses
> 225 mg/mL
> 2 mL diluent for a volume of 2.2 mL in a 500-mg single-dose vial

Order: 50 mg/kg/day divided q 6 h
Patient weight: 155 lb
How many mg will be administered per dose?

a. 116 mg

b. 875 mg

c. 3500 mg

d. 350 mg

___ **35.** Use the product label from question 34 to find the answer for this question.
Order: 50 mg/kg/day divided q 6h IM
Patient weight: 155 lb
What amount will be administered per dose?

a. 1167 mL

b. 225 mL

c. 4 mL

d. 1.2 mL

___ **36.** A 1-gram vial needs to be reconstituted with 2.5 mL NS for a concentration of 330 mg/mL. The recommended dosing is 24 mg/kg/day in 4 divided doses. How many milliliters (mL) would a 174-lb patient receive per dose?

a. 1.4 mL

b. 1 mL

c. 330 mL

d. 1896 mL

___ **37.** A 1-gram vial needs to be reconstituted with 2.5 mL NS for a concentration of 330 mg/mL. The recommended dosing is 24 mg/kg/day in 4 divided doses. How many milligrams (mg) would a 174-lb patient receive per dose?

a. 1896 mg

b. 330 mg

c. 24 mg

d. 474 mg

___ **38.** Use Young's rule to determine the pediatric dose.
Adult dose: Prednisone 10 mg po qd
Patient age: 7 years
How many mg should the child receive?

a. 10 mg

b. 0.37 mg

c. 3.7 mg

d. 12 mg

___ **39.** Use Young's rule to determine the correct dose.
Adult dose: Clindamycin 900 mg IVPB tid × 7 days
Patient age: 5 years
How many milligrams (mg) should the patient receive per dose?

a. 265 mg

b. 17 mg

c. 900 mg

d. 5 mg

___ **40.** Use the answer from problem 39 to determine how many grams the pediatric patient would receive for the prescribed therapy of 7 days.

a. 1.86 g

b. 795 g

c. 265 g

d. 5.6 g

___ **41.** Use Clark's rule to determine pediatric dosing.
Adult dose: Ceftriaxone 1 g IV
Patient weight: 40 lb

a. 0.266 mg

b. 1000 mg

c. 266 mg

d. 2.6 mg

___ **42.** Use Clark's rule to determine pediatric dosing.
Adult dose: Zantac 40 mg/4mL IV qd
Patient weight: 12 kg

a. 1.73 mg/mL

b. 17.3 mg/mL

c. 1040 mg/mL

d. 17.3 mg/4 mL

___ **43.** Prepare 1000 mL of dextrose 12% using dextrose 5% (D_5W) and dextrose 50% ($D_{50}W$). How many milliliters of each solution will you need?

a. 7 mL of 5% solution and 38 mL of 50% solution

b. 160 mL of 50% solution and 840 mL of 5% solution

c. 12 mL of 5% solution and 500 mL of 50% solution

d. 840 mL of 50% solution and 160 mL of 5% solution

___ **44.** The pharmacist asks you to dilute a stock solution. The volume needed is 250 mL.
Solution in stock 30% strength
Diluted to 2% strength
How many milliliters (mL) of the stock solution are needed to dilute to the pharmacist's request?

a. 250 mL

b. 16.67 mL

c. 500 mL

d. 30 mL

___ **45.** How much potassium should be added to a 100 mL mini bag to make a 1/10 strength?

a. 10 mL

b. 1 mL

c. 0.1 mL

d. 5 mL

___ **46.** A child weighs 55 lb. The physician orders Vancocin 250 mg po q 6h. The recommended dose is 25 mg/kg/day. Did the physician prescribe a safe dose?

a. no; the prescribed dose is too low; safe dose is 350 mg

b. no; the prescribed dose is too high; safe dose is 156 mg/day

c. yes; this is a safe dose

d. no; the prescribed dose is too high; safe dose is 625 mg/day

___ **47.** A TPN is ordered to run at 50 mL/hour for 24 hours. What volume is this TPN bag?

a. 2 L

b. 1 L

c. 2.2 L

d. 1200 mL

___ **48.** A patient fills a prescription for a medication that is to be taken in a dosage of 2 tsp tid for five days, then 1 tsp at hs for 5 days. How much should be dispensed to the patient for the full therapy?

a. 8 oz bottle

b. 4 oz bottle

c. 6 oz bottle

d. (2) 6 oz bottles

___ **49.** How many milliliters of medication should be given to a patient needing 160 mg of a drug if the concentration of the medication is 1:4?

a. 64 mL

b. 6.4 mL

c. 640 mL

d. 0.64 mL

___ **50.** A patient is to receive 200 mL of medication intravenously at a concentration of 125 mg/mL. It is to be administered over 2 hours. What will the flow rate be?

a. 1.6 mL/hr

b. 100 mL/hr

c. 200 mL/hr

d. 125 mL/hr

ANSWER SECTION

1. D

Normal Saline (NS) is also referred to as Sodium Chloride (NaCl). Therefore ½ NS is the same as ½ NaCl. We normally consider ½ to be equivalent to 50%; in this case ½ NS is worth 45% rather than 50%. NS is 0.9% NaCl. Therefore ½ NS is 0.45% NaCl (0.9 divided by 2 = 0.45). This means that NS contains 0.9 grams of NaCl dissolved in 100 mL of solvent and ½ NS is 0.45 grams of NaCl dissolved in 100 mL of solvent. The ratios can be converted to 9 grams of NaCL in 1 Liter of solvent and 4.5 grams of NaCl in 1 Liter of solvent.

2. C

Use the formula V/T = R

Convert 2 L to mL

2000 mL/24 hr = 83.3 mL/hr

3. B

Use the formula V/T × C = R, volume over time times the calibration equals the rate

100 mL/25 min × 20 gtt/mL = Rate

Cancel out the like labels (mL), which will leave you with an answer labeled in gtts/min

4. C

BSA ÷ 1.73 m² × adult dose

1.17 ÷ 1.73 × 15 mg = 10.1

5. B

The solute and the solvent add up to the total parts of the solution, which is the denominator

6. B

1/4 × 200 = 50 mL peroxide

Take the total amount of the solution 200 mL and subtract the solute (peroxide)

200 − 50 = 150 mL of solvent (water)

7. D

40 lb ÷ 2.2 = 18.18, round to 18 kg

8. A

15 mg × 18 kg = 270 mg/day

The dosing schedule is every 6 hours, which is 4 times a day

270/4 = 67.5 mg/dose

9. B

15 mg × 18 kg = 270 mg/day

10. D

The patient needs 67.5 mg/dose

Set the equation up as $\frac{D}{H} \times Q = X$

Or "have" on the right side and "need" on the left side

Have in stock	Need (Dr. Order)
$\dfrac{100 \text{ mg}}{5 \text{ mL}}$	$\dfrac{67.5 \text{ mg}}{X}$

Cross off like labels (mg), and your answer will be in mL

Cross multiply 100 × X = 100X

5 × 67.5 = 337.5

Divide by 100 to make X stand alone

100 ÷ 100 = 1X

337.5 ÷ 100 = 3.375

Round to the tenth place: 3.4 mL

Does this make sense? If there is 100 mg of medicine in 5 mL, does it make sense to need 3.4 mL for just 67.5 mg?

11. D
3.4 mL needed per dose
5 mL in 1 tsp
Not quite a teaspoonful is needed

12. D
Convert liter to mL 1 L = 1000 mL
Set up the problem:

$$\frac{1000 \text{ mL}}{X} = \frac{150 \text{ mL}}{1 \text{ hr}}$$

Cross off the like labels (mL), which will leave you with hours for your answer
Cross multiply: 1000 × 1 = 1000   150 × X = 150X
Divide each side of the equation by 150 so that X stands alone
150 ÷ 150 = 1X   1000 ÷ 150 = 6.67
Round this answer to the tenths place for 6.7 hours

13. C
Use the formula: $\frac{V}{T}$ = R, volume over time equals rate
100 mL ÷ 2 hr = 50 mL/hr

14. A
bid is 2 times a day
300 mg × 2 times a day = 600 mg/day
600 mg × 5 days = 3000 mg
3000 ÷ 150 mg tablet in stock = 20 tablets
Check your answer: 20 tablets × 150mg = 3000 mg

15. C
40 mg × 90 days = 3600 mg
3600 ÷ 20 mg tablets in stock = 180 tablets
Does this make sense? Yes. The patient will need to take 2 tablets a day for the 40 mg dose
2 tablets a day × 90 days = 180 tablets

16. C
Convert g to mg 0.275 g = 275 mg
Every 12 hours is twice a day
275 mg × 2 = 550 mg/day
550 mg/day × 7 days = 3850 total mg needed for the order
Now set up the equation to see how many mLs will need to be dispensed to reach the needed dose:

$$\frac{150 \text{ mg}}{5 \text{ mL}} = \frac{3850 \text{ mg}}{X}$$

Cross off like labels(mg), which will leave you with mL for your answer
Cross multiply: 150 × X = 150X   5 × 3850 = 19,250
Divide each side of the equation by 150 so that X stands alone:
150 ÷ 150 = 1X   19,250 ÷ 150 = 128.33
X = 128.3 mL to fill the order for 7 days supply

17. A
Convert g to mg   0.275 g = 275 mg
Set up the equation:

$$\frac{150 \text{ mg}}{5 \text{ mL}} = \frac{275 \text{ mg}}{X}$$

Cross off like labels (mg) and your answer will be in mLs
Cross multiply to solve for X:
150 × X = 150X   275 × 5 = 1,375

Divide each side of the equation by 150 to solve for X:
150 ÷ 150 = 1X   1375 ÷ 150 = 9.16, round to 9 mL

18. B
There are 5 mL in 1 tsp
9 mL/5 mL = 1.8 tsp round up to 2 tsp

19. C
Set up your equation:

$$\frac{4\ g}{200\ mL} = \frac{2\ g}{X}$$

Cross off like labels (g), which will leave you with mL for the answer
Cross multiply to solve for X:
4 × X = 4X   200 × 2 = 400
Divide both sides of the equation by 4 to solve for X:
4 ÷ 4 = 1X   400 ÷ 4 = 100
X = 100 mL

20. C
Using your answer from question 19 the patient needs 100 mL per dose
Every 8 hours is 3 times a day
100 mL × 3 times a day = 300 mL/day

21. A
Convert g to mg: 0.2 g = 200 mg
Set up the problem:

$$\frac{50\ mg}{5\ mL} = \frac{200\ mg}{X}$$

Cross off the like labels (mg) which leaves you with mL for the answer
Cross multiply to solve for X:
50 × X = 50X   5 × 200 = 1,000
Divide both sides of the equation by 50 to solve for X:
50 ÷ 50 = 1X   1000 ÷ 50 = 20
X = 20 mL

22. C
Convert g to mg: 0.2 g = 200 mg
Every 8 hours is 3 times a day
200 mg × 3 times a day = 600 mg/day
Set up the problem:

$$\frac{50\ mg}{5\ mL} = \frac{600\ mg}{X}$$

Cross off like labels (mg) which leaves mL for the answer
Cross multiply to solve for X:
50 × X = 50X   5 × 600 = 3000
Divide both sides of the equation by 50 to solve for X:
50 ÷ 50 = 1X   3000 ÷ 50 = 60
X = 60 mL

23. D
qid is 4 times a day
150 mg × 4 = 600 mg for the day
20 days supply 600 mg/day = 12,000 mg needed
12,000 ÷ 300 mg = 40 tablets needed of the 300 mg stock supply
Since these tablets are scored, the 300-mg tablet can be split to allow for the 150-mg prescribed dose

24. A
Convert the patient's weight from pounds to kilograms:
205 lb ÷ 2.2 = 93.18 kg, round to 93 kg
2.5 mg × 93 kg = 232.5 mg
Set up the problem:

$$\frac{10 \text{ mg}}{\text{mL}} = \frac{232.5 \text{ mg}}{\text{X}}$$

Cross off like labels (mg), which leaves you with mL
Cross multiply:
10 × X = 10X   232.5 × 1 = 232.5
Divide each side of the equation by 10 to solve for X:
10 ÷ 10 = 1X   232.5 ÷ 10 = 23.25
X = 23.25 mL

25. D
Use the "have" and "need" equation or use the $\frac{D}{H} \times Q = X$; dosage needed divided by what dosage is on hand, multiplied by the quantity needed
Set up the problem:
Remember when working with tablets, capsules, or other solid dosages, the quantity with this equation is 1

$$\frac{8 \text{ mg}}{4 \text{ mg}} \times 1 = 2 \text{ tablets needed per dose}$$

bid is two times a day
2 tablets needed per dose × 2 times a day = 4 tablets
4 tablets needed per day × 2 days = 8 tablets

26. A
Use the formula $\frac{D}{H} \times Q = X$

$$\frac{400 \text{ mg}}{100 \text{ mg}} \times 1 = 4 \text{ tablets needed for one dose}$$

TID is 3 times a day
4 tablets/dose × 3 times a day = 12 tablets/day
12 tablets/day × 5 days = 60 tablets

27. B
Convert lb to kg 162 ÷ 2.2 = 73.63 kg round to 74 kg
30 mg × 74 kg = 2220 mg/day
The order is in divided doses every 6 hours
Every 6 hours is 4 times a day
2220 mg ÷ 4 = 555 mg/dose
Set up the equation:
555 mg ÷ 500 mg × 100 mL = 111 mL

28. A
Use the answer from problem 27: 111 mL/dose × 4 doses = 444 mL/day

29. C
Use the formula $\frac{D}{H} \times Q = X$
Set up the problem:

$$\frac{200 \text{ mg}}{600 \text{ mg}} \times 4 \text{ mL} =$$

Cross off like labels (mg), which leaves you with mL for the answer

Calculate
X = 1.33, round to 1.3 mL

30. C
Use the answer from problem 29 of 1.3 mL/dose
Every 4 hours is 6 times a day
1.3 mL × 6 times a day = 7.8 mL

31. D
Use $\frac{D}{H} \times Q = X$ for the formula

$$\frac{1,000,000 \text{ U}}{5,000,000 \text{ U}} \times 1 \text{ mL} =$$

Cross off like labels and solve:
X = 0.2 mL

32. B
To solve this problem you need to find out the total amount of medication needed to fill the order
500 mg × 4 days = 2000 mg
Now we need to find out how many mLs we need to get our 2000 mg
Use D/H × Q = X

$$\frac{2000 \text{ mg}}{100 \text{ mg}} \times 5 \text{ mL} = \text{need 100 mL from a concentration of 100 mg/5 mL}$$
$$\frac{2000 \text{ mg}}{200 \text{ mg}} \times 5 \text{ mL} = \text{need 50 mL from a concentration of 200 mg/5 mL}$$

It will make more sense to dispense the 200 mg/5 mL concentration because this is less medicine for the patient to take.

33. B
Use the formula $\frac{D}{H} \times Q = X$

$$\frac{500 \text{ mg}}{100 \text{ mg}} \times 5 \text{ mL} = X$$

Cross off like labels (mg) and solve:
X = 25 mL
25 mL for 1 day × 4 days = 100 mL

34. B
Convert lb to kg   155 ÷ 2.2 = 70.4 kg, round to 70 kg
50 × 70 = 3500 mg/day
Every 6 hours is 4 times a day
3500 ÷ 4 = 875 mg/dose

35. C
Use the answer from question 34 of 875 mg/dose
Use the formula $\frac{D}{H} \times Q = X$

$$\frac{875 \text{ mg}}{225 \text{ mg}} \times 1 =$$

Cross off like labels and solve:
X = 3.88, round to 4 mL

36. A
Convert lb to kg   174 ÷ 2.2 = 79 kg
79 × 24 = 1896 mg/day

1896 ÷ 4 divided doses = 474 mg/dose

Use the formula $\frac{D}{H} \times Q = X$

$$\frac{474 \text{ mg}}{330 \text{ mg}} \times 1 = X$$

Cross off like labels and solve:

X = 1.43 mL, round to 1.4 mL

37. D

Convert lb to kg 174 ÷ 2.2 = 79 kg

79 kg × 24 mg = 1896 mg/day

1896 ÷ 4 divided doses = 474 mg/dose

38. C

Use the formula adult dose $\times \dfrac{\text{child's age in years}}{\text{child's age} + 12}$

Plug the numbers into the formula:

$10 \text{ mg} \times \dfrac{7 \text{ years}}{7 \text{ years} + 12 \text{ years}}$

10 × 0.37 = 3.7 mg

39. A

Use the formula: adult dose $\times \dfrac{\text{child's age}}{\text{child's age} + 12}$

Plug the numbers into the formula

$900 \text{ mg} \times \dfrac{5}{5 + 12}$

$900 \text{ mg} \times \dfrac{5}{17} = 264.7$, round to 265 mg

40. D

265 mg/dose

tid is 3 times a day

265 × 3 times a day = 795 mg/day

795 mg/day × 7 days = 5565 mg total

Convert mg to g: 5565 mg = 5.565 g, round to 5.6 g

41. C

Use the formula: adult dose $\times \dfrac{\text{weight of the child in pounds}}{150 \text{ pounds}}$

Plug in the numbers:

$1 \text{ gram} \times \dfrac{40}{150} = 0.266 \text{ g}$

Convert g to mg: 0.266 g = 266 mg

42. A

Convert kg to lb: 12 kg × 2.2 = 26.4 lb, round to 26 lb

Adult dose (40 mg/4 mL) × child's weight in pounds (26 lb) ÷ 150 lb

Multiply across = 1040 mg/600 mL and reduce = 1.73 mg/mL

43. B

Set up the tic-tac-toe grid

Put the desired solution in the center of the grid

The higher strength solution in the top left

The lower strength in the bottom left

50		7
	12	
5		38

Subtract diagonally to get $50 - 12 = 38$ and $12 - 5 = 7$

$7 + 38 = 45$

$7 \div 45 = 0.16$

0.16×1000 mL $= 160$ mL needed of 50% solution

$38 \div 45 = 0.84$

0.84×1000 mL $= 840$ mL needed of 5% solution

Check your answer by adding the quantities needed:

$840 + 160 = 1000$ mL

44. B

Use the formula:

$$\frac{\text{Stock solution volume}}{\text{desired dilution rate \%}} = \frac{\text{needed volume}}{\text{stock concentration \%}}$$

Plug in the numbers:

$$\frac{X}{2\%} = \frac{250 \text{ mL}}{30\%}$$

Cross off like labels (%)

Cross multiply:

$X \times 30 = 30X \quad 2 \times 250 = 500$

Divide each side of the equation by 30 to solve for X:

$30 \div 30 = 1X \qquad 500 \div 30 = 16.67$ mL

45. A

Set up the equation:

$$\frac{1}{10} = \frac{X}{100 \text{ mL}}$$

Cross multiply:

$1 \times 100 = 100 \quad 10 \times X = 10X$

Divide both sides of the equation by 10 to solve for X:

$100 \div 10 = 10 \quad 10 \div 10 = 1X$

$X = 10$ mL

Does the answer seem reasonable?

10 mL added to 100 mL to get a 1/10 strength 10/100 reduces to 1/10

46. D

Convert lb to kg $\quad 55 \div 2.2 = 25$ kg

Recommended safe dose: 25 kg $\times$ 25 mg $= 625$ mg/day

Every 6 hours is 4 times a day

The physician prescribed 250 mg $\times$ 4 times a day $= 1,000$ mg

The prescribed dose of 250 mg is too high

47. D

50 mL/hour $\times$ 24 hour $= 1200$ mL

48. C

1 tsp $= 5$ mL

tid is 3 times a day

2 tsp $\times$ 3 $= 6$ tsp/day

6 tsp $\times$ 5 $= 30$ mL $\times$ 5 days $= 150$ mL

1 tsp $\times$ 1 time a day $= 1$

1×5 mL $= 5$ mL

5 mL × 5 days = 25 mL
25 + 150 = 175 mL
30 mL in 1 oz
175 mL ÷ 30 = 5.83, round up to 6 oz.

49. C
1/4 means 1 mg to 4 mL
Set up the equation:

$$\frac{1\ mg}{4\ mL} = \frac{160\ mg}{X}$$

Cross off like labels and cross multiply to solve for X:
1 × X = 1X   4 × 160 = 640 mL

50. B

$$\frac{V}{T} = R$$

$$\frac{200\ mL}{2\ hr} = 100\ mL/hr$$

TEST F: PHARMACOLOGY

MULTIPLE CHOICE

Identify the choice that best completes the statement or answers the question.

_____ **1.** What would Lipitor (atorvastatin) be prescribed for?

a. pain

b. high cholesterol

c. high blood pressure

d. infection

_____ **2.** What drug class does Nexium (esomeprazole) belong to?

a. PPI

b. CCB

c. MAOI

d. NSAID

_____ **3.** Which medication would be prescribed for therapy of blood clotting?

a. Seroquel (quetiapine)

b. Prevacid (lansoprazole)

c. Plavix (clopidogrel)

d. Spiriva (tiotropium)

_____ **4.** The generic of Advair is

a. montelukast

b. fluticasone

c. salmeterol

d. fluticasone and salmeterol

_____ **5.** Which of these medications is an antipsychotic?

a. Seroquel (quetiapine)

b. Singulair (montelukast)

c. Actos (pioglitazone)

d. Aricept (donepezil)

_____ **6.** Abilify (aripiprazole) may be prescribed for

a. schizophrenia

b. asthma

c. blood clots

d. heartburn

_____ **7.** The generic for OxyContin is

a. oxy

b. codone

c. codeine

d. oxycodone

____ **8.** The physician prescribed Actos (pioglitazone) to help the patient with

a. depression

c. anxiety

b. controlling blood sugar

d. controlling high cholesterol

____ **9.** Many generic medications that end in "azole," such as lansoprazole, may belong to what drug class?

a. SNRI

c. MAOI

b. beta blockers

d. PPI

____ **10.** What drug class does Cymbalta (duloxetine) belong to?

a. antidepressant

c. anticonvulsant

b. diabetic

d. antipsychotic

____ **11.** What is the brand name for venlafaxine?

a. Cymbalta

c. Effexor XR

b. Zyprexa

d. Lexapro

____ **12.** Selective serotonin reuptake inhibitors (SSRIs) are part of what drug class?

a. antipsychotics

c. anti-inflammatories

b. anticonvulsants

d. antidepressants

____ **13.** Medications such as Crestor (rosuvastatin) where the generic ends in "statin" provide therapy for

a. high blood pressure

c. high blood sugar

b. high cholesterol

d. irregular heartbeat

____ **14.** Which of these medications may be prescribed for schizophrenia therapy?

a. Valtrex (valacyclovir)

c. Celebrex (celecoxib)

b. Lyrica (pregabalin)

d. Zyprexa (olanzapine)

____ **15.** Spiriva (tiotropium) is a

a. bronchodilator

c. diuretic

b. vasodilator

d. ACE inhibitor

____ **16.** Grandma Wilma is a resident of the nursing home suffering from Alzheimer's disease. Her prescribed medication is

a. Lyrica (pregabalin)

c. Aricept (donepezil)

b. Tricor (fenofibrate)

d. Valtrex (valacyclovir)

____ **17.** What is the brand name of valsartan?

a. Diovan

c. Januvia

b. Diovan HCT

d. Valtrex

____ **18.** Levaquin (levofloxacin) is used to treat

a. viral infections

c. mild dementia

b. bacterial infections

d. COPD

___ **19.** Concerta (methylphenidate) is a

a. sedative

b. local anesthetic

c. stimulant

d. anticonvulsant

___ **20.** The generic medication albuterol is used for

a. asthma

b. high blood pressure

c. high cholesterol

d. nasal congestion

___ **21.** Yaz (drospirenoneethinyl estradiol) is a contraceptive. What drug class does Yaz belong to?

a. vitamin therapy

b. CNS

c. hormone

d. steroid

___ **22.** Aleve, Tylenol, and Bayer are OTC

a. antacids

b. NSAIDs

c. analgesics

d. hormones

___ **23.** Claritin, Benadryl, and Mucinex are OTC

a. cold/allergy/sinus medications

b. antacids

c. analgesics

d. NSAIDs

___ **24.** An example of an OTC antacid is

a. Tums

b. Metamucil

c. Mucinex

d. Aleve

___ **25.** Generic medications that end in "olol," such as metoprolol and bisoprolol, oftentimes belong to what drug class?

a. CCB

b. beta blocker

c. diuretic

d. ACE inhibitors

___ **26.** Generic medications that end in "pril," such as enalapril, lisinopril, and benezepril, often-times belong to what drug class?

a. CCB

b. beta blockers

c. diuretics

d. ACE inhibitors

___ **27.** Diuretics, beta blockers, and vasodilators belong to what broader drug class?

a. gastrointestinal system

b. respiratory system

c. anti-infectives

d. cardiovascular

___ **28.** Diuretics are prescribed to

a. reduce inflammation

b. reduce pain

c. reduce edema

d. reduce heart rate

___ **29.** What body system do antacids, H_2 antagonists, and PPIs treat?

a. gastrointestinal system

b. respiratory system

c. central nervous system

d. cardiovascular system

___ **30.** A patient purchased a box of OTC Prilosec (omeprazole). What will this medication treat?

a. diarrhea

c. GERD

b. constipation

d. COPD

___ **31.** What larger drug class do glucocorticosteriods, xanthines, and bronchodilators belong to?

a. cardiovascular

c. gastrointestinal system

b. central nervous system

d. respiratory system

___ **32.** Generic medications that end in "mycin" and "cillin" will most likely belong to what drug class?

a. anti-infectives

c. MAOIs

b. CCB

d. cardiovascular

___ **33.** What drug class does SSRIs, MAOIs, and SNRIs belong to?

a. antiparkinson

c. antianxiety

b. antiseizure

d. antidepressant

___ **34.** A prescriber who orders a benzodiazepine for a patient may be treating

a. anxiety

c. nasal congestion

b. depression

d. recurrent pain

___ **35.** Analgesics are used to treat

a. anxiety

c. nasal congestion

b. depression

d. pain

___ **36.** A nonopioid analgesic:

a. acetaminophen

c. codeine

b. morphine

d. fentanyl

___ **37.** A common side effect of high blood pressure medications is

a. frequent urination

c. diarrhea

b. dizziness

d. nausea

___ **38.** Betty has been prescribed Vicodin (hydrocodone/acetaminophen). She may experience a common side effect of

a. weight gain

c. frequent urination

b. diarrhea

d. feeling tired

___ **39.** A common side effect of antibiotics is

a. upset stomach

c. dry mouth

b. weight gain

d. decreased sexual desire

___ **40.** Iodine may be prescribed for

a. vitamin deficiency

c. fertility treatment

b. cancer treatment

d. dehydration therapy

___ **41.** The "D" in Carinex D stands for

a. daytime

b. decongestant

c. dose

d. double

___ **42.** The "XR" in Augmentin XR stands for:

a. extra strength

b. extra long-acting

c. extended release

d. extended relief

___ **43.** What therapy is intravenous Zosyn (piperacillin/tazobactam) prescribed for?

a. chemotherapy

b. anemia treatment

c. anticoagulant

d. antibiotic

___ **44.** A hospitalized patient may be prescribed a dose of Diprivan (propofol) prior to

a. surgery

b. mealtime

c. discharge

d. physical therapy

___ **45.** Lovenox (enoxoparin) is used to treat

a. anemia

b. high blood pressure

c. Crohn's disease

d. blood clots

___ **46.** Aranesp (darbepoetin alfa) and Procrit (epoetin alfa) are both used to treat

a. anemia

b. high blood pressure

c. Crohn's disease

d. blood clots

___ **47.** Jacob has been diagnosed with rheumatoid arthritis. Which medication best fits his diagnosis?

a. Neupogen (filgrastim)

b. Remicade (infliximab)

c. Neulasta (pegfilgrastim)

d. Protonix (pantoprazole)

___ **48.** What therapy are methotrexate and fluorouracil prescribed for?

a. hormone therapy

b. reproductive therapy

c. AIDS therapy

d. chemotherapy

___ **49.** IV heparin is

a. an anticoagulant

b. a steroid

c. an emergency cardiovascular drug

d. an anti-infective

___ **50.** What is the generic name for Solu-Medrol?

a. methotrexate

b. dexamethasone

c. methylprednisolone

d. prednisone

ANSWER SECTION

1. B
2. A
3. C
4. D
5. A
6. A
7. D
8. B
9. D
10. A
11. C
12. D
13. B
14. D
15. A
16. C
17. A
18. B
19. C
20. A
21. C
22. C
23. A
24. A
25. B
26. D
27. D
28. C
29. A
30. C
31. D
32. A
33. D
34. A
35. D

36. A

37. B

38. D

39. A

40. B

41. B

42. C

43. D

44. A

45. D

46. A

47. B

48. D

49. A

50. C

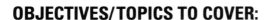

After Certification

OBJECTIVES/TOPICS TO COVER:

By completing this chapter, you will have an understanding of pharmacy technician:

- ✓ Recertification
- ✓ Reinstatement
- ✓ Revocation
- ✓ Continuing education
- ✓ Association membership

Once you have gained the title of Certified Pharmacy Technician, CPhT, you will be required to complete continuing education units to renew your certification. Your certification comes up for renewal every 2 years. Although the entity you are certified with (PTCB or ExCPT) should notify you by mail or e-mail to renew your certification, it's a good idea for you to mark your renewal date on your calendar and keep track of that date on your own. It is your professional responsibility to renew your certification in a timely manner. Please don't rely on PTCB (Pharmacy Technician Certification Board) or ExCPT (Exam for the Certification of Pharmacy Technicians) to send you a reminder. Your renewal date will be 2 years from the month and year listed on your certificate. You will never have to take the certification exam again as long as you keep current on your certification renewal!

CONTINUING EDUCATION

Continuing education units (CEUs) are easy to find and to complete. Typically, you will find an article on a topic that interests you. After you read the article, there are test questions for you to complete—usually 10–20 questions. Submit the test questions for grading, and you will receive a certificate of completion. Keep this certificate on file in the event that your certification board audits your continuing education units.

One of the best websites to find continuing education is www.powerpak.com. There are many articles to choose from. Find an article that is of interest to you and can help you be a better technician at your work setting. Print out the article and the accompanying test. By printing out the article, you can read and take the test at your leisure. You will have to access the website to submit your test answers. The test is graded immediately and a certificate of completion printed out.

POWER-PAK C.E. will keep a running log of all continuing education that you have completed from its site, which is very convenient and helpful for you in keeping track of your continuing education!

Your State Board of Pharmacy is also a good source for continuing education. The board will host an annual convention with seminars and guest speakers talking on a variety of topics. If you are someone who prefers attending a seminar rather than reading articles, this is a great way for you to get your required continuing education units. Your State Board of Pharmacy may also send out publications that offer continuing education articles.

Continuing education requirements for PTCB and ExCPT certification renewal are 20 hours of pharmacy-related continuing education every 2 years. One hour must be on pharmacy law.

The following list of websites can help you obtain pharmacy technician continuing education. Most of these websites offer free continuing education units.

www.cedrugstorenews.com

www.freece.com

www.theceinstitute.org

American Association of Pharmacy Technicians (AAPT) is a professional organization for pharmacy technicians that offers continuing education through publications and an annual conference.

What Do the Numbers Mean on Your Statement of Continuing Education Proof of Completion Certificate?

Your statement/certificate of education will show a series of numbers and letters. This is the ID for the continuing education. It should end in a "T," which denotes a pharmacy technician approved education.

The first set of numbers signifies the provider of the education. The second set of numbers signifies a cosponsor for the education. The third set of numbers signifies the year the education was created. The next set of numbers identifies the specific article or event in a series of articles or events created for the year. The last set of numbers before the "T" tells whether the continuing education was live, "L" (attending a seminar); home study, "H"; or both, "C." The numbers after this letter will signify whether the continuing education was 01 (drug therapy related), 02 (AIDs therapy related), 03 (law topic), 04 (general pharmacy topics), or 05 (patient safety).

You will not be tested on what each number signifies on your statement/certificate. This is good information to have but need not be memorized.

The Accreditation Council for Pharmacy Education (ACPE) and the National Association of Boards of Pharmacy (NABP) are in the process of developing a continuing pharmacy education tracking system. The tracking system uses a unique identification number issued to pharmacists and pharmacy technicians from NABP. ACPE and NABP hope to have the tracking system operational by year-end 2011.

PROFESSIONAL ORGANIZATIONS

It's always a good idea to become a member of an association that promotes your profession. In addition to providing continuing education, other membership benefits are networking opportunities, leadership roles, and career guidance. Membership in these organizations is not limited to pharmacists, even though the title of the group may signify so. I strongly urge each of you to become a member of your state's pharmacy association. Your state pharmacy association will help keep you abreast of changing laws, and, at times, you may become involved in the lawmaking process!

Some professional organizations for pharmacy technicians are

- ✓ American Association of Pharmacy Technicians (AAPT)
- ✓ State-specific pharmacist association, such as Iowa Pharmacist Association
- ✓ American Pharmacist Association (APhA)
- ✓ American Society of Healthcare Professionals (ASHP)

RECERTIFICATION

Renewal/recertification requirements:

- ✓ Renew every 2 years
- ✓ Complete and submit a recertification form
- ✓ 20 hours of CE must be completed prior to recertification deadline
- ✓ 1 of the 20 CE hours must be on pharmacy law

Cost to recertify:

- ✓ Payment and recertification form must be postmarked or received no later than the certification expiration date
- ✓ $40 online
- ✓ $50 paper application (PTCB)

REINSTATEMENT

Reinstatement occurs if the pharmacy technician misses his or her recertification deadline. The certification board will give the technician an extended amount of time from the certification expiration date to reinstate and renew to certified pharmacy technician, CPhT, status. If reinstatement is not completed by the deadline, the individual will no longer be a CPhT. The current cost to reinstate is $80.

- ✓ ICPT allows 18 months extension to reinstate
- ✓ PTCB allows 12 months extension to reinstate

REVOCATION POLICY

Each certification board, PTCB and ICPT, reserves the right to revoke an individual's CPhT status. This means that the board can take away your certification and credentialing as a certified tech. Any of the following may be reasons to revoke certification:

- ✓ Conviction of a felony, crime, or violation of state or federal laws regarding the practice of pharmacy or moral turpitude

Exhibit 19-1 Tips from a Certified Tech

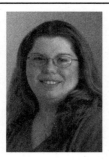

Tanya Smith, CPhT, MS
Vatterott College
Pharmacy Technician Instructor
Walgreens Pharmacy
Senior Technician

Being a certified pharmacy technician has been a great opportunity for me. It has led to job opportunities I wouldn't have gotten without my certification. Shortly after receiving my certification, I was promoted at Walgreens to senior certified pharmacy technician. The promotion gave me more job responsibilities as well as more money. Another opportunity that was opened up for me was to become employed as a pharmacy technician instructor at Vatterott College. Here is where I get to share my knowledge and skills with students.

Pharmacy is a growing field, so it is important to remain up to date on new technologies, drugs, and developments in the field. The easiest way for me to stay current is to make sure I complete my 20 hours of continuing education credits. As a certified technician you are required to complete 20 CE credit hours to maintain your certification. I have found that it is best to do 10 hours each year to keep up to date and make sure the certification remains intact. Without my certification I wouldn't be able to keep the current positions I have in my career field today. Becoming certified is definitely worth the time and effort.

- ✓ Documented gross negligence or intentional misconduct in the performance and of service as a pharmacy technician
- ✓ Revocation or suspension of a state-issued pharmacy technician license or registration
- ✓ Making false or misleading statements in connection with certification or recertification
- ✓ Cheating on or failing to abide by the rules regarding confidentiality of the certification examination (including postexamination conduct)
- ✓ Documented violation of the *Pharmacy Technician Code of Ethics* (http://www.nationaltech exam.org/pdf/code-of-ethics.pdf)
- ✓ Conviction of a felony or a crime involving prescription medications or controlled substances (including but not limited to the illegal use, sale, or distribution of prescription medications or controlled substances)

RESOURCES

1   Institute for the Certification of Pharmacy Technicians. *ExCPT Candidate's Guide: Exam for the Certification of Pharmacy Technicians*. Available at: register.nhanow.com/pics/.../ ExCPT%20Candidate%20Handbook.pdf. Accessed February 2011.

2   National Healthcareer Association: Institute for the Certification of Pharmacy Technicians. Pharmacy Technician Certification (CPhT). Available at: http://www.nhanow.com/pharmacy-technician.aspx. Accessed February 2011.

3   Accreditation Council for Pharmacy Education. Available at: http://www.acpe-accredit.org. Accessed February 2011.

4   Pharmacy Technician Certification Board. Available at: www.ptcb.org. Accessed February 2011.

Ethics

OBJECTIVES/TOPICS TO COVER:

- ✓ Show parallels in trust and professionalism.
- ✓ List elements of professionalism.
- ✓ Understand the importance of strong professional ethics.

TRUST

Pharmacists rank among the most highly regarded professions for honesty and ethics according to 2010 Gallup poll results. The confidence that the American public puts in pharmacists increased from 2009. A possible reason for the public's increase in trust of pharmacists may be due to the pharmacist's availability to the public and responsiveness in answering customer questions. Pharmacy technicians play a vital role in helping the profession remain honest and trusted.

The pharmacist is in charge of making sure the correct medication gets to the correct patient. Your pharmacist must have a level of trust in you—the pharmacy technician—to assist medication delivery by performing tasks correctly. This is an important trust that will have to be earned by acting and responding to situations in a professional manner.

PROFESSIONALISM

Professionalism directly ties in with honesty and trust. What are the expectations of your pharmacy manager? Your coworkers? Your community? Coworkers trust that you will arrive at work at the start of your shift. Of course, it's professional conduct to arrive to work in a timely manner and to work until the end of your shift. Patients trust that you have the skills and knowledge to fill their medication order accurately. Professionals make sure they have the skills and knowledge needed through training and by completing continuing education exercises.

Telepharmacy is one example of an area of pharmacy that demands a highly professional pharmacy technician. With telepharmacy, a remote pharmacy that serves an outlying rural area is staffed solely by a pharmacy technician; there is no pharmacist on site. Using technology, the pharmacist, who is at the home pharmacy, is able to monitor and check medication dispensing at the remote site via an automated machine. When the patient arrives at the remote pharmacy to pick up medication, the certified pharmacy technician has a huge responsibility in making sure the patient receives quality service. The technician helps to make sure the patient receives counseling from the pharmacist via video camera. The technician needs to be a well-trained professional to be able to serve the patient's needs without direct supervision from the pharmacist.

Becoming a certified pharmacy technician is a career choice. Certification distinguishes you as "having a career," not just "having a job." It's your professional responsibility to educate yourself continually on the constantly changing pharmacy trends.

Professionalism is more than having knowledge; it is about sharing your knowledge and skills in a meaningful way.

Professionalism 101

- Always use good manners.
- Show a successful attitude in your appearance, your words, your actions, and your body language.

Keep an updated electronic portfolio of your career accomplishments. Access rxportfolio.com to create a free electronic portfolio that will help you present yourself as a valued professional in the field.

Professional etiquette deals with your mannerisms and your outward appearance. Whether we like it or not, we are judged by the way we look and by our body language. Pharmacy is a reserved profession. While it may be acceptable for cosmetologists, for example, to have facial piercings, tattoos, and multicolored hair, this is not an acceptable or professional appearance for a pharmacy technician. Someday, perhaps, the pharmacy profession will evolve and become more accepting of liberal and unique styles, but for now, most pharmacy settings require a professional outward appearance of covered tattoos and no facial piercing. Remember, if you're working as a pharm tech in an aseptic compounding environment, jewelry (piercings) is not allowed per <797> standards.

As the pharmacy technician profession develops, the responsibilities of the technician will increase. At this time, a handful of states use a tech check program in which the certified pharmacy technician rather than the pharmacist has the final check on medications. With the increase in technician responsibilities, malpractice insurance should be considered.

ETHICS

Ethics are principles and standards that guide the way we conduct ourselves on the job. Having a solid set of ethics is crucially important, because ethics provide the standards of our work environment.

Oftentimes the morals and values that we're raised with influence decisions we make in our adult lives. As long as personal morals coincide with a strong work ethic, you will succeed in your career. If you are ever in doubt about a moral or ethical dilemma while on the job, your first concern should always be for the patient. The *Code of Ethics for Pharmacy Technicians* was developed by the American Association for Pharmacy Technicians (AAPT). Read the guidelines set forth in the Code of Ethics at www.nationaltechexam.org/pdf/code-of-ethics.pdf. Follow the *Pharmacy Technician Code of Ethics* to be the most professional pharmacy technician possible.

PHARMACEUTICAL ASSISTANCE PROGRAMS

Your first concern is for the care of the patient. Patients may wait to get their prescriptions filled because they don't have the finances to pay for the medications. Help your patients out by referring them to the website of the manufacturer of their new medication. Familiarize yourself with the information needed on the forms so you can help the patient fill out the forms. Most often the patient will need to supply financial information along with basic demographic information.

RxOutreach	www.rxoutreach.org
RxAssist	www.rxassist.org
Partnership for Prescription Assistance (PPARx)	www.pparx.org
Medicare	www.medicare.gov
State Programs	www.ncsl.org/programs/health/drugaid.htm

Exhibit 20-1 Tips from a Certified Tech

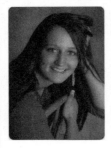

Emma Wickland CPhT, BS
Story County Hospital
Nevada, Iowa

As a pharm tech, you are not allowed to counsel patients. Your work *must* be checked by a pharmacist before leaving the pharmacy. Techs are the glue that holds it all together, just filling in wherever the pharmacist needs you at any given time.

Technicians have to be computer literate and preferably fast learners. Take notes; it's hard to memorize how to do everything!

In your daily duties, you will fill prescriptions; matching the NDC numbers is the best way to know you picked the correct drug, and make sure you double-count controlled drugs. Some pharmacies allow techs to enter the prescriptions in the computer, but others keep that as a pharmacist-only task.

My favorite duty is filling nursing home meds. There are a multitude of packaging types and sizes like cassettes or bubble packs.

Also, I think it is important for people to know that in the retail world it is super important to have good customer service skills. There are going to be some more difficult customers, and the people helping them need to know to just get it done and move on—don't dwell on the negative.

In any work environment, you need to be able to get along with the people you work with. Having a positive attitude will help you through your own day and probably help the people around you as well.

This is your checklist to make sure you understand what you need to know for the certification exam. Review chapter content if there is a topic you're uncertain of.

I know:

√	…how to demonstrate professionalism to patients and members of the healthcare team.

RESOURCES

1   Judson K, Hicks S. *Glencoe Law and Ethics for Medical Careers*. 3rd ed. Columbus, OH: McGraw-Hill; 2003.
2   www.gallup.com

Exam Content Checklist

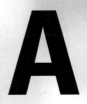

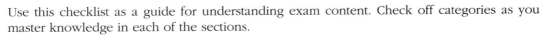

Use this checklist as a guide for understanding exam content. Check off categories as you master knowledge in each of the sections.

Pharmacy Technician Duties
The role of pharmacists and pharmacy technicians
Inventory control: Stocking medications, identifying expired products
Functions that a technician may and may not perform
Pharmacy security and diversion
Pharmacy layout and workflow
Quality assurance and quality control for pharmacy practices
Policies and procedures
Infection control
Controlled Substances
Difference among the controlled substances schedules
Refill regulations and prescription transfers
Correct procedures for handling schedule V sales
Controlled Substance Act
Drug Enforcement Agency (DEA) numbers
Filing hard copies
Required record keeping
Pharmacy Laws and Regulations
HIPAA
Generic substitution (including brand vs. generic products)
Professionals with prescribing authority (and acronyms)
Child-resistant packaging
Role of government agencies (Board of Pharmacy, DEA, Food and Drug Administration, etc.)
Labeling for over the counter (OTC) and Rx
Proper disposal and/or destruction of medications
Reporting medication error

Drugs and Drug Therapy	
	Major drug classes
	Dosage forms (types, characteristics, and uses)
	OTC products
	National Drug Code number
	Proper storage
	Durable medical equipment, prosthetics, orthotics, and supplies (DMEPOS)
	Reference books used in pharmacy practice
Know the Following for the Most Frequently Prescribed Medications	
	Brand and generic names
	Basic mechanism of action (MOA) and drug classification
	Primary indications
	Common adverse drug reactions, interactions, and contraindications
Prescription Information	
	Information required on a valid prescription form/inpatient order
	How to handle telephoned, faxed, and electronic prescriptions
	Refill requirements
	Required patient profile information (age, gender, etc.)
	Patient information needed for medication therapy management (MTM)
	Interpretation
	Recognizing and using common prescription abbreviations
	Calculating quantity needed to fill order; days supply
Preparing/Dispensing Prescriptions	
	Avoiding errors (such as sound-alike/look-alike names)
	Systems for checking prescriptions
	Automated dispensing systems
	Data entry
	Steps in filling the medication order
	Labeling prescriptions properly
	The purpose and use of patient records
	Proper packaging and storage
	Procedures to use for hazardous, radiopharmaceutical, and investigational drugs
	Third-party payers: Prior authorizations (PA), rejected claims
	Automated dispensing machines/robots
Calculations	
	Conversions/systems of measurement used in pharmacy
	Calculating the amounts of prescription ingredients
	Calculating quantity or days supply to be dispensed
	Calculating individual and daily doses
	Calculations used in compounding
	Calculating dosages and administration rates for IVs
	Business calculations (pricing, markup, inventory control)

	Compounding Sterile and Nonsterile Products
	Routes of administration for parenteral products
	Equipment used and calibration /maintenance
	Drug distribution systems used in hospitals and nursing homes
	Correct procedures for maintaining the sterile product environment
	Aseptic technique and the use of laminar flow hoods
	Special procedures for chemotherapy
	Types of sterile products
	Accurate compounding and labeling and record keeping of sterile and nonsterile product prescriptions
	Unit Dose and Repackaging
	Procedures for repackaging medications
	Record keeping for repackaged medications
	Prescription compliance aids, such as pillboxes

Suggested Readings and Videos

Documentary

Chasing Zero: Winning the War on Healthcare Harm
www.safetyleaders.org/pages/chasingZeroDocumentary.jsp
Approximately 53 minutes in length.

Online Video

60 Minutes

This is a segment on a medication error that affected Dennis Quaid's family.
www.cbsnews.com/stories/2008/03/13/60minutes/main3936412.shtml
Approximately 13 minutes in length.

20/20

This segment documents a medication error that cost a stay-at-home mother her life.
abcnews.go.com/blogs/headlines/2007/08/258-million-ver/

USA Today

"A Prescription's Path Through a Pharmacy"
www.usatoday.com/money/graphics/rx_error/flash.htm

Online Webcasts

Baxa Webinars
www.baxa.com/webinars
　　I strongly recommend watching these webinars to gain a better understanding of the subject matter on each topic. A picture is worth a thousand words, and these webinars will clear up questions you may have about a pharmacy setting or a piece of equipment that you're unfamiliar with. These webinars will be especially beneficial for you if you want to learn more about hospital pharmacy and sterile compounding. Some of the available topics are listed:

> *Alternatives to Bar Coding*
> *It's Not Just Food: The Importance of TPN for Patient Outcomes*
> *Regulatory Challenges to a Hazardous Drug Safety Program*

Improving Sterile Compounding Quality Through Automation

Implementing a Regional Compounding Program for Compounded Sterile Preparations

A Culture of Safety in Pharmacy: Lessons Learned

DoseEdge™: Changing Pharmacy Practice Through Workflow Management

The Clinical Advantages of Custom Parenteral Nutrition

Confronting the Challenges of Neonatal and Pediatric Medication Safety

The FDA Video Webcast Center has a large assortment of short webcasts. Access the list of webcasts at www.accessdata.fda.gov or search FDA Webcast.

A suggested list of webcast segments to help review for your certification exam:

Medical Errors from Misreading Letters and Numbers

Never Use Parenteral Syringes for Oral Medications

Dosing Errors with Certain Oral Syringes

Reporting Adverse Events to MedWatch

New Formulation for OxyContin

Avoiding Maalox Mix-Ups

Important Changes for Heparin

Update on Precipitate Formation with Ceftriaxone and Calcium-Containing Products

FDA Approves First Human Drug from Genetically Engineered Animals

Don't Overdo It with Acetaminophen

Avoiding Medication Errors with Multiple Brand Names

Books

Incomprehensible Demoralization by Jared Combs
A quick read in which a pharmacist tells about his addiction to alcohol and drugs and his journey to recovery. True story.

Dangerous Dosages by Katherine Eban
A true story about how counterfeit drugs get into America's drug supply. This investigative story tells about involvement in counterfeit drugs by big pharmaceutical wholesalers as well as corner pharmacies.

Movies

Extraordinary Measures

Inspired by a true story, a father tries to find a cure for his two young children who have been diagnosed with Pompe disease. This movie shows the trials and triumphs of researching a new drug and the steps involved to bring it to market.

Lorenzo's Oil

This is a 1992 movie starring Susan Sarandon and Nick Nolte. The couple's son develops a rare disease and the two work through controversies to develop a medicine to cure the child's illness.

Awake

A young man suffers from anesthesia awareness while receiving a heart transplant. This movie depicts (lack of) professional ethics and personal morals. A real thriller starring Hayden Christensen, Jessica Alba, and Lena Olin.

Common Endings and Classes

APPENDIX

C

Cardiovascular	-alol	Beta Blockers
	-olol	Beta Blockers
	-azosin	Antihypertensive
	-pril	ACE inhibitors
	-tiazem	CCB
	-thiazide	Diuretics
Cholesterol Lowering	-fibrate	Antihyperlipidemics
	-statin	Antihyperlipidemics
Gastrointestinal	-prazole	Antiulcer
Psychotics	-azepam	Antianxiety agents
	-peridol	Antipsychotics
Antiinfectives	-cef	Cephalspoins
	-cillin	Penicillins
	-conazole	Antifungals
	-cycline	Antibiotics
	-mycin	Antibiotics
	-sulfa	Antibiotics
	-oxacin	Antibiotics
Chemotherapy	-mustine	Antineoplastics
	-rubicin	Antineoplastic antibiotic
Anesthetic	-caine	Anesthetic
Hormone	-pred, pred-	Prednisone derivative

Vitamins

Vitamin	Derivative	
A	Retinol and Beta carotene	Fat Soluble
B1	Thiamin (thī-ə-mēn)	Water Soluble
B2	Riboflavin	Water Soluble
B3	Niacin, Nicotinic Acid	Water Soluble
B12	cyanocobalamine (sigh-an-oh-koe-BAL-uh-min)	Water Soluble
C	Ascorbic Acid	Water Soluble
D		Fat Soluble
E		Fat Soluble
K	phytonadione (fī-tō-nə-dī-ōn)	Fat Soluble
Folic Acid	Folate	Water Soluble

Index

Figures and tables are indicated by f, t and e following the page number.

Metric system of measurement, 206, 207–209, 208–209t
Military health plans, 42
Milligram per kilogram equations, 224–225
Mixed number fractions, 190
Molds, 163
Monoamine oxidase inhibitors (MAOIs), 61
Mortars and pestles, 162, 163f, 165
MSDS (Material Safety Data Sheets), 144, 156
MTM. *See* Medication therapy management
Multidose vials, 174, 176, 180
Multiplication, 192, 196

N

NA/DRIs (noradrenaline dopamine reuptake inhibitors), 61
Narcotic Addiction Treatment Act of 1974, 124
Narcotics. *See* Controlled substances
National Association of Boards of Pharmacy (NABP), 306
National Drug Code (NDC) numbers
　barcode technology and, 21, 32, 69
　defined, 148, 148f
　reference materials for, 134
　rejected claims and, 43
National Provider Identifier (NPI) numbers, 43
National Quality Forum, 133
Naturally occurring drugs, 54
NDAs (new drug applications), 38
NDC numbers. *See* National Drug Code numbers
Needles, 153, 155, 156, 169, 174–176, 175–176f
Negligence, 107
Nervous system, 54, 61, 73, 78f
Network providers, 42
New drug applications (NDAs), 38
Nomograms, 231, 232f
Noncompliance to medications, 28
Nonprescription drugs. *See* Over-the-counter (OTC) drugs
Nonsterile compounding. *See* Extemporaneous
　　　　compounding
Noradrenaline dopamine reuptake inhibitors (NA/DRIs), 61
Normal saline (NS), 172, 173
NOW medication orders, 26
Nuclear pharmacies, 65–66, 142
Nuclear Regulatory Commission (NRC), 66

O

Occupational Safety and Health Administration (OSHA), 107
Ointment slabs, 163
Omnibus Budget Reconciliation Act of 1990 (OBRA), 103
Online adjudication, 20, 43
Online pharmacies, 106
Onset of action, 51
Open formularies, 142
Ophthalmic route of absorption, 49
Oral contraceptives, 23
Orange Book (FDA), 51, 134
Orphan Drug Act of 1983, 102
OSHA (Occupational Safety and Health Administration), 107
OTC drugs. *See* Over-the-counter drugs
Otic route of absorption, 49
Out-of-pocket expenses, 38
Outpatient pharmacies. *See* Retail pharmacies
Over-the-counter (OTC) drugs
　interactions and, 52
　laws and regulations, 100–101, 105, 121
　reference materials for, 134

supplements, 103
top-selling, 69, 79t

P

Packaging
　laws and regulations, 22, 23, 101, 102, 107
　patient package inserts, 23
　prescription drugs, 22, 23, 32
　repackaging, 145–148, 146–147f, 161
　tamper-resistant, 107
　unit dose medications, 26–27, 26f, 145–148, 161
Pain management devices, 177, 179f
PAR (periodic automatic replenishment), 142
Parata Robotic Dispensing System, 29, 30f
Parchment paper, 163
Parenteral medications, 169, 173, 173t, 182–183, 223
Part D. *See* Medicare
PAs (prior authorizations), 43
Patent protection, 102
Patient assistance programs, 40, 42
Patient-controlled analgesia (PCA) pumps, 177, 179f
Patient package inserts (PPIs), 23
Patient profiles, 27–28
Patient safety. *See* Laws and regulations; Medication safety
PBMs (pharmacy benefit managers), 44
PDR (*Physicians' Desk Reference*), 134
Pearson Vue, 10, 11
Pediatric patients
　compounding and, 161
　dosage calculations for, 231–234
　laws and regulations, 104
　safety and, 22, 102, 104, 133–134
Percentages, 197, 205–206
Periodic automatic replenishment (PAR), 142
Perpetual inventory, 141
Personal protective equipment (PPE), 155, 156, 163, 170, 183
Pestles, 162, 163f, 165
pH, 164
Pharmaceutical alternatives, 51
Pharmaceutical assistance programs, 310
Pharmaceutical equivalence, 51, 52
Pharmacies
　hospital. *See* Hospital pharmacies
　nuclear, 65–66, 142
　online, 106
　retail. *See* Retail pharmacies
　telepharmacies, 309
Pharmacodynamics, 50–52
Pharmacogenomics, 52
Pharmacokinetics, 49–50
Pharmacology, 49–85
　dispensing guidelines, 67–69
　drug classification, 52–54, 55–60t, 61, 73, 74–78f, 319
　interactions, 52, 53t
　pharmacodynamics, 50–52
　practice examinations, 298–304
　principles of, 49–50
　radiopharmaceuticals, 65–66, 66t, 142, 144
　restricted drugs, 66, 67t
Pharmacy benefit managers (PBMs), 44
Pharmacy management and administration, 37–47, 131–138.
　　　　See also Business calculations; Inventory control;
　　　　Prescription processing

Photo Credits

Openers © Evon Lim Seo Ling/ShutterStock, Inc.

Dedication
Courtesy of Tanya Smith, CPhT, MS

Chapter 3
3-4 © Pharmex/Precision Dynamics Corporation. Pharmex Original Copyrighted Warning Labels were copied/printed with authorization by Precision Dynamics Corporation.; 3-5 Courtesy of DFL Enterprises, Inc. www.dfl-enterprises.com; 3-6, 3-8 Courtesy of Judy Neville; 3-9–3-12 Courtesy of Care Fusion

Chapter 10
10-1–10-6 Courtesy of MediDose

Chapter 11
11-1, 11-2 Courtesy of NuAire, Inc.

Chapter 12
12-1 © Photodisc

Chapter 13
13-1 Courtesy of Judy Neville; 13-2, 13-3 Courtesy of Care Fusion; 13-4 © Africa Studio/ShutterStock, Inc.; 13-6, 13-7 Courtesy of Medidose; 13-8 The Alaris System Image is © 2012 CareFusion Corporation; Used with permission.; 13-10 Courtesy of Pfizer; 13-11 Courtesy of B. Braun Medical Inc.

Chapter 16
16-1 Courtesy of Pfizer; 16-2 © Jones & Bartlett Learning. Photographed by Gina Licata;
16-3 Reprinted From: Boyd, E. Nelson Textbook of Pediatrics. 1983. Copyright Elsevier;
16-4–16-7 Courtesy of Pfizer

Chapter 19
19-1 Courtesy of Tanya Smith, CPhT, MS